BARRON'S
DAT®
DENTAL ADMISSION TEST

2ND EDITION

Richard A. Lehman, DDS

Contributing Authors

Edwin H. Hines, DDS
Professor and Chairman
Department of Pediatric
Dentistry
Meharry Medical
College, School of
Dentistry

Allen S. Otsuka, Ph.D.
Associate Professor
School of Dental
Medicine
Southern Illinois
University

Donald L. Chi, DDS
Resident, Pediatric
Dentistry and Dental
Public Health
College of Dentistry
University of Iowa

Sophia G. Saeed, DMD
Assistant Clinical
Professor
University of California,
San Francisco
School of Dentistry

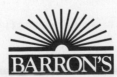

BARRON'S

All inquiries should be addressed to:
Barron's Educational Series, Inc.
250 Wireless Boulevard
Hauppauge, NY 11788
www.barronseduc.com

Library of Congress Catalog Card No. 2008053472

ISBN-13: 978-0-7641-9384-2 (Book/CD package)
ISBN-10: 0-7641-9384-8 (Book/CD package)

Library of Congress Cataloging-in-Publication Data

Lehman, Richard A.
    DAT / Richard A. Lehman ; contributing authors, Donald L. Chi . . . [et al.]. — 2nd ed.
    p. ; cm.
    Rev ed of: How to prepare for the dental admission test (DAT) / Richard A. Lehman ;
contributing authors Suzanna L. Kahlil . . . [et al.]. c1999.
    Includes bibliographical references.
    ISBN–13: 978–0–7641–9384–2 (Book/CD Package)
    ISBN–10: 0–7641–9384–8 (Book/CD Package)
    1. Dental Admission Test—Study guides. 2. Dental schools—United States—Entrance
examinations—Study guides. 3. Dentistry—Ability testing. 4. Dentistry—Examinations, questions, etc.
I. Lehman, Richard A. How to prepare for the dental admission test (DAT).   II. Title.
    [DNLM: 1. Dentistry—Examination Questions. 2. Aptitude Tests—Examination Questions.
3. Educational Measurement—Examination Questions. WU 18.2 L523d 2009]

RK76.L44 2009
617.60076—dc22   2008053472

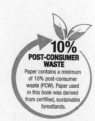

10% POST-CONSUMER WASTE
Paper contains a minimum of 10% post-consumer waste (PCW). Paper used in this book was derived from certified, sustainable forestlande.

Contents

Acknowledgments

Special thanks to Dr. Jayne S. Reuben, Assistant Professor at the Texas A&M Health Science Center Baylor College of Dentistry, for her contributions to the biology section of Barron's *DAT,* 2nd edition.

The author would like to thank the following individuals for their contributions to the text of the 1st edition of Barron's *DAT*: Suzanne L. Khalil, Sharon Joyce, Scott M. Blyer, Brian Stern, A. W. Whitehead, Jason L. Burak, Assaf T. Gordon, and Thomas J. Meals.

The author would like to thank the following for permission to reprint excerpts in this book and on the CD-ROM:

The Compendium of Continuing Education in Dentistry, 1997. Vol. 18, No. 10: 1002, 1006–1007.

Clinical Periodontology, 8th Edition. Fermin A. Carranza, Jr. et al. © copyright 1995 by W. B. Saunders Company.

"Addressing Tobacco-Related Health Disparities," [Moolchan ET, Fagan P, Fernander AF, Velicer WF, Hayward MD, King G, Clayton RR], *Addiction,* 2007 (Vol. 102, Supp. 2). © copyright *Addiction.* Reprinted with permission.

"Gastrointestinal Complications of Diabetes," [Shakil A, Church RJ, Rao SS], *American Family Physician,* June 15, 2008 (Vol. 77. No. 12). © copyright American Academy of Family Physicians. Reprinted with permission.

"Hereditary Dentin Defects," [Kim JW, Simmer JP], *Journal of Dental Research,* 2007 (Vol. 86, No. 5). © copyright *Journal of Dental Research.* Reprinted with permission.

"Reiter's Syndrome: The Classic Triad and More," [Wu IB, Schwartz RA], *Dermatology,* April 24, 2008. © copyright American Academy of Dermatology, Inc. Reprinted with permission.

"Rural-Urban Differences in Acute Stroke Management Practices: A Modifiable Disparity," [Leira EC, Hess DC, Torner JC, Adams HP], *Archives of Neurology,* July 2008 (Vol. 65, No. 7). © copyright *Archives of Neurology.* Reprinted with permission.

"Ultrastructure of Dentine Carious Lesions," [Zavgorodniy AV, Rohanizadeh R, Swain MV], *Archives of Oral Biology,* February 8, 2008 (Vol. 53, No. 2). © copyright by Elsevier, Ltd. Reprinted with permission.

A NOTE TO THE TEST TAKER

You have purchased a comprehensive DAT review written specifically for the dental school applicant. The review chapters are tailored to the scope of the examination established by the ADA Department of Testing Services. Much effort has gone toward including only the most relevant material, that which has the highest probability of appearing on the exam.

You will find that some other concerns and questions of many applicants are addressed in the chapter titled "Dental Education and Practice." Information about the American Association of Dental Schools Application Service (AADSAS), letters of recommendation, the Personal Statement, and interviews, as well as some material on career options and dental organizations, are included in this chapter.

Good luck on the DAT and in your dental career.

Introduction

CHAPTER 1

ABOUT THE DAT

The American Dental Association Department of Testing Services annually reports on the *appropriateness* of the DAT. It has been proved through statistical analysis that the test battery is a significant indicator of success in dental school as well as a valuable indicator of performance on Part I of the National Board Dental Examinations. The DAT is also used as a method of standardizing and quantifying the undergraduate preparation received at various academic institutions.

The Dental Admission Testing Program is administered by the ADA Department of Testing Services. It consists of *four timed sections*:

- **Survey of the Natural Sciences (SNS)**

- **Perceptual Ability Test (PAT)**

- **Reading Comprehension Test (RCT)**

- **Quantitative Reasoning Test (QRT)**

Although there are only four timed sections, there are six scored sections. Notice in the list below that the Survey of the Natural Sciences has three scored sections that are administered in one timed section. *You will receive the following **eight** score reports*:

- **Biology** (Questions 1–40 of the Survey of the Natural Sciences)

- **General Chemistry** (Questions 41–70 of the Survey of the Natural Sciences)

- **Organic Chemistry** (Questions 71–100 of the Survey of the Natural Sciences)

- **Quantitative Reasoning**

- **Reading Comprehension**

- **Total Science** (a combination of the biology, general chemistry, and organic chemistry raw scores)

- **Academic Average** (a composite score that is an average of the quantitative reasoning, reading comprehension, biology, general chemistry, and organic chemistry scores)

- **Perceptual Ability** (a score that is not incorporated in the other composite/combination score reports; it is always reported separately)

The specifics regarding the number of questions and the time allotted for each section are as follows for the Dental Admission Testing Program:

Section	Questions	Time Average	Average Time Per Item
Survey of the Natural Sciences	100 questions; (40 Biology, 30 General Chemistry, 30 Organic Chemistry)	90 minutes	54 seconds/question
Perceptual Ability Test	90 questions (composed of 6 different sections)	60 minutes	40 seconds/question (see section for specifics on timing)
BREAK		15 minutes	
Reading Comprehension Test	50 questions (three passages with 16–17 questions following each passage)	60 minutes	20 minutes/passage
Quantitative Reasoning Test	40 questions	45 minutes	1 minute 7 seconds/question
TOTAL	**280 questions**	**4 hours 30 minutes (start to finish)**	

SCORING

The DAT is scored on a 30-point scale with 30 being the highest mark and 1 being the lowest. *There is no penalty for wrong answers.* The total number of correct answers on each section is the raw score. The score on each section that is reported to you and to the dental schools you select is your *standard score*. It is the standard score that is used to compare one administration of the exam to another. The actual derivation of the standard score is quite complex: it utilizes a log ability scale based on the Rasch psychometric model. What you need to know is that a score of 17 is about the national average on most sections of the DAT. You should aim to get above this national average on all sections. A composite score of 18–19 is currently the average of enrollees in the first-year classes. *Therefore, a score of 18–19 should be your goal.* A standard score of 18–19 converts roughly to a raw score of 65–75% of questions answered correctly, so of 40 biology questions, for example, you should be able to answer approximately 30–33 correctly.

A NOTE TO CANADIAN STUDENTS

There are some distinct differences between the American Dental Admission Test (DAT) and the Canadian Dental Aptitude Test (DAT). The following major differences should be noted:

- **The Canadian DAT is administered in the written format, as opposed to the computerized American DAT.**

- **The Canadian DAT includes a *Carving Dexterity* Test; the American DAT does not.**

- **The Canadian DAT does not include *organic chemistry* in the Survey of the National Sciences Test, nor does it have a *Quantitative Reasoning Test*. The American DAT has both.**

The Canadian Dental Association (CDA) and the ADA sample exams included in the test preparation materials of these two bodies are *identical*, word for word, for the following sections: perceptual ability, biology, general (inorganic) chemistry, and reading comprehension. Therefore, this book is well suited for review of the sections tested on the Canadian DAT battery with the exception of the Carving Dexterity Test. A lengthy explanation, including helpful hints, of exactly what is tested in the soap-carving section is included in *Preparation Manual: Dental Aptitude Test*, published by the CDA.

Practice for this section of the Canadian DAT is essential, and you can purchase practice materials directly from the CDA at the following address:

The Dental Aptitude Test Program
c/o Canadian Dental Association
1815 Alta Vista Drive
Ottawa, Ontario K1G 3Y6
E-mail: *datecda-adc.ca*

Specific information regarding the administration of the CDA can readily be obtained from the Ottawa office of the DAT program or from faculty of the 10 Canadian dental schools.

THE ART OF TEST TAKING

In order to take the Dental Admission Test (DAT), you need only to pay the required fee, register, show up at the testing site, and spend several hours answering the battery of test questions. Alternatively, you have chosen to do more than just take the test. By purchasing this book, you have begun a commitment to something much greater. Your decision to engage in test preparation is a sign that you seek to take control of the test and that you believe that performance is largely a result of preparation. Hopefully, the following comments regarding test preparation for the DAT will prove useful.

Studying and Preparation Strategies

STUDY WHAT YOU *DON'T* KNOW

After a few weeks of studying for this exam, you will find that much of the material looks familiar. Concentrate on acquiring the information you don't have rather than continuously reviewing the information that you've read before. This tip seems obvious, but failure to follow it is the downfall of many test takers.

UTILIZE ALL YOUR SENSES

Read the material, write the material, and speak the material to maximize the experience of learning. If you enhance the learning experience, you will enhance your ability to recall that experience.

USE REPETITION

Read, write, and speak the information for 6 weeks, and you will be able to recall important facts with greater ease.

DON'T STUDY JUST THE SCIENCES

Any single low score on any section could be reason to *not* accept you, whereas a single high score will *not* greatly help your application. High scores across *all* sections are what is desired.

FOR THE SNS, CREATE MNEMONICS

For an easier way to remember unfamiliar or unrelated science information, make up mnemonics. Major corporations that rely on phone orders usually spell out a familiar word to make it easier for their customers to remember their phone number (1-800-GO FEDEX is a lot easier to recall than 1-800-463-3339). Make up phrases and words that stand for difficult to remember items of information in biology, chemistry, and organic chemistry.

ALLOW SUFFICIENT TIME

Do not schedule your examination before you can realistically be prepared to take it. Only you will know how much time you will need to spend reviewing. Use the model exams in this book/CD package to gauge your proficiency with the subject matter. Schedule a date that will permit you to critically and thoroughly review all the material for the exam. Usually 6 weeks is sufficient for the average student; but, depending on how much time you will dedicate to studying each day, you may require only 4 weeks, or as many as 8, to fully cover all the material.

BE DISCIPLINED

This is the common strategy of all test takers who score in the top few percentiles. It is through hard work that high marks are achieved. Discipline yourself to a regimented schedule of studying for the DAT. Do not let anything come between you and the scores you desire. Between now and your test date, many things will try to distract your attention from your studies, but *be disciplined*!

Test-Taking Strategies

ANSWER *EVERY* QUESTION

On the DAT, unlike the SAT, you are *not* penalized for wrong guesses. You will have a 20% chance of guessing the correct answer if you respond randomly.

BEWARE OF *ALL* AND *NONE*

The ADA Department of Testing Services does not want to have to rescore examinations and answer inquiries regarding ambiguous questions. Therefore, "gentle" words, such as *usually*, *often*, and *rarely*, are preferred in answer choices. "Harsh" words—*always*, *never*, *all*, *none*—can prove disastrous if any one exception can be argued. If you are really baffled on a question, steer clear of choosing an answer containing a "harsh" word.

BE KNOWLEDGEABLE ABOUT DISTRACTERS

The wrong answer choices to a question are termed distracters because their purpose is to distract the test taker from the obvious correct answer. The ADA Department of Testing Services does not really want to confuse you; rather, it wants the correct answer to blend in with the wrong answers. The distracters lure the test taker from the correct answer by presenting possible answers that may be partially correct. On any given question, the distracters will be similar in their "degree of distraction." The following example will illustrate how to identify and eliminate distracters.

1. What is the first day of the week?

   A. January
   B. Monday
   C. Saturday
   D. 1st
   E. Sunday

It is obvious that Sunday, answer E, is correct. However, this simple example clearly shows how difficult science answers will be structured. Answers A and D test to see whether you can identify the days of the week. January is the first month of the year, and the 1st is the first day of the month. If you did not know the days of the week but you knew the months of the year, you might be distracted because January is the first month of the year. Answer C not only is a day of the week, but also starts with the same letter as the correct answer. This could distract the test taker who could identify the days of the week and who may have read once that Sunday is the first day of the week. The last distracter, answer B, Monday, is the type that you will find on the most difficult questions. Even if you know the days of the week and their sequence, you may still accidentally choose this distracter if little thought is put into selecting the answer. While Monday is the first day of the work week, it is not the first day of the calendar week.

Supplemental information must be used to eliminate the wrong answers. Do not get caught in the trap of choosing the most familiar and comfortable answer. On a difficult organic chemistry question involving an obscure reaction that you are not familiar with, undoubtedly at least two familiar reactions will appear in the answer choices as distracters. You will want to choose one of these as the correct response because we all like to feel comfortable with our answers. Use any knowledge you possess about any answer choices to identify distracters and thus eliminate them.

DRAW IT

You will almost always be able to more clearly understand what is being asked if you can sketch a chart, a figure, or some other graphical representation of the question you are asked. You will be given erasable scratch boards and markers upon request; use them to your advantage.

KNOW THE PAT DIRECTIONS

Before the test date, be sure that you know exactly what you will be asked to do in each section of the Perceptual Ability Test. For the other tests, the directions are rather straightforward; for the PAT, however, they are not as clear-cut. A sufficient review of the material presented in this book should clear up any confusion as to what will be required of you on the PAT's six sections.

BE SENSIBLE ABOUT SLEEP, EATING, AND EXERCISE

To give a peak performance on the day of the test, you will need to take care of yourself in the days prior. Eat right, get plenty of sleep, and exercise the week before the test. Getting adequate sleep the night before will not compensate for a series of late nights. Also, it is generally difficult to sleep the night before the test.

GET READY THE NIGHT BEFORE

The night before the test, you should have everything accounted for so that no last-minute stresses will distract you on test day. Be sure that everything you need is in order and that plans are set for your timely arrival at the test site. Again, your focus on the test is reinforced by a general sense of control over the situation. Have clear plans for the test day that include what you will eat, wear, and take to the center.

BE PREPARED TO SUCCEED

At the test site, remain calm. Don't be concerned about sweaty palms or a slightly racing heart. You know that you are prepared, and your body is reflecting the excitement that you feel—you are ready to peak!

ABOUT ANXIETY

By viewing your future goals as intimately connected to your actions in the present, you will undoubtedly acknowledge the value of engaging in preparative measures to ensure future success. You will possess a sense of control over your performance. Control will help you to stay focused, to remain in the present, and to use the mental tools that you have worked hard to refine. When you possess a high level of self-control, anxiety can serve you positively in two ways: It can help to keep you motivated as you actively prepare and it can even help boost performance on the day of the test.

It is normal to be anxious about the DAT. In fact, it would probably be a sign of concern if you had no qualms about the test. The fact that you possess a degree of anxiety suggests that you respect the difficulty of the test, the importance of peaking on test day, and the value of a high score. Anxiety will be your mentor, reminding you to actively prepare for this test. Anxiety will help to ensure that you have taken care of important details, such as verifying that you have the proper identification and familiarizing yourself with the best way to get to the test site. On the day of the test, if you maintain a sense of being in control of your own destiny, as discussed above, you will walk into the testing center confident that your hours of preparation will pay off. During the test, your slightly rapid heart rate will serve to keep you working at a productive pace. You will remain alert, and you will perform to your best ability.

BECOME COMFORTABLE WITH THE COMPUTERIZED FORMAT

Because the test will be administered on computer, you should be certain to clear up any concerns about the computer format prior to your test date. It is strongly suggested that you order the computer tutorial from the ADA Department of Testing Services. This will help you to know what the test will look like on the computer screen and how you can register your answers appropriately. You should also consider ahead of time how you will use your erasable boards and markers.

Dental Education and Practice

CHAPTER 2

THE APPLICATION PROCESS

Timeline of Events

Understanding the sequence of events in the application process should reduce the confusion and alleviate some stress. However, it should be noted that there is no correct sequence. You should use this timeline as a suggestion; then create your own timeline tailored to your individual situation.

When should you take the DAT? With the computerized format, you are now able to take the test at your convenience, so, the best answer is as soon as you are adequately prepared. Schedule time to review for the DAT, and then arrange an appropriate date with your local Sylvan Technology and Learning Center. You should try to take the DAT before the fall semester of your senior year (or the fall of the year prior to matriculation if you are not currently enrolled).

Note: You do not have to take the DAT before applying through the American Association of Dental Schools Application Service (AADSAS). Filling out and submitting your application early is imperative to maximizing your chances for acceptance. When you take the DAT, your scores will be sent directly to the dental schools to which you are applying through AADSAS.

The following timeline is a suggestion of when events should occur for the typical undergraduate who is seeking admission to dental school. Some extra suggestions have been included; however, they are not essential and are indicated with an asterisk (*).

Junior Year—Fall

- Start saving money for AADSAS fees and interviews.*
- Informally visit and tour the dental schools you have an interest in attending.*
- Keep your grades up.
- Intern with a dentist.*

Junior Year—Spring

- Register for the DAT (or summer between junior/senior year).

- Schedule a meeting with the Pre-Health Professions Advisor in your college or with faculty members to lay the groundwork for your letters of recommendation.

- Practice a mock dental school interview with your Pre-Health Professions Advisor, a faculty member, or a dentist.

- Start drafting your Personal Statement and have it reviewed by an on-campus writing specialist.

- Complete the Personal Statement.

Junior/Senior Summer

- Apply through AADSAS.

- Make sure you have appropriate clothes for an interview.

- Ask yourself these questions: Have you paid all necessary secondary processing fees to the schools to which you have applied? Have you submitted any additional information that was requested?

Senior Year—Fall

- Check your application status at the schools to which you have applied. A school will notify you if you are invited for an interview. Not all candidates are interviewed; only those who pass the first round of reviews from the Admissions Committee are invited to the school. It can't hurt, though, to inquire about your application status; and if your application is missing anything, the director of admissions will let you know.

- After an interview, send a follow-up thank you note to your interviewer.

- Keep in mind that the agreed national notification date for the AADS is December 1.

- If (When) you are accepted, remit a deposit to the school of your choice and withdraw your application from the others.

- Complete all necessary paperwork.

- Notify your Pre-Health Professions Officer of your decision, and thank him or her for help. Or, if you used individual faculty members and health practitioners, let them know of your decision and express your appreciation.

- If you plan to apply for financial aid, file your taxes as soon after January 1 as possible, as this will facilitate the process of awarding financial aid.

Senior Year—Spring

- Receive and complete financial aid paperwork provided by your school's Financial Aid Office.

- Complete orientation forms, and take care of predental school tasks, such as collecting teeth and getting your hepatitis shots.*

Senior Year—Summer

- Find housing accommodations.

- Try to network with current dental students, who can give you advice regarding books to buy, the best place to set up your bank account, and other details to make your transition to dental school as easy as possible.

American Association of Dental Schools Application Service (AADSAS)

In order to apply to most dental schools, you must use a universal application that is offered through the American Association of Dental Schools Application Service (AADSAS). The AADSAS application enables a student to apply to several schools with greater ease and has helped Admissions Committees to efficiently process and review applications.

AADSAS serves merely as a clearinghouse for applications; this service plays no role in the evaluative aspect of the admissions process. Students who apply through AADSAS submit transcripts, a Personal Statement, a list of intended future coursework, information regarding participation in activities, financial aid requests, and letters of recommendation. For a fee, AADSAS processes all of this information and then disseminates it in a profile folder and on diskette to each school that the candidate has indicated an interest in attending. Thus, with one AADSAS application, a student can apply to several schools.

After all required documents and fees have been submitted to AADSAS, the service generally takes from 3 to 6 weeks to process an application and send it to all of the candidate's requested schools. Upon receipt of your official AADSAS identification number, you can be confident that your materials are on the way to the schools you indicated.

Once the AADSAS profile folders and diskettes are received by a dental school, the Admissions Committee reviews them and then selects candidates for interviews. The main items of information from the AADSAS application that the Admissions Committee will weigh are your grades (science and nonscience), Personal Statement, letters of recommendation, and DAT scores.

It should be mentioned that, although most schools rely solely on the information provided by the AADSAS application, some schools also have secondary applications. It is important, therefore, that you find out exactly what is required in the application process for each individual school.

Common mistakes to avoid in filling out the application include not following the specific directions provided by AADSAS and leaving blanks. If you are not sure how to answer something on the AADSAS application, call the service directly or call a dental school admissions officer for advice. Mistakes made on the AADSAS application can hold up your application for weeks. As time is of the essence, avoid submitting an AADSAS application with errors.

In the event that you become aware of an error made on an application that has been submitted to AADSAS and disseminated to the schools you indicated, you must request AADSAS to complete the paperwork needed to issue a revised application to each school to which you are applying.

Although not required, it is suggested that you submit an AADSAS application prior to your senior year. In the event that you do apply earlier, however, you will need to update your application with current grades (up to and including fall grades from your senior year) and note any other additions or changes by using the revised application form provided by AADSAS.

AADSAS applications are usually made available in the middle of the summer.

In addition to providing the application service, the American Association of Dental Schools provides a useful guide that is recommended for review by prospective dental students. Published yearly, *Admission Requirements: United States and Canadian Dental Schools* includes each school's most recent incoming class profile (average DAT scores, GPAs, etc.). Additionally, information is given about the program offered by each dental school, and the composition of the student body is described.

Letters of Recommendation

Letters of recommendation play a key role in Admissions Committees' decision-making process. They serve as an analysis and critique of your abilities and true desire to attend a school of dental medicine. Most dental schools require a minimum of three letters of recommendation for your file to be considered complete. These letters should come from faculty members, preferably in the sciences, of your college.

Admissions Committees prefer to review letters that not only comment on your intellectual abilities but also address your personal demeanor. Because you are attempting to enter a profession that requires patient interaction, your communicative skills and compassion should be critically assessed. Furthermore, as the competitiveness for positions in dental schools escalates, Admissions Committees are adamant about selecting students who have experience in dental medicine, whether this be observational or hands-on. Recommendations can serve to address any experience you have had in the field of dentistry.

Generally speaking, if you and another applicant appear similarly qualified on paper—same grades, DAT scores, and the like—your letters of recommendation could be the deciding factor between your admittance and the other candidate's.

If you are serious about attending dental school, it is suggested that you start finding possible recommenders during your undergraduate studies. This means that you should attend classes, be prepared, sit in the front row, ask questions, and approach faculty members early on to disclose your desire to study dentistry. Although you will not formally need to secure your letters until your junior year, if you identify yourself—favorably, of course—early, you will be remembered later.

The type of institution you attend may dictate the type of recommendation letter dossier you will compile. Some colleges have Pre-Health Profession Committees. If you attend a large university, more than likely there is an on-campus Pre-Health Professions Office. This office is specifically designed to advise and assist students whose goal is to attend a graduate health professions school, whether it be medical, dental, physical therapy, or other. (Some smaller colleges also have these resources.)

Undergraduate students are often unaware that a Pre-Health Professions Office exists at their college or university, or they assume that this office is only for students preparing to gain admittance to medical school. If you are unsure as to whether your undergraduate college or university has a Pre-Health Professions Office, check with your academic advisor.

The Pre-Health Professions Office is responsible for compiling and mailing out your letters of recommendation, thereby helping to ensure their confidentiality. Whether or not you make use of a Pre-Health Professions Office, you will be asked to sign a statement that you waive the right to read your letters of recommendation. Although you have the option to retain this right, the norm is to waive it. The person you ask to write a letter for you may not give an entirely reflective and honest account of your abilities if you have access to his or her statement.

Some colleges have the Pre-Health Profession Committee write a profile on you that is mailed to the schools you wish to attend. If your school adheres to this practice, you probably will need to make a formal appointment for an interview with the Pre-Health Profession Committee. You should take this interview very seriously; it will be similar to any formal interview you will have at a dental school. The individuals who comprise the Pre-Health Profession Committee are professionals who either have been selected or have volunteered to serve as reviewers of the potential pre-health professions candidates at their particular college or university. There will be faculty from the sciences, student service personnel, and the chair of the Pre-Health Professions Office, who may be either a faculty member or a student service professional.

Appearing before the Pre-Health Profession Committee is a rigorous process. Prior to your interview, the members will often request to review a Personal Statement (this can be the same statement that you submit to AADSAS) and your official college transcripts. During your scheduled formal interview, they will review your grades and ask you about your desire to attend dental school, your exposure to dental medicine, and your hobbies and activities (see "The Interview," page 20). After you meet with the Pre-Health Profession Committee, the members will review your candidacy, draft a comprehensive letter, or complete a Likert scale form that assesses your abilities. The committee then assigns a recommendation rank. Usually the rank represents some variation of "Highly Recommend;" "Recommend;" "Recommend with Reservation;" or "Do Not Recommend."

Given that this can be an arduous process, why would a student choose to go through the Pre-Health Profession Committee? *A letter of recommendation from the Pre-Health Profession Committee is preferred over individual letters from faculty.* This is not to say that you will be penalized if your school does not have a Pre-Health Profession Committee. However, Admissions Committees are aware that the Pre-Health Profession Committee is an assemblage of persons who possess the knowledge base and skills to accurately assess future health care practitioners.

While some Pre-Health Professions Offices actually issue the recommendations, others make it the student's responsibility to approach faculty recommenders for the written assessment. The faculty submit their recommendations directly to a Pre-Health Professions Office, which, in turn, will compile the letters and mail them out at the student's request.

It is obviously in your best interest to approach professors with whom you have had some interaction, even if limited, or for whom you performed well in their course(s). Ideally, your recommenders are professors who know you well and have seen your potential. After selecting these professors, you should arrange individual meetings with them to discuss your goals and reasons for selecting the dental schools you have chosen.

If your hands-on or observational experience in dentistry has been only with family members, it is suggested that these persons not write recommendations. Given the familial connection, such endorsements are not appropriate and will not be given serious consideration.

Regardless of whether you are using a Pre-Health Profession Committee or an assemblage of faculty recommenders, you should provide these persons with your personal statement, resume, and transcript. The more documentation you provide, the easier it will be for them to write strong letters.

When you meet with the Pre-Health Profession Committee or with your faculty recommenders to discuss your goals and reasons for applying to dental school, you should also address your strengths and weaknesses. Be honest about any shortcomings in your academic record. Nobody but you can provide the personal insight that is often needed to humanize data and to account for any blemishes that appear in your file. It is important that you state what you have done to overcome setbacks or how you have dealt with adversity.

Once you have completed the appropriate meetings, be sure that the committee or individual faculty members have all they need to complete the recommendation. Find out when your committee letter or individual faculty letters will be complete. If you are not making use of a Pre-Health Profession Committee, and individual faculty members are writing the recommendations, it is suggested that you collect and mail them. These recommendations *must* be sealed and bear the instructors' signatures across the seal of the envelopes.

Lastly, acknowledge the time and effort that went into writing the recommendations by sending thank you letters to the committee or your individual faculty recommenders. Also, once a decision has been made concerning your dental schooling, you should notify those who offered you their support.

SUPPLEMENTAL LETTERS OF SUPPORT

In some circumstances it is appropriate to submit more than the required number of letters of recommendation. If you have spent time observing or assisting in a dental office or have performed some type of noteworthy community service, you may also submit supplementary letters of recommendation. Although most schools request only three letters of recommendation, *it is acceptable to go over this limit* within reason. If you are going through the committee process and its members are writing your formal letter, you may ask to have a supplemental letter or supplemental letters added. Generally, the committee will readily comply with this request.

A SPECIAL NOTE TO NONTRADITIONAL STUDENTS

If you have made the decision to attend dental school after being in the work force for a number of years, you may also submit supplemental letters from your employer(s). However, it is still advisable to follow the protocol of submitting letters from faculty members, preferably in the sciences. If your alma mater has a Pre-Health Professions Office, you should still, as an alumnus/alumna, have access to its services. Otherwise, you should follow the recommendations for traditional students in this situation.

PERSONAL STATEMENT

Your essay is the first form of personal contact that the Admissions Committee has with you. It is of utmost importance, therefore, that you write an essay that is truly reflective of your motivation to attend dental school. This essay serves as a unique personal window that only you can open for your readers.

In all strong essays, candidates use this opportunity not only as a means of introduction, but also as a way to highlight personal strengths and, where applicable, address any weaknesses that may have a bearing on their candidacy.

The Personal Statement is an appropriate vehicle to describe any honors you may have been awarded, whether academic or civic, and to tell why you were so recognized. Furthermore, any experiences you have had in the field of dentistry, such as an internship with a general practitioner, should be highlighted and explained in the Personal Statement. It is not enough to write that you have had "hands-on" experience. What did you do? What did you learn? Why did this experience or these experiences solidify your decision to attend dental school?

Also, you may describe any leadership positions you held during your undergraduate tenure, write about clubs you have been involved with, and/or discuss practical work experiences you have had. The point of providing this information is to demonstrate to the Admissions Committee that you are a well-rounded individual.

Address the depth of your experiences. For example, how did being a class officer help you to learn to work with others? Has your involvement in civic organizations heightened your compassion for others? Give concrete evidence as to why these activities have been meaningful to you, and also explain how they have contributed to your candidacy for dental school.

If you are applying to dental school after being out of college for a number of years, you should focus on your life experiences after earning your undergraduate degree. This out-of-school time will not be seen as a weakness in your essay if you compose a thoughtful statement integrating your recent activities with your aspirations. What wisdom and insight have you gained since leaving school? More importantly, why have you decided to pursue dental medicine; what has made you decide to change your career track? Or, if you are already working in the field of dentistry, as a hygienist, for example, why is it now important for you to further your education?

In addition to writing about your strengths, you may also wish to address any weaknesses in your overall application. For example, if your grades suffered during a particular semester, explain why. Perhaps a parent died or you were ill. In addressing your weaknesses, you should not elaborate in great detail; the gravity of a situation such as the death of a parent is well understood. Nor should weaknesses be the focus of your Personal Statement. You have only one page in which to clearly and concisely present yourself, so strategically compose your essay with an emphasis on the positive.

Because the Personal Statement serves as the Admissions Committee's first assessment of you as an individual, it is important to attract their attention at the outset. An opening paragraph that begins "Ever since I was a young child I have wanted to attend dental school" is trite and probably untrue. Approach this component of your application as an opportunity to be creative.

Brainstorm some experiences that you have had within the field of dentistry. Think of quotations to incorporate that summarize you as a person, embody your ethics, or have been of particular inspiration to you. Have a theme to your essay. Use humor with care—don't become too comedic, and be sure to avoid sarcasm. Most important, what have you accomplished in your life that sets you apart from the other 1,000 candidates applying to dental school? Don't trivialize your successes; be proud of your achievements while maintaining a sense of humility.

As the Personal Statement is part of your application to graduate school, it should be flawless and presented in a professional manner. Essays that are handwritten or contain many errors in spelling or grammar are unacceptable. Before submitting your final draft, proofread it several times. Also, find someone in your school's writing center who will critique and, where necessary, correct your Personal Statement. You might ask the faculty members writing your letters of recommendation or perhaps someone in a Pre-Health Professions Office to give you feedback on your essay.

It is expected that the Personal Statement be formally presented in a black, easy-to-read font. Before you print out your statement on the official form provided by AADSAS, make duplicates of the form and test-run your final essay through the computer's printer. You may discover that you need to adjust your margins to fit within the AADSAS format.

However you choose to approach the writing of your Personal Statement, try to readily embrace the task, rather than viewing it as an arduous chore. Remember that the words you write serve as a precursor to any interviews you wish to secure. A well-written, well-executed Personal Statement should pique the Admissions Committees' curiosity about you as a candidate and make them want to learn more during an interview.

Three Personal Statements from successful applicants are reprinted here to provide you with examples of well-written essays. Proper names have been omitted, but the essays are otherwise reprinted as they appeared on the AADSAS form. Examine how each statement contains details that shed light on the uniqueness of the applicant.

PERSONAL STATEMENT 1

Science and artistry, two seemingly unrelated terms, share a harmonious relationship with each other. I believe that dentistry reveals this intrinsic and unconstrained association, allowing the two terms to be juxtaposed in a natural way. I have devoted 16 years to the piano and 12 years to the flute; the two instruments have become prominent defining factors in my life. With the many required hours of practice each day and with the number of different performances, I have acquired a deep happiness and satisfaction in producing the art forms with my hands and fingers. Because of the emphasis I have placed on the development of manual dexterity, I feel that the career that I choose should in some way incorporate my hands to a large degree. I am a steadfast believer that the hands have an amazing power to heal.

I liken the practice of dentistry to the learning of a new musical piece: both facilitate the satisfaction of beginning a project and having a final product to show at the end. In dentistry, a problem is recognized; then certain skills are employed to remedy it. Whether it be filling a cavity or replacing a crown, the acquired techniques and skills are utilized and directed toward the specific situation. With the piano and flute, I slowly work each key, measure by measure, from the beginning, until the time tuning of the piece is accomplished. Both dentistry and the playing of an instrument require the mechanical skill that develops through years of training. The idea of focusing my mind on something specific and then applying a certain technique to achieve the desired goal appeals greatly to me.

Many people question health practitioners about the reasons they choose their certain profession. The answer "I want to help people" has been stated so frequently that it almost seems cliched; however, I truly believe that the words warrant greater respect. When I was seven, a tragic accident ended my brother's life. From that episode of my life, a seed was implanted within my mind to one day serve others and help them in some way, whether by performing music, saving lives, aiding in the betterment of health, or by other means. With involvement in activities that serve the community—soup kitchens, ministry within the church, performances at hospitals and geriatric homes, volunteering at the local hospitals, and charity concerts—I have realized that I ultimately want a profession that enables me to serve others. Because of my combined need to help people and love for science, I have found that dentistry has the special characteristics that many other occupations do not afford.

I hope that one day, as a practicing dentist, I will be able to help people feel better about themselves. I want to help people attain a beautiful smile and increase their level of self-esteem and confidence. Having grown up in Taiwan in the 1930's and 40's, my parents were not so fortunate as to have had the dental treatment that the present generations receive. I see how, in every photo, there is always embarrassment at being unable to show a nice smile because they are so ashamed of their teeth. I see the suffering and the pain that they go through, having received numerous crowns, bridges, and root canals. It is important to inform people that maintaining personal health and caring for one's teeth and gums are vital to everyday life. I want to show people that they can exercise control over their own health. Dentistry undoubtedly allows the possibility of achieving this goal.

PERSONAL STATEMENT 2

At the age of eleven, I possessed the facial structure of the nation's favorite TV horse, Mr. Ed. People were forced to duck whenever they came face to face with my teeth. Fortunately, my parents eagerly placed me in the hands of my would be hero, Dr. [omitted], who gave me not only a smile to be proud of but also the self-confidence and courage to venture into the most terrifying stage of life: adolescence. Amazing! The truth is, dentistry had fascinated me long before my braces came into existence. My lifelong exposure to the health care field, my innate interest in dentistry accompanied by the hands on experience I have gained in the profession throughout the years, and finally my desire to dedicate my life to the service of others are some of the reasons I have decided to pursue a career as a dentist.

As the daughter of a physician, the hard work, sacrifice, and devotion involved in the delivery of quality health care are well known to me. I was first exposed to patient care and interaction at the age of fifteen when my father asked me to work for him as an office clerk, and a short time later as a medical assistant. After seeing my father skillfully and confidently helping other human beings, I knew my future work would be in the health care field. Although many of my summers were spent working as a medical assistant, never did I stray from my lifelong desire to become a dentist. Given my profound interest in dentistry, I contacted my regular dentist, Dr. [omitted], in [omitted], Georgia, and asked for the opportunity to observe him at work. My fascination lead me to advance from the status of "tourist," to volunteer worker, and finally to part-time employee during the summers of '91, '93, and '96. Currently I am volunteering six to eight hours a week at his office while I also work part-time as a medical assistant at my father's surgical practice. Not only does a career in dentistry give me the ability and freedom to establish my professional independence, but also the ongoing scientific and technical advancements in the field ensure continuous challenges and motivation, while allowing me the opportunity to enrich my life through humanitarian service to my community. I anticipate with much excitement the intellectual and personal challenges the dental field will provide throughout my years of practice.

At this time my primary interest lies in the field of pediatric dentistry. Because of the absence of a pediatric dentist in [omitted], I have had the delight of working with the many children who come into Dr. [omitted] office. For me, children are magical. I vowed to dedicate my future work to children in the summer of 1994 when I volunteered at the [omitted] Oncology Clinic for Children in [omitted], Georgia. Here I devoted my time to the entertainment and supervision of the children (patients and siblings) in the playroom. This experience reinforced the profound and innate joy the ability to help others as well as working with children gives me.

The highlight of my undergraduate studies at [omitted] University occurred during my senior year when I was granted the privilege to do research in the field of reproductive biology at the [omitted] Primate Research Center of [omitted] University. During the course of the year I studied the effects of certain cryoprotective additives on the biological and biophysical parameters of human embryos, and cow and rhesus monkey oocytes. Dissecting cow and rhesus monkey ovaries and extracting and recovering oocytes, along with their subsequent handling through the use of special pipettes, not only sharpened my mechanical abilities but also showed me how much I enjoyed the mechanical challenge of precision work. Thus, while patient care is to be my primary focus as a dentist, I nonetheless intend to actively engage in research while in dental school. Having lived in a rural area for almost ten years now, I know from firsthand experience the lack of and need for qualified and specialized health care professionals. I enjoy the life-style small towns have to offer, and as a result I plan to settle down in a rural area following my dental education. My ultimate goal is to better serve the more underprivileged communities with little or no access to dental care.

I would like to give back to dentistry what it has given to me: dedication, excellence, and compassion. There are currently five physicians, three physical therapists, three nurses, one speech therapist, and one optometrist in my family. I have had sufficient exposure to every single one of these areas, and not one of them has been able to captivate my interest as has dentistry. The beauty of dentistry lies within its power to coalesce the sciences, arts, and humanities to make it the unique vocation that it is. I desire more than anything the opportunity to be part of a field that allows me to help my fellow human beings while offering me the challenge and satisfaction necessary to lead a fulfilled and productive life.

PERSONAL STATEMENT 3

From my first retainer, to braces, to oral surgery, my teeth and I have experienced many of the services of the dental profession. No matter how physically uncomfortable a procedure, the dentists always treated me and their other patients with a compassion and devotion that instilled a certain resolve in me to pursue the field of dentistry.

My exposure to the dental profession has mostly been from the chair, and it was not until about a year ago that I came to the realization that dentistry was the perfect career for me. Past experiences and current visits to my own dentist to view the inner workings of the field have encouraged my desire, and everything about my decision began to fall into place. My attraction to dentistry began about seventeen years ago with my PlayDoh Dental Set. I spent many fun-filled hours making teeth, drilling, and pulling. At age five I remember discussing setting up a dental office with my friend. Of course, then it would have been a "you hold them down and I'll yank" type of practice. Luckily, I've become more sensitive since then! I know that my quest to become a dentist is real. I am adamant about committing to this intense, yet rewarding path.

To make sure that my choice was the right one, I spent a number of days in my dentist's office. The doctors there amazed me, not only by the technology used, but also by giving me a glimpse into the doctors' rapport with their patients. I was fascinated that children who are normally apprehensive about spending time in a dentist's chair could leave the office with a shine on their teeth and a smile on their faces. I spoke to a number of people in the field, and they were all dedicated, sincere professionals who left me feeling confident about my decision to attend dental school.

Apart from the actual dental work, I know that the doctor must have a trusting, caring relationship with each patient. This interaction is not something that can be obtained from books. My experience with community service both in high school and at [omitted] University has helped me to develop a greater understanding of people.

As a college freshman, I began with a volunteer organization and tutored a high school senior who read at a first grade level. While pleased with his progress, I realized that he needed more structured assistance than I could offer. I expressed my concerns to his guidance counselor and teacher, and succeeded in getting him into the school's special program. I was instrumental in starting an after school study program at an area high school. During my sophomore year, I assisted a graduate by teaching high school ESL students. This class was very rewarding. I taught half the students by myself, which gave me greater confidence speaking in front of people and articulating my ideas. For the past three years, my roommate and I have been a part of Project [omitted]. We pick up perishables from local businesses and deliver them to various shelters in the area to aid the homeless.

My greatest achievement as a volunteer has been working for "[omitted]." I have contributed a lot of time and effort to this program, ultimately serving as president for the past two years. "[omitted]" distributes donated furniture to those in the greater Providence area who cannot afford to buy their own. When out on a shift, I meet many people who directly benefit from "[omitted]." I have had many memorable experiences as a member of this organization.

In addition to these volunteer organizations, other extracurricular activities include intramural soccer and ice-skating. I played hockey for many years and take advantage of the time I can spend in an ice rink. From a teaching assistant in immunology, to an ice-skating instructor, to president of "[omitted]," my extracurricular activities have broadened my perspective and enriched me as a person. I especially enjoy interacting with children and had a job as a camp counselor for the past three summers.

This summer I am involved in research at [omitted] Cancer Center. Interning in the Human Immunogenetics Laboratory affords me the opportunity for intellectual growth and increased technical aptitudes. Not only am I gaining a great deal of knowledge from assisting in the lab on a groundbreaking study, but also the molecular biological protocol involves manipulating DNA and bacteria, which requires a delicate, exacting hand—excellent practice for dentistry.

I am excited at the prospect of embarking on a career in dentistry. I hope to incorporate my desire to work with children, and participate in current research along with my dental education and career. I look forward to it with great anticipation.

The Interview

Much preparation is required for an interview. The 20 to 30 minutes you spend in an interview may be the final contributing factor determining your acceptance to dental school. Interviewers are continually amazed at the number of applicants who drift into admissions interviews without any apparent preparation and only the vaguest idea of what they are going to say. Since the interview plays such a critical role in the selection process, you should prepare for it as you would for any other examination on which you would be evaluated.

In preparation for an interview, research the dental school that you will be visiting. Then prepare a short personal history that will help you focus on the important aspects that you would like to convey during the interview. Review the highlights of your undergraduate experience, summer jobs, research, volunteer work, and experience with dentistry. It is important to be able to relate some personal experiences and history in the interview in order to establish a rapport with the interviewer. The picture you provide to the interviewer must convince him or her that you are the best candidate for admission. Be ready to state why you chose the field of dental medicine and what unique perspectives you can bring to that particular school. Having a strong sense of oneself and taking adequate time to prepare will help the dynamics of the interview.

Applicants who have thoroughly prepared will enter into the interview process with focus and confidence. Be aware that the interview will start the moment you walk into the room. Your posture and manner will create a first impression. For this reason you should practice how to enter a room, sit, and stand. Maintain eye contact and a pleasant look. Positive facial expressions and body language set the mood for a constructive interview and can help conversation flow. You will want to manage the interview through posture, voice, and manner and to engage the interviewer by conveying thoughts and feelings with enthusiasm throughout the interview.

Listed below are some questions that interviewers frequently ask. Practicing your responses to these questions out loud will help you to become a more articulate and polished speaker.

- Why do you want to be a dentist?

- What originally stimulated your interest in dental medicine?

- What steps have you taken to acquaint yourself with what a dentist does?

- What do you do in your spare time?

- With so many well-qualified candidates, why should we invite you to enroll at our school of dental medicine?

- As an interviewer, what should I look for in a candidate?

- What prompted you to apply to our school?

- How would your plans differ if we were now under socialized medicine?

- What do you think is the most pressing issue in dental medicine today?

- What was the last book that you have read? Or favorite book?

- Have you previously applied to other educational programs (i.e., medicine, public health, or M.S. program)?

- How has your undergraduate major prepared you for dental school and a career in dentistry?

- What are your biggest fears?

- What are your strengths? Weaknesses?

- Is there anything else you would like us to know that hasn't yet been conveyed in your application?

Throughout the entire interview process, speak about those areas that you know best or feel passionately about. Your enthusiasm and interest, shown in your voice and accompanying facial expressions, will engage the interviewer. With proper preparation and confidence, you will have a successful interview.

Most interviews will have a traditional one-on-one format. Some schools, however, use a committee interview, which can be a bit more daunting than just meeting with one faculty member or dental school administrator. Prior to your interview, contact the Admissions Office and ask which format that particular school uses. If the answer is a committee format, you may want to practice before a simulated committee of friends or family. Generally speaking, the questions will be the same as in a one-on-one interview, but being questioned by more than one person can be a nerve-wracking experience. If you prepare for a committee interview, it will pose no greater challenge than the one-on-one format. Try to remember to address all interviewers rather than focusing on the person who asked you a particular question. If you stumble over a question, ask whether you can come back to it later; the interviewers know that you are human and it's normal to be a bit nervous.

An interview is your opportunity to view the school as a prospective applicant who may become an enrolled student. Not only are you being interviewed; this is your turn to interview the school. Therefore, be prepared to ask some questions of the interviewer regarding the dental school or even the dental profession. This will convey the message that you have a serious interest in the particular school or the future of dentistry.

Listed below are some commonly asked questions from prospective students:

- What is the faculty/student ratio? What percentage of the faculty is full-time? Part-time?

- What is the male/female ratio of the dental student body? Minority student enrollment? In state/out-of-state enrollment?

- What were last year's statistics for your incoming class? GPAs? DATs?

- How many of your graduates specialize in ortho, perio, endo, oral surgery, etc.?

- How many attended GPRs or AEGDs? How many went into the military?

- How much is tuition? How much are instruments, supplies, and other expenses? Is financial aid available? Are scholarships, grants, and fellowships available?

- What is the average student indebtedness at graduation?

- Are there opportunities for research?

- Can I pursue any other degrees, such as an M.P.H. or M.B.A., while I am a dental student here?

- How did your students perform on the National Boards last year?

- What can you tell me about the patient pool and how patients are assigned?

- Where do most of the dental students live? What is an average figure for the cost of living?

- Is the school located in a safe area?

- How are curriculum problems addressed and are there any?

- Do the students have any participation in the decision-making process for the school?

- What clubs, student dental organizations, and fraternities exist?

- With all of the school requirements, is it difficult to participate in extracurricular activities?

Most interviews are scheduled so that you will have the opportunity to meet current dental students, admissions staff, financial aid officers, and, of course, faculty members. You should also be provided with a tour of the facilities so that you can view the clinics and preclinics, library space, computer facilities, and the like. While you are visiting the dental schools where you have been invited to interview, ask questions! In particular, take time to speak frankly with one or more dental students. It is through your communication with the student body that you will gain the most insight into the real inside workings of the school. For example, a stressed and tired dental student will not hold back on revealing what he or she perceives as inadequacies in the system. Listen closely, and note the school's weaknesses as well as its strengths.

Remember: The purpose of an interview is not to line you up in front of a firing squad. Rather, the goal should be a positive exchange of information between you and the interviewer(s). Ultimately you are looking for a good fit between your expectations of a dental program and the reality of what that particular school offers. The Admissions Committee is likewise looking for confirmation that you would be successful at this institution and that it would benefit by having you as a member of their next incoming class.

Financial Aid—A Brief Overview

There are two major types of financial aid, *gift aid*, which refers to scholarships and grants, and *nongift aid*, which refers to loans. Unfortunately, at the graduate school level, there are no grants similar to what you may have had as an undergraduate student, such as the federal Pell Grant, or a state-sponsored grant. Scholarships are available: some are merit based; others are not. More than likely, the dental school you attend will award merit-based scholarships once you have matriculated and are a dental student. These merit-based awards will be disbursed based on grades and class rank, so be sure to work hard in dental school. Other scholarships may be based on involvement in research, clubs, and other activities, or on other criteria, such as representation of a minority group in the field of dentistry.

The first step in applying for financial aid, if you intend to take out student loans, is to file a Free Application for Federal Student Aid (FAFSA). Anyone who plans to apply for student loans *must* have this application on file with the federal government. In order to file the FAFSA, if you worked you should complete your federal income tax return as soon after January 1 as possible. This is also the date when the FAFSA forms for the upcoming school year become available.

Keep in mind that, by virtue of the fact that you will be a graduate student, you are now independent for financial aid purposes. *Do not* report parental/guardian information on the FAFSA unless otherwise requested by your dental school's financial aid office. We suggest that you submit your completed FAFSA to your financial aid office so that a professional financial aid officer can check for errors; corrections can take up to 6 weeks.

The FAFSA is a tool used by the federal government to calculate students' Expected Family Contribution (EFC). This is not as intimidating as it sounds; rather, it is a number used in calculating your need for financial aid.

After the FAFSA has been filed, within 4 to 6 weeks, you will receive a Student Aid Report (SAR) in the mail. It is always printed on colored paper and is typically five pages long. The SAR is simply a printed-out report of all the information you provided on the FAFSA. The second step in applying for financial aid is to submit your SAR to the dental school you will be attending. The financial aid office needs the SAR to obtain your EFC.

The third step in applying for financial aid (if you plan to borrow funds) is to obtain and complete a Stafford Loan application. After the federal government has processed your FAFSA, you will receive a Stafford Loan application in the mail. By then, you should also receive from your dental school financial aid office an award letter that will notify you of how much, if any, funds you will need to borrow for school. Your award letter is a simple equation:

$$\text{Budget Amount} - \text{EFC} = \text{Need}$$

After you have received your award letter and have completed your Stafford Loan application, return the loan application(s) to your financial aid office to double-check the material for accuracy. Your financial aid office also has a responsibility to "certify" all loans, that is, approve you for the funds requested on your loan application(s).

Once the loan application process has been completed, you have finished—for one financial aid cycle. You will have to complete all necessary paperwork on a yearly basis, however, while enrolled in school. Keep in mind, too, that if you need to defer payment on student loans obtained when you were an undergraduate, you will need to do that every semester while in dental school. Your financial aid office should have all the appropriate deferment forms.

The Stafford Loan Program is the most comprehensive and accessible loan to dental students who are U.S. citizens or permanent residents. However, even with the maximum total award through the Stafford Loan Program, some dental students find that they are still short of funds for school. Most of those students will apply for a

DEAL Loan, which has rates similar to those of the Stafford Loan while the student is enrolled; however, the interest rates fluctuate while the borrower is in repayment. Finally, another loan is the Health Professions Loan (HPL), which is subsidized while the dental student is in school; but the amounts awarded are usually low compared to the amounts available through the Stafford or DEAL Program. Also, even though a student is independent for financial aid purposes, for the HPL parents must submit a signed tax return and complete a school-specific supplemental application.

A Note to Foreign Dental School Applicants

A major problem for foreign applicants is that the formula AADSAS uses for calculating grades is not always comparable to a foreign scale. If you have determined that AADSAS calculated your foreign transcripts incorrectly, you will want to approach the individual dental schools to rectify the problem. One possibility is to provide each dental school you wish to attend with a notarized copy of your transcript. The school, in turn, can have the transcript evaluated by the on-campus office that works specifically with international students.

One of the most serious problems associated with foreign students who choose to pursue an education in the United States is the lack of financial aid that is available to them. Generally speaking, unless a student holds a green card/is a permanent resident, he or she is ineligible for financial aid programs such as the Stafford loan. Also, in order to apply for studies in the United States, students have to provide proof of sponsorship. There are a few sources of loans to foreign students, which you should investigate.

If English is your second language, some dental schools may require that you take the TOEFL (Test Of English as a Foreign Language) test. This varies from school to school: some schools use the DAT reading comprehension score to ascertain language ability, others do not. Therefore, check with the dental schools to which you are applying to see what their policies are toward non-native language speakers.

Most dental schools with English prerequisites do accept Grade 13 English and the Canadian DAT. However, to be sure, you should call all the dental schools in the United States that you are interested in attending to check their individual requirements.

DENTAL SCHOOL

In almost all dental schools, the first 2 years are primarily devoted to courses in the basic sciences and preclinic dental sciences. Most courses have both a didactic (lecture format) and laboratory component. All schools teach the following courses within the first 2 years as they are tested subjects on Part I of the National Board Dental Examinations:

- Anatomic Sciences
- Biochemistry
- Physiology
- Microbiology
- Pathology
- Dental Anatomy and Occlusion

Although pharmacology is not tested on Part I, it is often taught in the second year so that the students may begin practice in the clinic by their third year.

The third and fourth years are taught mostly in the clinic. The emphasis is on radiology, operative dentistry, anesthesia, and the clinical specialties of periodontics, endodontics, prosthodontics, pedodontics, orthodontics, and oral surgery.

Some schools have unique programs integrating the science disciplines, whereas others teach via a "problem-based learning" format or a "case-based learning" format. Some schools have condensed the basic science curriculum into 14–18 months. Some of these alternative curricula are very interesting and should be fully investigated if you are considering a school that provides such an education.

The following is a sample schedule similar to most dental school curricula:

First Year

General Histology

Embryology

Oral Histology

Biochemistry

Dental Materials

Dental Anatomy

Amalgam Restoration

Functional Waxing

Gross Anatomy

Neuroanatomy

Head and Neck Anatomy

Preventative Dentistry

Occlusion

Composite Restoration

Physiology

Cast Restorations

Second Year

Pathology

Oral Radiology

Anesthesia

Microbiology

Pharmacology

Pediatric Dentistry

Removable Partial Dentures

Periodontology

Occlusion

Behavioral Science

Nutrition

Radiology

Oral Surgery

Orthodontics

Endodontics

Dental Materials

Complete Dentures

Fixed Partial Dentures

Third Year

Oral Pathology

Oral Medicine

Anesthesia

Oral Surgery

Prosthodontics

Orthodontics

Endodontics

Abnormal Psychology

Geriatrics

Esthetic Dentistry

TMD Management

Electives

Periodontics

Pediatric Dentistry

Radiology

Fourth Year

Ethics	Oral Surgery
Practice Management	Pediatric Dentistry
Dental Public Health	Prosthodontics
Oral Medicine	Restorative Dentistry
Emergency Care Clinic	Periodontology
Implantology	Orthodontics
Diagnosis and Treatment Planning	Electives
Maxillofacial Prosthodontics	

THE PROFESSION OF DENTISTRY

Dentistry is the branch of the healing arts devoted to maintaining and treating the oral cavity and maxillofacial complex. A dentist is a scientist dedicated to providing a high quality of health care through prevention, diagnosis, and treatment of oral diseases. The dentist contributes enormously to the state of a person's health and quality of life. Through prevention of decay, periodontal disease, malocclusion, and oral-facial anomalies, dentistry provides an invaluable service to the public.

The opportunities and responsibilities of the dental profession in today's society are dynamic and make the field one of the most exciting, challenging, and rewarding professions. The dental profession includes involvement in research, public health, and patient care. Each discipline contributes to the overall general welfare of the public.

Dentistry offers many challenges and rewards. The profession is one of autonomy; becoming a dentist allows you the freedom to be your own boss. Today's private-practice dentist is more than a clinician. Dentists also must be businesspeople and managers. As a manager, you must constantly be aware of the consumer, the government, and third-party representatives. Your knowledge and ability as a businessperson is as important as your clinical skills.

Dentists need a thorough understanding of how to manage themselves, their staff, and their patients. Strong communication skills are essential in this management process. Communication skills include interpersonal skills, listening skills, speaking skills, and nonverbal skills. No matter how good a dentist's clinical skills may be, the quality of his or her communication skills will greatly impact the dental practice. The ability to provide dental services depends on the ability to inform patients about their dental needs. Uninformed patients will not perceive the importance of good dental health. Excellent patient relationships help ensure the best treatment for the patient and also will benefit the dental practice, leading to increased patient referrals and recommendations. Strong interpersonal communicative skills promote the sort of caring, friendly atmosphere vital to a successful practice.

Dentistry is both an art and a science. The outstanding dentist possesses both superior manual dexterity and technical expertise. A dentist restores a patient's dentition to be both functional and aesthetically pleasing. Restoring teeth, especially cosmetic dentistry, improves the self-esteem of patients. For most dentists, the greatest satisfaction is derived from improving patients' self-esteem through restoring their smiles.

Dentistry offers various opportunities from which an individual can choose based on his or her personality and career objectives. The following are some of the options that should be anticipated and considered:

- Solo practice
- Associateship
- Academics
- Dental research
- Service in the federal government
- Public health care

Because of the dynamic state of U.S. health care, new career options are being developed every year. New opportunities for dental health care providers are being created in private practice, industry, government, dental societies, national scientific organizations, and educational institutions.

A basic question that a recent graduate must ask him or herself is whether to pursue a solo or an associate practice. Historically, one of the factors in selecting dentistry as a career has been the opportunity to be one's own boss. Approximately 150,000 dentists are practicing in the United States. Most dentists have been trained as general dentists. General dentists may choose a solo or an associate (group) practice.

The solo practitioner is independent and has complete autonomy in making decisions and in setting practice policy. He or she can make choices that influence the day-to-day operations of the practice and the potential for financial reward. The dentist is responsible solely for all decisions and takes a greater financial risk. A solo practitioner must be a self-starter. The daunting tasks of selecting a community, deciding on a location, securing a lease, designing an office, selecting equipment and supplies, hiring and training staff—thousands of important and minute details are all part of starting a practice.

An associateship position gives the recent graduate an opportunity to gain more knowledge in all aspects of dental practice. An associate agrees to work in a practice for a certain period of time as either an independent contractor or as an employee. The vast majority of new graduates who go directly into private practice are doing so as associates. This is also true for dentists completing residency or graduate programs. The high financial investment and uncertainty involved in starting a solo practice are the main reasons for recent graduates to choose an associateship. Rising educational debt may also preclude the graduate from starting a solo practice. Moreover, an associateship position helps to facilitate the transition from the academic environment to clinical practice, increases clinical knowledge and speed, and, in some cases, allows the associate to buy into a practice. Being an associate requires flexibility in treatment planning and the ability to practice in someone else's office. The associate has less discretion and decision-making authority than solo private practice affords. Associateship agreements are varied and should be structured to fit the needs of all parties. Some associateships are based on the current owner's retiring and phasing out of the practice; some are simply an employer-employee situation; and in some a new practitioner is considered an independent contractor.

A dental general practice residency (GPR) is an excellent opportunity to gain additional knowledge beyond dental school. The challenges of providing quality dental care to the medically compromised, the mentally and physically handicapped, and the dental phobic attract many graduates to apply for a GPR. A GPR may offer training in anesthesiology, medicine, and emergency and trauma cases and is usually a one-year residency program that offers a stipend or small salary. This valuable experience provides the student with additional knowledge and skills that may motivate a decision to specialize in some area of the dental profession.

In addition to general practice, there are eight recognized specialties: dental public health, endodontics, oral and maxillofacial pathology, oral and maxillofacial surgery, orthodontics and dentofacial orthopedics, pediatric dentistry, periodontics, and prosthodontics. Specialties require additional training after receiving a dental degree and are very competitive. The cost and the number of years required for a particular program vary from institution to institution. Specialty programs enable an individual to concentrate in one field of dentistry and to perfect his or her clinical skills in that area. Generally, a specialist's services are more costly; therefore, these practitioners have higher incomes than general dentists.

Following are brief descriptions of the procedures dentists perform in each specialty field, the additional education required beyond dental school, the length of the program, and the number of programs available:

- **Dental public health:** Individuals who enter the dental public health field are involved in developing policies and programs that affect the community at large. The individual may earn a certificate or a master's or doctoral degree. Most of the programs are between 12 and 24 months long, and there are currently 22 programs.

- **Endodontics:** Endodontists diagnose and treat diseases and injuries specific to the dental nerves, pulp, and tissues that affect the vitality of the tooth. Programs offer certificates or master's degrees. The lengths of the program vary but are usually 24 months, and there are currently 47 programs.

- **Oral and maxillofacial pathology:** Oral pathologists are dental scientists who study and research the causes, processes, and effects of diseases with oral manifestations. These diseases may be confined to the mouth and oral cavity. Oral pathologists do not deal with patients directly. They provide critical diagnostic and consultative biopsy services to dentists and physicians in the treatment of their patients. Programs offer certificates or master's and/or doctoral degrees. The length of the program is usually 36 months, and there are currently 15 programs.

- **Oral and maxillofacial surgery:** Oral surgeons provide a broad range of diagnostic services and treatments for diseases, injuries, and defects of the neck, head, jaw and associated structures. Programs offer certificates or master's and/or doctoral degrees and most are at least 48 months long. Currently, there are 109 programs.

- **Orthodontics and dentofacial orthopedics:** Orthodontists treat problems related to irregular dental development, missing teeth, and other abnormalities. Orthodontists establish normal functioning and appearance for their patients. Some programs offer certificates; others, master's degrees. Most of the programs are 24 to 36 months in length, and there are 53 programs.

- **Pediatric dentistry:** This field specializes in treating children from birth to adolescence. Also, practitioners may treat disabled patients beyond the age of adolescence.

The programs may offer certificates or master's and/or doctoral degrees. Most of the programs are 24 to 36 months in length. There are currently 57 programs.

- **Periodontics:** Periodontists diagnose and treat diseases of the gingival tissue and supporting bone of the teeth. Some programs offer certificates; others, master's or doctoral degrees. Most programs are 36 months in length, and there are 52 programs.

- **Prosthodontics:** Prosthodontists replace missing teeth with fixed or removable substitutes. Again, some programs offer certificates; others, master's or doctoral degrees. Training may be from 12 to 36 months, and there are currently 70 programs.

The decision as to what to do after receiving a dental degree takes as much thought as making the initial decision to enter the dental profession. Recent graduates must take into consideration their financial situations upon graduation and their personal and career goals.

There was a time when almost any professional could walk into a bank, spend less than a half-hour with a loan representative, and be approved for a large loan. This situation came to an abrupt halt in the 1980s. Although it is not impossible to obtain a loan, approval is far from automatic. Factors such as credit rating, positive cash flow, net asset value, and other criteria are considered. Although professionals, dentists no longer are treated any differently than small business owners when applying for a loan. With the exception of service in the federal government and an associateship, however, applying for a bank loan is usually inevitable.

The level of prior indebtedness plays a major role in the path that the recent graduate follows. Whether right out of school or after completing a general residency program, most recent graduates become associates or buy existing practices. Starting a solo practice from scratch is very risky and entails a large financial burden that few students can afford.

To enjoy dentistry, one must be happy with his or her personal and professional choices. An imbalance leads to unhappiness and stress. Since the dentist wears many hats, dentistry can be a very stressful profession. Mitigating the burden involved in fulfilling the many obligations of dentistry must be a general sense of contentment and well-being that comes from satisfaction with the profession.

The future of dentistry is bright. The professional rewards of being a dentist are numerous. Dentists obtain personal satisfaction from helping others and are highly regarded by the community. In addition, dentists are well paid. The average income for a dentist is in the upper 8 percent of family incomes in the United States. The increasing public awareness of the importance of oral health has resulted in a greater demand for dental insurance. The number of persons who have dental insurance has grown from fewer than 5 million to more than 100 million. Increases in preventive, geriatric, and cosmetic dental care also have contributed to growth in the demand for dental services.

We are in the age of high technology, and the dental profession is continually changing with new advances. The CAD/CAM, computer-generated radiographs, improved restorative materials, and new antiplaque agents and vaccines are only a few of the recent advances in dentistry. A dentist's education is not completed after earning a dental degree, which is only the beginning. With the advances in technology, a dentist must continually enroll in continuing education classes, review dental journals, and participate in the local dental society. The opportunities for continuing education are numerous; courses are offered in everything from practice management seminars to dental materials and are available from universities, private industry, and national and local dental societies.

Dentistry is an exciting and rewarding profession. As a healing art, the profession continues to advance at a rapid pace, changing the day-to-day operations of the dental practice. Thanks to modern miracles, people are living longer and the need for continued preventive and restorative dentistry will continue to rise.

Paradoxically, as the demand for dental services has increased, over the last decade or more, there has been a steady decrease in the number of dentists graduating in the United States. This has led to a decrease in the ratio of dentists to patients in the population. The American Dental Association has predicted that by the year 2010 the patient/dentist ratio will be approximately 1,800/1.

The dental profession has been fortunate that managed care has not affected dentistry as much as medicine. It is true that dentists are now working harder for the same income, but they still enjoy a very comfortable life. In summary, dentistry provides many opportunities for an individual and can be very fulfilling professionally and personally.

Interviews

Three transcribed interviews with practicing dentists follow. Each interviewee offers a different perspective on the field of dentistry. These interviews are included, not to provide a comprehensive picture of the entire profession, but rather to inspire you to call your local practitioners and interview them. Tailor your interviews to your own needs by asking questions relevant to your interests in dentistry. Almost all practitioners respond well to aspiring dentists; let them relate their success stories to you. They will be able to convey the real-life struggles and triumphs of dentistry better than any text.

Dr. Roberta Doyle

Q. *How long have you been in practice?*

A. About 16 years.

Q. *Do you own your practice?*

A. Yes.

Q. *What factors made you want to pursue dentistry as a career?*

A. My parents wanted me to be a physician, but that wasn't exactly what I wanted. I'm artistic, and dentistry is a good combination of medicine and art.

Q. *Please describe your practice (location, staff, hours, etc.).*

A. My practice is in downtown suburbia. I have 12 employees. My regular hours are 7:45 A.M.–5:15 P.M. Monday through Friday, with lunch hours available.

Q. *What have been the most rewarding aspects of dentistry for you?*

A. I like to see my patients walk out feeling good—I like to change their perspectives.

Q. *What have been the biggest challenges in your practice?*

A. Owning my own business and being the one to take care of people, I'm running the show.

Q. *Were you given training for the business aspect of your work?*

A. No, but I knew a lot about it.

Q. *What have been the most significant changes in dentistry that you have seen?*

A. The big changes have been in bonding.

Q. *What about the social changes you've seen?*

A. Better dental health.

Q. *Would you do it all over again?*

A. Yes, definitely.

Q. *What qualities do you think make an excellent dentist?*

A. You need ethics and good communication skills, and you must be good at working with people. It's really a people-oriented job.

Q. *What advice would you convey to dental school applicants?*

A. It's a lot of hard work, so be prepared. You have to also be willing to do a lot of different things; you won't just come out of dental school and be a hit.

Q. *How has being a woman influenced your career?*

A. In school, it was harder to be a woman, but once I got out I found it to my advantage. I'm a general dentist, so I go directly to the public. People perceive that I am more gentle, so they come and seek treatment more readily. I don't know how I would feel if I were a specialist because then I'd be relying on men for referrals.

***

Dr. Ben Williamowsky

Q. *Where did you go to dental school?*

A. University of Maryland–Baltimore.

Q. *When did you graduate?*

A. 1948.

Q. *Did you do a postdoctoral program? GPR, AEGD, Specialty?*

A. No, I was a general dentist.

Q. *How long were you in practice?*

A. I was in practice for 48 years, but I have been retired for many years.

Q. *What factors made you want to pursue dentistry as a career?*

A. If there was anything definitive, I would say it was that my cousin was a dental student. He took me to NYU and showed me around. I was 13 or 14 years old at the time, and I thought I wanted to be a physician. When I saw what my cousin Sam was doing, I wanted to be like him.

Q. *Please describe your practice (location, staff, hours, etc.).*

A. There were many changes during my 48 years. In the last 25 years of practice, at first I had one partner. We were multidisciplined—we did some of everything other than orthodontic care. We did some surgery, some periodontal work, and general dental work. No HMOs. The staff consisted of nine full-time and a few part-time employees besides the dentists. Later there were two partners, and then a third a couple of years prior to my retirement. There were eight operators.

Q. *What have been the most rewarding aspects of dentistry for you?*

A. The relations with people. I really miss that.

Q. *What have been the biggest challenges in your practice?*

A. Keeping up with all of the new things.

Q. *What have been the most significant changes in dentistry that you have seen?*

A. The sophistication of dental practices, I would say. It used to be "Fill 'em and drill 'em," but now there's reconstruction and implants. In the last 10–15 years of my practice, I didn't do more than a couple per year of denture sets on new patients.

Q. *What changes do you anticipate? Where is dentistry headed in your opinion?*

A. Well, the biggest problem on the horizon is insurance—HMOs. In the ending years of my practice, I was discouraged by the need to focus on how to deal with insurance, rather than concentrating on actual dentistry. Maybe that's just a phase, though, I don't know.

Q. *What qualities do you think make an excellent dentist?*

A. A good dentist relates well to people and has artistic or visual-conceptual abilities. Also, a good dentist, when faced with disease and pain, sees it as a challenge to heal the ailment.

Q. *What advice would you like to convey to dental school applicants?*

A. A lot of dental schools have changed in that they realize their job is to help the students graduate, not challenge them to fail. If there is a choice of schools, go to them and talk with some students and see how their professors treat them. Also, everyone seems to think that it's 4 years and then, BOOM!—you're a dentist. Plan to spend at least one year in residency.

***

Dr. Steven Marsh

Q. *What have been the most significant changes in dentistry that you have seen?*

A. The dental materials have changed greatly. I don't use amalgam or silver in my practice anymore. We not only restore teeth and make them stronger, but they look a lot better. There is much more emphasis on cosmetic dentistry now.

Q. *What changes do you anticipate? Where is dentistry headed in your opinion?*

A. I anticipate an even greater emphasis on cosmetic dentistry.

Q. *Would you do it all over again?*

A. Absolutely. It's been a wonderful experience.

Q. *What qualities do you think make an excellent dentist?*

A. You have to have what we call a "good eye" for aesthetics, you must be terrific with your hands, and probably the #1 quality is the ability to have good relations with people, be it with patients or staff.

Q. *What advice would you like to convey to dental school applicants?*

A. You can control your own destiny with this career. It's one of the few fields left where you assume all of the responsibility. You can practice and market yourself however you desire. It's the kind of career where you can support your family, and you won't be traveling all over the country like some salespeople.

Survey of the Natural Sciences Review

 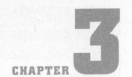

The following chart shows the expected number of questions, by major subject area, in each of the three parts of the Survey of the Natural Sciences section of the Dental Admission Test. For a detailed listing of content in each subject area, see the outline at the beginning of each review section. Remember that this review is not intended to be a substitute for a comprehensive 1-year course in each of these subjects.

Content Specifications for Biology, General Chemistry, and Organic Chemistry

1. Biology (40 questions)

Subject Area	Expected Number of Questions
Origins of Life, Cell Metabolism, Enzymology, Cellular Processes, Thermodynamics, Organelle Structure and Function, Mitosis/Meiosis, Cell Structure, Experimental Cell Biology	13
Biological Organization and Relationship of Major Taxa (Five Kingdom System)	3
Structure and Function of Vertebrate Systems	9
Fertilization, Descriptive Embryology, Developmental Mechanisms, Experimental Embryology	4
Molecular/Human Genetics, Classical Genetics, Chromosomal Genetics	7
Natural Selection, Population Genetics, Speciation Cladistics, Population and Community Ecology, Ecosystems, Animal Behavior	4

2. General Chemistry (30 questions)

Subject Area	Expected Number of Questions
Atomic and Molecular Structures	3
Periodic Properties	2
Stoichiometry	4
Gases	3
Liquids and Solid	1
Solutions	3
Acids and Bases	3
Chemical Equilibrium	3
Oxidation Reduction Reactions	3
Thermodynamics and Thermochemistry	2
Chemical Kinetics	2
Nuclear Reactions	1

3. Organic Chemistry (30 questions)

Subject Area	Expected Number of Questions
Bonding, Aromaticity	3
Nomenclature	2
Stereochemistry	3
Chemical and Physical Properties of Molecules, Organic Analysis	3
Acid-Base Chemistry	3
Mechanisms (Energetics, Structure, Stability)	6
Reactions of the Major Functional Groups, Synthesis	10

BIOLOGY REVIEW OUTLINE (SNS Q1–Q40)

I.   OVERVIEW

II.   BUILDING BLOCKS

III.   ORIGINS OF LIFE
    A. First Living Cells
    B. Theories

IV.   ENZYMOLOGY
    A. Chemical Reactions
    B. Lock and Key Model

V.   CELL METABOLISM
- **A.**   Chemical Pathways
- **B.**   Cellular Respiration: Glycolysis, the Krebs Cycle, and the Electron Transport Chain
- **C.**   Photosynthesis

VI.   THERMODYNAMICS
- **A.**   Kinetic and Potential Energy
- **B.**   First and Second Laws of Thermodynamics

VII.   CELL AND ORGANELLE STRUCTURE AND FUNCTION
- **A.**   Cell Membranes
- **B.**   Prokaryotic Cells—Bacteria and Archaea
- **C.**   Eukaryotic Cells
    - Nucleus
    - Ribosomes
    - Endoplasmic Reticulum
    - Golgi Apparatus
    - Lysosomes and Endocytosis
    - Peroxisomes
    - Vacuoles
    - Mitochondria
    - Choloroplasts
    - Cytoskeleton and Microfibers

VIII.   CELLULAR REPRODUCTION
- **A.**   Overview
- **B.**   Mitosis
    - Prophase
    - Metaphase
    - Anaphase
    - Telophase
    - Cytokinesis
    - Differences in Plants
    - Control of Cell Division
- **C.**   Meiosis

IX.   BIOLOGICAL ORGANIZATION AND RELATIONSHIP OF MAJOR TAXA
- **A.**   Taxa and Taxonomy
- **B.**   Binomial Nomenclature
- **C.**   Domains
- **D.**   Five Kingdom Classification
- **E.**   Animalia Phyla
    - Lower Invertebrates
    - Higher Invertebrates
- **F.**   Plantae
- **G.**   Fungi
- **H.**   Protista
- **I.**   Monera

I. Brain and Nervous System
   Anatomy and Function of the Neuron
   Types of Neurons
   Transmission of Information
      Resting Potential
      Action Potential
      Propagation of the Impulse
      Transmission Between Cells
      Processing Information
   Central and Peripheral Nervous Systems

J. Endocrine System
   Hypothalamus and Pituitary Gland
   Hormones
   Regulation

K. Reproductive System
   Gametes
   Male Reproductive System
   Female Reproductive System
   Hormones and the Reproductive Pattern

XI. DESCRIPTIVE EMBRYOLOGY AND DEVELOPMENTAL MECHANICS
   A. Cleavage
   B. From Morula to Gastrula
   C. Development of the Fetus

XII. CLASSICAL GENETICS
   A. Genes
      The Principle of Segregation and the Principle of Dominance
      Genotype versus Phenotype
      Independent Assortment
   B. Degrees of Dominance

XIII. CHROMOSOMAL GENETICS
   A. Chromosomes
   B. Sex Chromosomes

XIV. ASEXUAL AND SEXUAL REPRODUCTION
   A. Asexual Reproduction
   B. Sexual Reproduction

XV. MOLECULAR AND HUMAN GENETICS
- **A.** Independent Assortment
- **B.** Linkage
  - Sex-Linkage
- **C.** Gene Structure
  - DNA Replication
- **D.** DNA Transcription and Translation

XVI. EVOLUTION
- **A.** Natural Selection
- **B.** Cladistics
- **C.** Analogous and Homologous Evolution

XVII. POPULATION GENETICS
- **A.** Hardy-Weinberg Equilibrium
- **B.** Mutations or Random Events
- **C.** Reproductive Isolation
  - Allopatric Speciation
  - Parapatric Speciation
  - Sympatric Speciation

XVIII. POPULATION AND COMMUNITY ECOLOGY
- **A.** Populations
- **B.** Communities
  - Succession
  - Niche
- **C.** Interspecific Interactions Within a Community
  - Competition ($-/-$)
  - Predation—Predator/Prey Oscillations ($+/-$)
  - Symbiosis
- **D.** Ecosystems

XIX. ANIMAL BEHAVIOR
- **A.** Ethology
- **B.** Social Behavior and Kin Selection

OVERVIEW

The first section of the DAT is the Survey of Natural Sciences, comprised of 100 multiple-choice questions in three subject areas. There is no division between the subject areas within the Survey of Natural Sciences, but the format is 40 biology questions followed by 30 general chemistry questions and 30 organic chemistry questions. Most questions in the biology section are conceptual, testing your understanding of processes, functions, and organization of biological systems. Pure recall questions are mostly limited to long-established and unchanging concepts in biology such as cell cycle and cellular processes.

Biology can be overwhelming because of the vast amount of material that it covers, along with its ever-changing nature. The text of this book matches the most recently published sections for the DAT. Some sections require significant background information, but the take-home points are few; other sections will require you to memorize much more. Some figures present in this section are purely to help you visualize, while others contain information that you will need to become very familiar with. The latter will be obvious through the text.

Some mnemonic devices are provided throughout this section. You may find your own memorization techniques just as helpful. And do not hesitate to search the Web for interesting songs or images that help you remember the information you need to know.

Your time will be best spent learning the major biological concepts first and then filling in detailed information. Also, realize what types of information you are more likely to be tested on. Given the topic of histological layers of arteries and veins, you *may* be asked on the DAT what layers (or tunics) are adjacent to Auerbach's plexus in arteries. But you are far more *likely* to be asked *why* arteries have a thicker layer of musculature than do veins. The answer to the latter question incorporates more information. Again, focus your review on learning the concepts; they are the subject matter of the questions most frequently asked. When you are ready for the sample questions, work on your ability to strategically eliminate "bad" or "distracting" answer choices in order to help you to select the best answer choice.

BUILDING BLOCKS

Our discussion of biology begins with the building blocks of life. Though you are unlikely to be tested on the chemical structure of individual molecules on the biology portion of the exam, a basic understanding of these structures will help you grasp the concepts, and will also help you prepare for the chemistry sections. Living things are made up mostly of carbon-based compounds. Carbon has the unique chemistry to form the large, complex, and diverse macromolecules of life. In fact, carbon compounds are studied in their own special field—organic chemistry. The macromolecules that play key roles in biological functioning are lipids, carbohydrates, nucleic acids, and proteins. The formation of each of these molecules requires a chemical reaction called dehydration synthesis. For each covalent bond that is formed, a molecule of water is lost. Similarly, the addition of water to a system will break a bond in a reaction called hydrolysis.

Lipids are a diverse group of molecules that are insoluble in water. Many lipids are made up of fatty acids, or

TIP
Vocabulary
organic = carbon-containing
inorganic = noncarbon-containing

long hydrocarbon chains, each with a carboxyl group at one end. Lipids have a variety of uses: fats store energy, phospholipids are principal components in cell membranes, and steroids, such as estrogen and testosterone, play key roles in hormonal regulation.

(a) Components of a fat molecule

$$H_2C \!-\! OH \qquad HO \!-\! \overset{\displaystyle O}{\overset{\displaystyle \|}{C}} \!-\! CH_2 \!-\! CH_2 \!-\! CH_3$$

A saturated fatty acid

$$HC \!-\! OH$$

$$H_2C \!-\! OH \qquad HO \!-\! \overset{\displaystyle O}{\overset{\displaystyle \|}{C}} \!-\! CH_2 \!-\! CH_2 \!-\! CH \!=\! CH \!-\! CH_3$$

Glycerol

An unsaturated fatty acid

(b) Synthesis of a fat molecule

$$H_2C \!-\! O \!-\! H \qquad HO \!-\! \overset{\displaystyle O}{\overset{\displaystyle \|}{C}} \!-\! CH_2 \!-\! CH_2 \!-\! CH_3$$

$$HC \!-\! OH$$

$$H_2C \!-\! O \!-\! H \qquad HO \!-\! \overset{\displaystyle O}{\overset{\displaystyle \|}{C}} \!-\! CH_2 \!-\! CH_2 \!-\! CH \!=\! CH \!-\! CH_3$$

(c) Product of synthesis

$$H_2C \!-\! O \!-\! \overset{\displaystyle O}{\overset{\displaystyle \|}{C}} \!-\! CH_2 \!-\! CH_2 \!-\! CH_3$$

$$HC \!-\! OH$$

$$H_2C \!-\! O \!-\! \overset{\displaystyle O}{\overset{\displaystyle \|}{C}} \!-\! CH_2 \!-\! CH_2 \!-\! CH \!=\! CH \!-\! CH_3$$

$$+ 2H_2O$$

A display of fats showing (a) the composition of a molecule of fat; (b) dehydration synthesis; and (c) the new fat molecule.

Carbohydrates, commonly called sugars, are carbon compounds that fit the formula ration of 1:2:1 for carbon, hydrogen, and oxygen. An individual sugar molecule, such as glucose, is called a monosaccharide or simple sugar. A molecule formed from two joined sugars is a disaccharide, a group that includes the ordinary table sugar, sucrose. Complex carbohydrates, or polysaccharides, are compounds with varying numbers of covalently bonded sugars. This group includes such compounds as starch (energy stored in plants), cellulose (a major component of plant cell walls), and chitin (exoskeleton of insects).

A display of monosaccharides. (a) Glucose is the most frequently encountered monosaccharide in anatomy and physiology and metabolism. It exists both in a chain form and a ring form, as shown. (b) Two other monosaccharides, galactose and fructose, have the same number and type of atoms, but the arrangements are different.

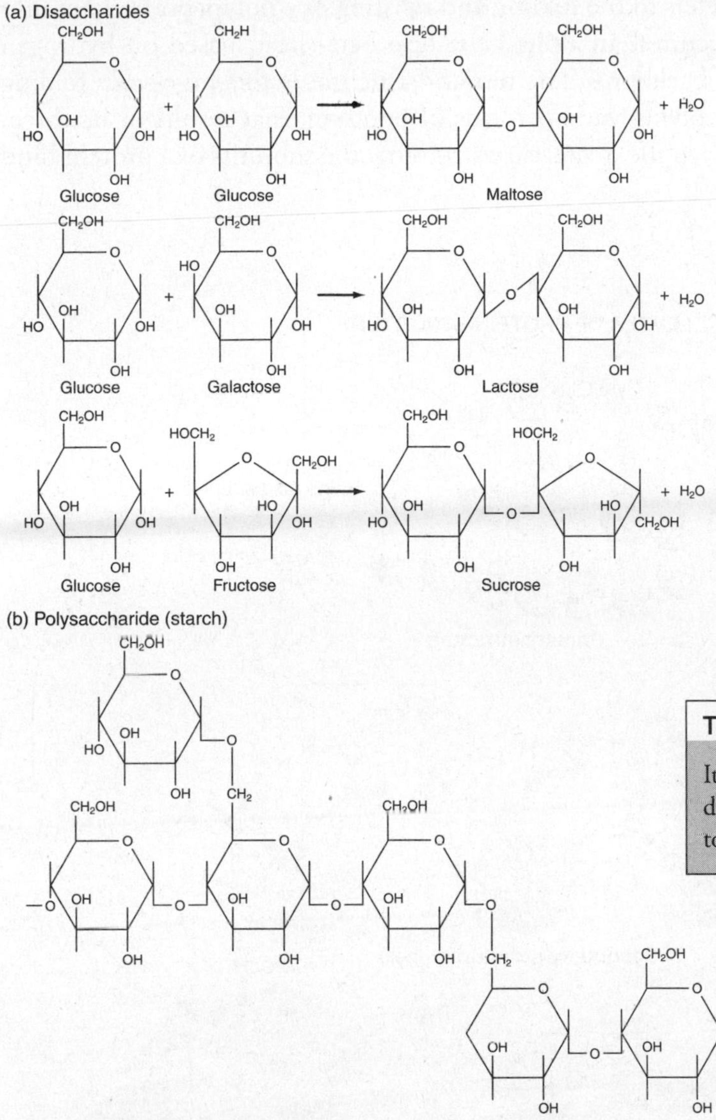

(a) Disaccharides

CH₂OH CH₂H → CH₂OH CH₂OH + H₂O

Glucose Glucose Maltose

Glucose Galactose Lactose

Glucose Fructose Sucrose

(b) Polysaccharide (starch)

> **TIP**
>
> It is more important to remember that maltose is a disaccharide made of two glucose molecules than it is to remember its chemical structure.

Disaccharides and the polysaccharide starch. (a) The disaccharides maltose, lactose, and sucrose are formed from their constituent monosaccharides. (b) Starch is formed from numerous glucose units. Note that the carbohydrates are shown in their ring forms. Water molecules are formed in the synthesis of disaccharides and polysaccharides.

Proteins are another very diverse group of macromolecules; they are instrumental in almost all processes in an organism. Humans, for example, have tens of thousands of proteins, each with its own specific structure and function. Protein functions include support (keratin in hair), transport (hemoglobin in blood), movement (actin and myosin in muscle), and hormonal coordination (insulin in the pancreas). A large number of proteins are enzymes, or catalysts, without which many of the processes in living organisms could not occur. We will discuss enzymes separately in a later section. The architecture of protein molecules is highly variable and very complex. Proteins are made up of amino acids, simple carbon compounds that link together through peptide bonds to form polypeptide chains. The sequence of amino acids in the polypeptide chain is programmed in genes and is called the primary structure.

The secondary structure refers to the folding and twisting of a polypeptide chain into one of two patterned structures, an alpha-helix or a beta-sheet, based on hydrogen bonds of the polypeptide backbone. The tertiary structure is the large-scale folding pattern of the protein, involving various forms of bonding, that results in its three-dimensional shape. Finally, in the quaternary structure, the subunits of a protein bind together in a specific way.

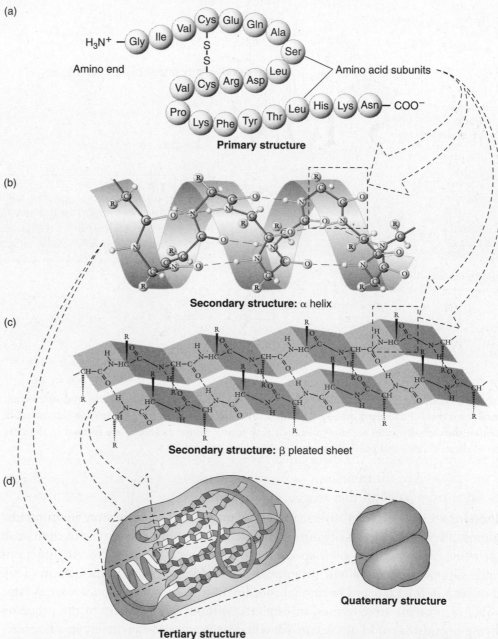

Protein structure. (a) Primary structure—amino acid sequence; (b) Secondary structure—alpha helix and beta sheet formation through hydrogen bonds; (c) Tertiary structure—three-dimensional shape with hydrogen bonds, disulfide brides, ionic bonds, and van der Waals interactions; and (d) Tertiary structure—subunit arrangement.

Nucleic acids are macromolecules that carry genetic information. There are two types of nucleic acids: deoxyribonucleic acid (DNA) and ribonucleic acid (RNA). Nucleic acids are made of chains of nucleotides, each of which is composed of a five-carbon sugar, ribose or deoxyribose, covalently bonded to a phosphate group and one of five nitrogenous bases. Further discussion of nucleotides will occur in a later section.

The basic structure of a nucleotide includes a five-carbon sugar, a phosphate group, and a nitrogenous base.

ORIGINS OF LIFE

First Living Cells

How did life begin on Earth? There are many scientific theories and much disagreement. Most biologists agree, however, that because there was no free oxygen in the ancient atmosphere, the first living cells were anaerobic; that is, they lived in the absence of oxygen. These cells were autotrophs, able to capture energy from their environment, and were one-celled and prokaryotic, similar to the bacteria of today.

Theories

Spontaneous generation, the theory that living organisms arise from nonliving material, was adhered to for thousands of years. For instance, it was widely believed that frogs came from soil and that maggots arose from rotting flesh. In 1668, however, Francseco Reidi challenged the theory of spontaneous generation by showing that larvae appear only in carcasses that have been exposed to air, thereby demonstrating that maggots cannot originate solely from meat.

A more scientifically sound theory is that, under primordial conditions, inorganic material accumulated and synthesized to form organic molecules, such as amino acids. These organic molecules joined to form larger molecules, for example, proteins or nucleic acids, which isolated themselves from their environment, developed heredity, and slowly evolved into many other types of molecules. Stanley Miller demonstrated this synthesis in 1953, when he showed experimentally that inorganic materials organized themselves into amino acids when maintained under ancient atmospheric conditions.

ENZYMOLOGY

Chemical Reactions

During a chemical reaction, bonds are either made or broken. Reactions that release energy are exergonic; reactions that require energy are endergonic. In living cells, the exergonic reactions usually provide the energy to perform the endergonic reactions. However, even exergonic reactions requires require a small amount of energy, called activation energy, to get them started. Often activation energy comes as heat, which, if not available, prevents the reaction from taking place.

In chemistry, catalysts are the chemical compounds that lower the activation energy to make it easier for a reaction to occur. Catalysts do not affect the energy transfer of the reaction and are not consumed by the reaction. Enzymes are proteins that act as biological catalysts. They are very important for the functioning of cells, as we will see in subsequent sections, because they allow necessary reactions to take place at ordinary temperatures. Enzymes can also speed up or slow down reactions.

> **TIP**
>
> **Vocabulary**
> exergonic—reaction that releases energy
> endergonic—reaction that requires energy

Lock and Key model

There are thousands of enzymes in the living cell, each specific to a certain compound. Imagine the enzyme as a lock into which only one type of molecular "key" can fit. This key, with a very specific shape, is called the substrate. The place on the enzyme where the substrate binds is called the active site. As binding takes place, the active site of the enzyme slightly changes shape to better fit the substrate; this new fit is called the induced fit. Now, at an accelerated rate, the substrate undergoes a chemical reaction.

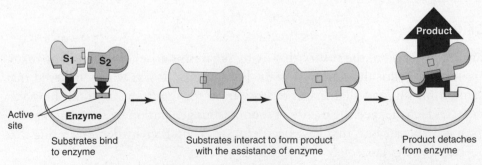

The activity of enzymes. An enzyme has a specific active site where a pair of substrate molecules bind. The product detaches, and the enzyme is freed to participate in another reaction.

Many enzymes require an additional molecule to function. If this helper is inorganic, it is called a cofactor. A cofactor usually is an atom of metal such as zinc, copper or iron. If the helping molecule is an organic molecule, it is called a coenzyme. Vitamins are examples of coenzymes that aid in various enzymatic reactions in the body. On the other hand, certain compounds inhibit enzyme function. Molecules that mimic the substrate and reversibly block the enzyme's active site are called competitive inhibitors. Noncompetitive inhibitors are molecules that bind irreversibly to the active site or bind to a site other than the active site, thereby altering the shape of the enzymes' active site and making it unusable. Sites other than the active site that are involved in enzyme activity are called allosteric sites. Molecules that bind at allosteric sites may stimulate or inhibit the enzyme's activity.

Enzymes can be thought of as reaction machines. It is important to control these machines in order for metabolic pathways to operate correctly. Enzyme regulation is based on the principle that an enzyme pathway can fluctuate between active and inactive. The most common mode of enzyme regulation is feedback inhibition, where the product of the reaction also acts as an inhibitor. As a result, when low amounts of a compound, such as an amino acid, are present, the enzyme pathway switches "on." When there are sufficient amounts, the pathway switches "off." Feedback inhibition is an example of allosteric regulation, in which varying concentrations of allosteric activators (molecules that stimulate enzyme function) and allosteric inhibitors (those that inhibit enzyme function) can determine the rate and duration of enzyme activity.

CELL METABOLISM

Chemical Pathways

Just as cars need fuel to run, so cells need energy to survive. Cells create, store, and release energy in various forms through carefully arranged reactions called chemical pathways. These pathways continuously transfer energy from one form to another for use by the cell. There are thousands of reactions and many pathways within the cell; metabolism can be thought of as a map that tracks the movement of energy through these transformations.

There are two main types of reactions: anabolic and catabolic. Anabolic reactions require energy in assembling larger molecules from smaller ones. Catabolic reactions, on the other hand, release energy by breaking down large molecules into smaller ones. Cells, for instance, use catabolic reactions to break down the organic molecules in food to simpler products. In the process, the cell harvests some of the potential energy stored in the food for use in cellular work (the rest is released as heat). The following subsections provide a summary of the catabolic pathways that provide energy for cellular life.

> **TIP**
>
> **Mnemonic**
> **A**nabolic
> **A**ssembles
> **C**atabolic
> **C**rushes

Cellular Respiration: Glycolysis, the Krebs Cycle, and the Electron Transport Chain

We usually associate respiration with breathing. On a cellular level, two forms of respiration occur: aerobic and anaerobic. Aerobic respiration is many times more efficient in producing energy than anaerobic respiration (respiration in the absence of oxygen), which is why plants and animals primarily use aerobic respiration to produce energy.

The types of energy in organic compounds vary, but the most representative source of energy is the simple sugar glucose. Respiration breaks down the C—H bonds of

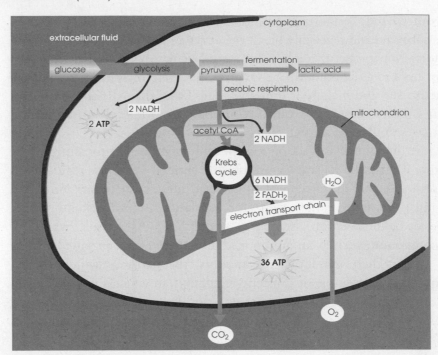

Overview of Cellular Respiration

glucose, releasing energy to change adenosine diphosphate (ADP, a low-energy molecule) into adenosine triphosphate (ATP, a high-energy molecule). ATP is a nucleotide that is an excellent source of immediate energy for the cell. Aerobic respiration can be summarized by the equation:

$$C_6H_{12}C_6 + \quad O_2 \quad \rightarrow H_2O + \quad\quad CO_2 \quad\quad + \text{ATP}$$

Glucose + Oxygen → Water + Carbon Dioxide + Energy

Aerobic and anaerobic respiration begin in the cytoplasm of the cell in a process called glycolysis. This series of reactions breaks glucose down into smaller organic compounds and releases a small amount of ATP. In the presence of oxygen, the two subsequent stages of respiration—the Krebs cycle and the electron transport chain (ETC)—occur in and around a specialized structure called the mitochondrion. These stages yield a large amount of ATP. In the absence of oxygen, the products of glycolysis are further fermented into lactate or ethanol; however, no additional ATP is produced. Fermentation occurs in simple organisms such as yeast and bacteria, in oxygen-deficient environments, and in vertebrate muscle cells after strenuous activity has exhausted oxygen resources. A simple overview of anaerobic and aerobic respiration can be seen in the diagram above.

Glycolysis, the "splitting of sugar," is a series of ten steps converting glucose, a six-carbon sugar, into pyruvate, a three-carbon compound. Enzymes catalyze each step of glycolysis; however, it is unnecessary to memorize these details for the DAT so they have not been included here. Glycolysis can occur with or without the presence of oxygen in the environment. The process is exergonic, releasing energy. The ten steps are divided into two stages: energy investment and energy payoff. In the energy investment phase, two ATP are expended, and glucose passes through several steps until it is catabolized into two three-carbon molecules. It is important to remember that each subsequent step occurs twice, once with each three-carbon molecule. This is illustrated in the figure. In the energy payoff steps, ADP is phosphorylated by direct enzymatic transfer of a phosphate group in a process called substrate-level phosphorylation, yielding four ATP and two NADH, a high-energy electron carrier. The net products of glycolysis are two pyruvate, two ATP, and two NADH.

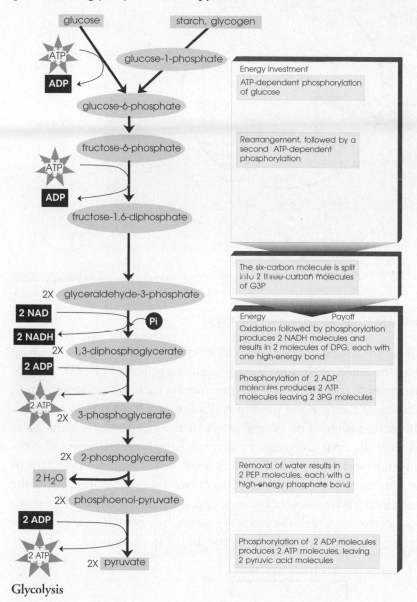

Glycolysis

If oxygen is present in the cell, the Krebs (or Citric Acid) cycle is the second step in glucose energy release. The two molecules of pyruvate generated during glycolysis enter the mitochondrial matrix where they undergo further transformation yielding six NADH, two $FADH_2$, CO_2, and GTP (an ATP-like compound whose energy is used to phosphorylate ADP into ATP). Again, enzymes catalyze each step.

The last step in aerobic respiration is the electron transport chain, which occurs in the inner membrane of the mitochondrion and results in the greatest production of ATP molecules. In this step, the high-energy electron products of the Krebs cycle

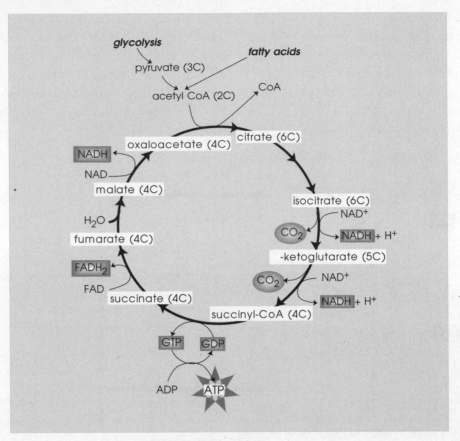

The Citric Acid Cycle (Krebs Cycle, Tricarboxcylic Acid Cycle)

(NADH and FADH$_2$) are passed down a series of electron acceptors. Most of these electron acceptors are proteins, including large protein complexes I, II, III, and IV embedded in the membrane, as well as mobile transporters such as the cytochromes. The only electron acceptor that is not a protein is ubiquinone (coenzyme Q), which is a small hydrophobic molecule. The energy levels of the electrons are reduced at every step and end with the final acceptor of electrons—oxygen. The series of reactions in the electron transport chain are called redox (short for reduction-oxidation) reactions. Reduction refers to the acceptance of electrons by one compound in the reaction. The loss of electrons by the other compound is called oxidation. The compound that donates electrons is called the reducing agent, but is itself oxidized. That which accepts electrons is called the oxidizing agent, but is itself reduced:

$$\text{becomes oxidized}$$
$$X \;+\; Y \;\rightarrow\; X^{+} \;+\; Y^{-}$$
$$\text{becomes reduced}$$

X is the reducing agent; Y is the oxidizing agent. An increase in oxidation state is oxidation. A decrease in oxidation state is reduction. In the electron transport chain, oxygen is the final acceptor of electrons: it is therefore reduced. The electron energy released from the cascading reactions of the electron transport chain drives a highly efficient production of ATP from ADP, called oxidative phosphorylation.

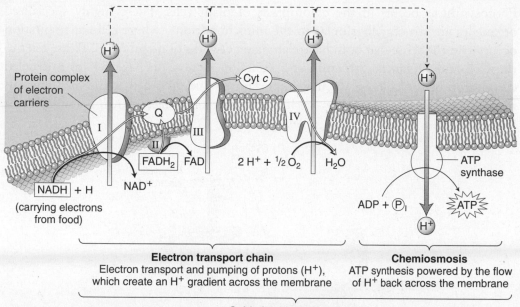

Electron transport chain
Electron transport and pumping of protons (H⁺),
which create an H⁺ gradient across the membrane

Chemiosmosis
ATP synthesis powered by the flow
of H⁺ back across the membrane

Oxidative phosphorylation

Electron Transport and Oxidative Phosphorylation in Mitochondria

Photosynthesis

An autotroph is an organism that sustains itself by making its own organic materials (e.g., sugars, amino acids, and fats) from inorganic resources. This mode of acquiring energy is different from that used by a heterotroph, which relies on the consumption of other organisms for food. Plants are autotrophs, synthesizing organic compounds from light and carbon dioxide in a process called photosynthesis. Photosynthesis can be considered the opposite of respiration. During photosynthesis, CO_2 reduces to form a sugar; in respiration, a sugar oxidizes to form CO_2.

The reaction of photosynthesis is:

$$6H_2O + 6CO_2 + ATP \rightarrow C_6H_{12}C_6 + 6O_2$$

Water + Carbon Dioxide + Energy → Glucose + Oxygen

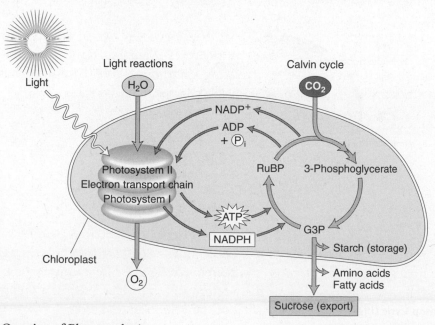

Overview of Photosynthesis

Photosynthesis occurs in the chloroplasts of plant cells. These highly specialized organelles are structurally similar to the mitochondrion—where cellular respiration occurs—in the sense that both have elaborate networks of membranes. Please refer to the Cell and Organelle Structure and Function section on page 54 for a detailed description of the chloroplast. It is important to understand that the membranous networks create distinct spaces within this tiny organelle, allowing for different "microclimates" within the chloroplast.

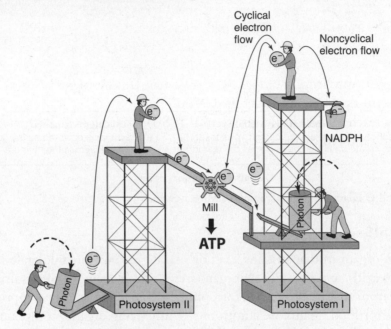

Electron Transport and Photophosphorylation in Chloroplasts

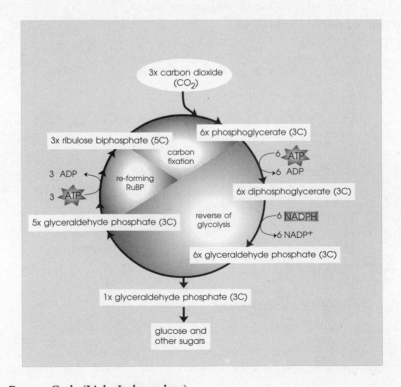

The Calvin-Benson Cycle (Light Independent)

There are two main stages of photosynthesis: the light reactions, which occur in the thylakoid membrane, and the Calvin-Benson cycle (light-independent reactions), which occurs in the stroma of the chloroplast. The light reactions occur only in the presence of the sun's energy; they convert the light energy into chemical energy in the form of ATP and NADPH. The Calvin-Benson cycle requires the chemical energy of ATP and NADPH to convert carbon dioxide into food molecules.

In the light reactions, chlorophyll in the thylakoid membranes absorbs light energy from the sun in the unit of a photon. The photon is passed around from one to the next pigment molecule until it reaches a special pigment molecule called chlorophyll *a*, which is surrounded by a specialized structure called the light-harvesting complex. There are two main types of light-harvesting complexes whose chlorophyll *a* molecules absorb slightly different wavelengths of light: Photosysytem II's chlorophyll *a* is called P680 and Photosystem I's chlorophyll *a* is called P700.

The photon first reaches P680 in Photosystem II (PSII), exciting the chlorophyll's electrons, which are captured by the so-called primary electron acceptor. This leaves the P680 chlorophyll as a strong oxidizing agent. A molecule of water is enzymatically split into two electrons, two hydrogen atoms, and an oxygen atom. The oxygen immediately combines with another oxygen atom, creating molecular oxygen, O_2. The two electrons are supplied to P680.

The electrons that reach the primary electron acceptor are then shuttled to Photosystem I (PSI) via an electron transport chain similar to that seen in the last step of aerobic respiration, producing ATP along the way.

A separate photon excites electrons in the P700 chlorophyll of PSI, which are captured by its own primary electron acceptor. The electrons shuttled from PSII replace the excited electron in P700, just as the electrons from a water molecule replaced the excited electrons of P680.

When electrons reach the primary acceptor in PSI, they can follow one of two routes. Noncylical electron flow is the dominant route whereby the electrons are transferred to $NADP^+$ forming NADPH. In the alternate route, cylical electron flow, the electrons are shuttled back to the electron transport chain, producing more ATP, but not producing NADPH. This is important because the Calvin-Benson cycle requires more ATP than NADPH.

Moving now to the stroma, where the ATP and NADPH have been released, the Calvin-Benson cycle uses the energy from these molecules to convert carbon dioxide into food molecules through a series of steps. Three carbon dioxide molecules, six ATP, and six NADPH are utilized to produce six molecules of glyceraldehyde-3-phosphate, one of which exits the cycle and is utilized for food. The remaining five molecules are recycled in the cycle, using three more molecules of ATP. In summary, for one molecule of sugar to be produced, nine ATP and six NADPH are expended.

THERMODYNAMICS

Kinetic and Potential Energy

Energy, defined as the capacity to do work, comes in many forms. Kinetic energy is the energy of a moving object. For instance, water flowing down a stream contains energy that can turn a turbine that powers a windmill. Energy also can be stored as potential energy. A pencil lying on a desk has potential energy. It is not moving, so it does not have kinetic energy. If the pencil falls off the desk, however, its energy will be released as it falls to the ground. In biology, potential energy comes in a special form called chemical energy, which is contained in the bonds that hold molecules together. As seen in the metabolic pathways, energy can be converted from one form to another and then back again. Energy changes are studied in a field called thermodynamics.

First and Second Laws of Thermodynamics

The first law of thermodynamics states that energy in the universe is neither created nor destroyed. Energy stays constant; it just changes forms. This law is sometimes referred to as the *principle of conservation of energy*. When a bullet is fired from a gun, the chemical energy of the gunpowder is converted into the kinetic energy of the moving bullet. The gunpowder's potential energy converts to the work of moving the bullet.

The second law of thermodynamics is involved with such energy transformations. When energy is transferred or transformed, some small amount is lost as unusable energy. In other words, when the chemical energy of the gunpowder is converted into the chemical energy of the moving bullet, a small amount is released as heat. The heat dissipates quickly into the environment and is not available to perform work. Such loss of usable energy increases the disorder, or *entropy*, of the universe.

CELL AND ORGANELLE STRUCTURE AND FUNCTION
Cell Membranes

Membranes are extremely important to the functioning of the cell. They separate the cell from its environment, divide the cell into different compartments, and control the passage of substances. The basic structure of a membrane is a lipid bilayer. The lipids that compose the bilayer, called phospholipids, have a hydrophilic polar group (water-loving head) on the outside of the membrane and an oily hydrocarbon chain (water-fearing tail) in the membrane's center. Dispersed throughout the lipid bilayer are membrane proteins, which may serve as selective transporters of molecules through the membrane.

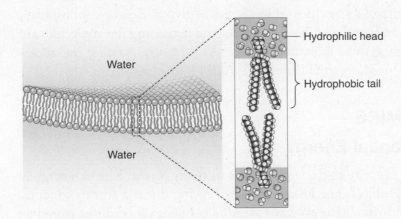

Phospholipid bilayer (cross section).

Membranes are not rigid bodies with their many components locked into place. Rather, they are fluid, flexible, and changing, with proteins, lipids, and other elements able to move about freely in the plane of the membrane. This dynamic model of membrane structure is called the fluid mosaic model. Membrane fluidity is important for the membrane to work properly and can change with such factors as temperature, electrical charges, and the presence of various electrolytes (e.g., sodium and calcium) in the immediate environment.

Membranes are selectively permeable; that is, some molecules can pass through them easily and some cannot. The passage of molecules through a membrane on their own, without any energy exerted by the cell, is called passive transport. One type of passive transport is diffusion, which is the tendency of particles to spread from areas of higher concentration to those of lower concentration. A second type of passive transport is osmosis, which is the movement of water across a semipermeable membrane. As with diffusion, a concentration gradient has to exist for osmosis to take place. Water will flow from areas of high water concentration (low solute concentration) to areas of low water concentration (high solute concentration) until equilibrium is reached. It is the semipermeable membrane that prevents the solutes themselves from moving down their gradient, so water moves down its own gradient.

For instance, if a bag of salt water is placed in a beaker of fresh water, and the bag is permeable to water but not to salt, the fresh water will flow into the bag of salt water. If unable to reach equal salinity, the bag will eventually rupture. The fresh water is considered hypotonic to the cell. Now imagine the opposite scenario: a semipermeable bag of fresh water placed in a beaker of salt water. Water will leave the bag of fresh water and move into the hypertonic salt water.

TIP
Vocabulary   hypotonic = lower concentration of solute   isotonic = same concentration of solute   hypertonic = greater concentration of solute

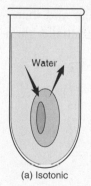 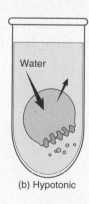 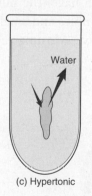

(a) Isotonic   (b) Hypotonic   (c) Hypertonic

The process of osmosis in three different environments. Imagine the same cell being placed in three different solutions: (a) A solution with an equal concentration of solutes to the cell is considered isotonic. There is no *net* movement of water. (b) A solution with a lower concentration of solutes compared to the cell is called hypotonic. There is a net movement of water into the cell. (c) A solution with a greater concentration of solutes compared to the cell is called hypertonic. There is a net movement of water out of the cell.

The force generated by the osmotic movement of particles is called osmotic pressure. Cells must counteract this osmotic pressure; otherwise, they will keep taking in water and burst in a hypotonic environment or lose water and shrivel in a hypertonic environment. The cell's process of balancing its water concentrations, called osmoregulation, is extremely important to cell functioning. Some cells "bail out" excess water through specialized contractile vacuoles. In larger organisms, the microenvironment around the cell is maintained as an isotonic solution, one having water concentration equal to that within the cell. For many plants, bacteria, and algae, the answer is to have a cell wall, which is a rigid layer surrounding the membrane that prevents the cell from expanding. Only plants, fungi, and bacteria have cell walls.

Some molecules diffuse through membranes with the help of transport proteins. In a process called facilitated diffusion, these molecules are "carried" through the membrane by the action of carrier proteins. It is important to note that facilitated diffusion speeds up particle movement but does not change the direction of transport. The direction can only be changed in a process known as active transport, which uses the energy of the cell to move particles against a concentration gradient, or from low concentrations to higher concentrations. An example of active transport is the sodium-potassium pump, which uses energy from ATP molecules to pump three sodium ions out of the cell for each two potassium ions it pumps in.

> **TIP**
>
> **Vocabulary**
> **Passive transport**—movement of solute (diffusion) or water (osmosis) down its gradient. No energy used.
> **Facilitated transport**—movement of solute down its concentration gradient through specialized "carrier" protein. No energy used.
> **Active transport**—movement of solute against its concentration gradient through specialized carrier proteins. Energy used.

Prokaryotic Cells—Bacteria and Archaea

Every organism is composed entirely of either prokaryotic or eukaryotic cells. Prokaryotic cells have no true nucleus and no membrane-bound organelles. In the five-kingdom classification, they are found only in the kingdom Monera, which consists of bacteria and cyanobacteria. In the newer domain classification, the domains of bacteria and archaea are entirely prokaryotes. All other plants and animals are made up of eukaryotic cells, which have true nuclei and organelles that have membranes. Prokaryotic cells are far simpler and smaller than eukaryotic cells and therefore are thought of as more primitive. Most bacteria are 10 to 100 times smaller than a typical eukaryotic cell.

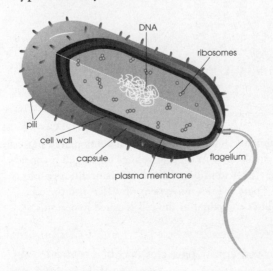

Generalized Prokaryotic Cell

Prokaryotic cells contain cytoplasm bound by a plasma membrane. Within the cytoplasm, genetic material is contained in a dense ball of DNA called the nucleoid. Ribosomes are also suspended throughout the cytoplasm. Prokaryotic cells can also contain a cell wall, pili, flagella, and outer capsule.

Eukaryotic Cells

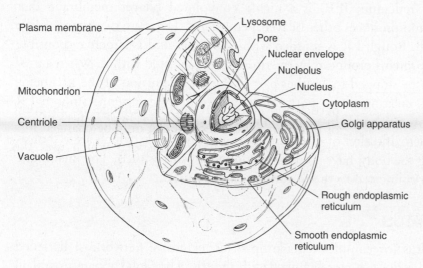

A diagram of a typical human cell showing certain organelles. Some of the smaller organelles have been drawn larger than their normal relative size to show their detail.

Eukaryotic cells are, by definition, those that contain a membrane-bound nucleus. Such cells also contain a number of other organelles, which are suspended within the cell in the protein-rich cytoplasm. Cytoplasm can change from a liquid state in which the cell's macromolecules disperse, to a semisolid gel state, where the particles interact to form a network. Most organelles are surrounded by membranes and perform specialized tasks for cell processing. While reviewing the organelles, keep in mind that there are some differences between plant and animal eukaryotic cells. Animal cells can contain lysosomes, centrioles, and flagella. Plant cells can contain chloroplasts, central vacuoles and tonoplasts, cell walls, and plasmodesmata.

NUCLEUS

The nucleus is the organelle that contains almost all of the cell's DNA and is responsible for several cellular activities, such as cellular reproduction, DNA replication, RNA synthesis, and responses to changes in the cell's environment. The condensed material inside the nucleus, called chromatin, consists mostly of DNA and protein. The nucleus may contain one or more nucleoli (singular = nucleolus), which are specialized areas within the nucleus that produce ribosomal RNA and help assemble proteins.

RIBOSOMES

Ribosomes are small particles, not bound by membranes, that consist of ribosomal RNA and protein. They are abundant in cells that have high rates of protein synthesis, as this is their role. A ribosome consists of a small and a large subunit and is either bound to the membrane of the endoplasmic reticulum or free in the cytoplasm. Proteins produced by free ribosomes generally remain in the cytoplasm; proteins produced by bound ribosomes generally are destined to fuse with membranes of organelles. Ribosomes are also found in prokaryotic cells.

ENDOPLASMIC RETICULUM

The endoplasmic reticulum (ER) is a highly convoluted bilayer membrane that secretes enzymes and produces other bilayer membranes. There are two types of ER: rough and smooth. Rough ER is studded with ribosomes and is largely responsible for exporting the proteins produced by the ribosomes associated with it. When a protein is destined to be shipped to another part of the cell, a portion of the ER membrane pinches off, creating a transport vesicle containing the protein. Smooth ER does not have ribosomes and is involved in the synthesis of lipids, metabolism of carbohydrates, and detoxification of drugs and poisons. Liver cells, which are responsible for detoxifying the body, have abundant amounts of smooth ER. The membrane of the ER is often connected to the membrane of the nucleus.

GOLGI APPARATUS

The golgi apparatus (or complex), made up of an extensive network of flattened membrane-bound vesicles, is closely linked with the ER. The Golgi apparatus and all of its budded vesicles contain a bilayer membrane. There is a *cis* face to this flattened stack, which receives transport vesicles from the rough ER. The Golgi apparatus sorts, modifies, and stores the proteins made by the ER. When the protein is ready to be secreted, a portion of the Golgi membrane on the *trans* side buds into a vesicle and transports the protein to its final destination. If the protein is to be excreted from the cell altogether, the bud is called a secretory vesicle rather than a transport vesicle. Its membrane binds with the lipid bilayer plasma membrane of the cell and releases its contents to the extracellular space in a process called exocytosis.

LYSOSOMES AND ENDOCYTOSIS

Lysosomes are vesicles that contain hydrolytic enzymes that can digest macromolecules into smaller compounds that the cell can more easily use. The enzymes and vesicle originate from the rough ER, are modified by the Golgi apparatus, and are then released into the cytoplasm. If another organelle is damaged, it is encapsulated into a vesicle, which then binds with a lysosome. The lysosome breaks down the organelle and allows the byproducts to be recycled. The process of bringing substances into the cell is called endocytosis. In some cells, the substance that is endocytosed may be digested by lysosomes.

PEROXISOMES

Bound by only a single membrane, the peroxisome is another small saclike organelle. Peroxisomes contain enzymes that create hydrogen peroxide (H_2O_2), which can catabolize large molecules and toxins. If left alone, the hydrogen peroxide would be toxic, but the peroxisome also contains enzymes that convert the H_2O_2 to water. Peroxisomes do not bud from the ER.

VACUOLES

Vacuoles are large membranous sacs that store food, minerals, waste, and other chemical products in plant cells. They are similar to lysosomes in that they originate from the ER, and they carry out hydrolysis. In plant cells, a large vacuole called the central vacuole, is enclosed by a membrane called the tonoplast. The larger vacuoles arise from coalescence of several smaller ones. The number of vacuoles in a cell and the compounds stored vary from cell to cell. Vacuoles can contract and expel water out of the cell, or expand and play a role in cellular elongation.

MITOCHONDRIA

Mitochondria are the sites of many of the steps of cellular respiration. For example, ATP synthesis occurs in the mitochondria. Since ATP is an essential, high-energy molecule, the mitochondria are regarded as the energy powerhouses of the cell. The number of mitochondria in a cell varies from one to thousands, depending on the cell's energy needs. These organelles are composed of a deeply folding inner membrane surrounded by an outer membrane.

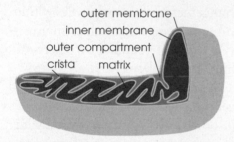

The mitochondria is the site of cellular respiration. The Krebs cycle occurs within the matrix, while the components of the electron transport chain are embedded within the inner membrane.

CHLOROPLASTS

In plants and photosynthetic cells, solar energy is converted into chemical energy by organelles called chloroplasts. Chloroplasts contain chlorophyll and other molecules that absorb the radiant energy of sunlight. This energy drives the light-dependent reactions of photosynthesis, which produce high-energy compounds for use by the cell. The chloroplast, like the mitochondria, has two membranes. In addition, the chloroplast has a number of thylakoids, which are flattened membrane-bound sacs, separating the chloroplast into two main spaces: the thylakoid space and the stroma.

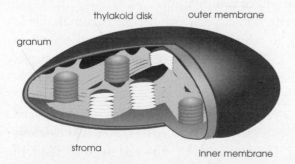

The chloroplast is the site of photosynthesis. The light reactions occur on the membrane of the thylakoids. The Calvin-Benson cycle occurs in the stroma.

CYTOSKELETON AND MICROFIBERS

The cytoskeleton is the support structure of the cell. It is a network of criss-crossing fibers that help to maintain and change the cell's shape. The cytoskeleton is composed of three types of fibers: microtubules, intermediate filaments, and microfilaments.

Microtubules are the largest and are thick, hollow rods found mostly in the cytoplasm. The centrosome is the microtubule organizing center in the cell; in some cells it contains a pair of centrioles. In cross section, a centriole is composed of nine sets of triplet microtubules arranged in a ring. Centrosomes and centrioles are the components of the cytoskeleton that play a role in the separation of chromosomes during cell division. Other microtubules within the cytoplasm create tracks along which transport vesicles from the ER and Golgi can move. Microtubules also compose cilia and flagella, specialized organelles used for locomotion by some cells. As opposed to the nine triplets of centrioles, cilia and flagella are comprised of nine doublets arranged in a ring, with two single microtubules in the center of the ring. This arrangement is commonly called the "9 + 2" arrangement.

Intermediate filaments are midsize protein fibers that maintain the structural integrity and the shape of the cell, as well as the arrangements of the organelles within the cell. While microtubules and microfilaments often rearrange themselves, intermediate filaments are more permanent. The nucleus is often surrounded by a network of intermediate filaments holding it in place within the cytoplasm.

The smallest fibers are microfilaments composed of a twisted double chain of a protein called actin. Microfilaments help the cell change shape. In muscle cells, microfilaments are responsible for contraction. In other cells that move by crawling along their surface, microfilaments are responsible for the pseudopod formation. Lastly, microfilaments form the cleavage furrow in cell division.

CELLULAR REPRODUCTION

Overview

Cells have several stages in their life history. These stages repeat, leading to the term "cell cycle." Ninety percent of the total time in the cell cycle is spent in interphase, a time when the cell grows, maintains itself, and metabolizes energy sources. There are three parts to interphase: the S phase and two gap phases (G1 and G2) before and after the S phase. During all three phases, the cell grows by producing proteins and organelles; however, it is only during the S phase that DNA replication occurs. The remaining 10% of the life cycle is the period of cell division.

All cells reproduce to make new cells. Prokaryotic cells (e.g., bacteria) divide through a process called binary fission, in which DNA is replicated and there is a systematic compartmentalizing of DNA into two cells. The genetic material disperses throughout the cytoplasm, and a membrane forms in the middle of the cell and continues to extend until there are two daughter cells.

Most eukaryotic cells divide through a process called mitosis, which is far advanced to binary fission but results in the same: two identical, diploid daughter cells. Meiosis takes place only in reproductive cells. The products of meiosis are four haploid cells, called gametes. These gametes meet and combine the genetic material in sexual

reproduction. Mitosis and meiosis are processes that include the mechanics of nuclear disassembly and reassembly and are more complicated than simple fission because of the presence of nuclei and multiple chromosomes.

Mitosis

The DNA of a cell is organized into structures called chromosomes. Each eukaryotic cell has a defined number of chromosomes. All human cells, except gametes, have 46 chromosomes. As a reminder, the chromosomes are duplicated in the S phase of interphase. In mitosis, there are several stages that prepare, line up, and separate the genetic material of the cell for reproduction.

PROPHASE

During this stage, the nuclear envelope begins to disintegrate and the chromosomes condense. Each chromosomes consists of two duplicated DNA strands called chromatids. These strands are held together at the center by a centromere forming an X-shaped structure. Microtubules appear, forming the mitotic spindle near the centrioles.

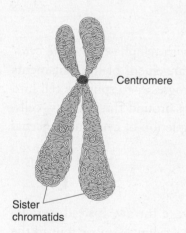

Centromere

Sister chromatids

A Chromosome and its Components

METAPHASE

During this stage, the centrosomes gravitate to opposite ends of the cell. The mitotic spindle, composed of microtubules extending from the centrosomes, attaches to the centromere of each chromosome. The spindle helps align the chromosomes in the middle of the cell.

> **TIP**
>
> **Mnemonic**
> In **M**etaphase, the chromosomes line up at the **M**idline of the cell.

ANAPHASE

When the chromosomes begin to separate, anaphase begins. The centromeres split, and the spindle fibers pull the chromatids apart to opposite ends of the cell.

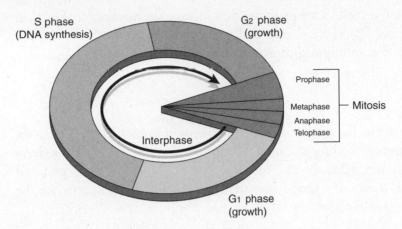

The cell cycle. The two major periods of interphase and mitosis are shown.

TELOPHASE

When the chromatids are at opposite ends of the dividing cell, they become less condensed and the mitotic spindles disappear. Nuclear membranes begin to form in each daughter cell, completing mitosis.

CYTOKINESIS

It is in this stage, which usually occurs simultaneously with telophase, that the cytoplasm is divided between the two daughter cells. Rearrangement of microfilaments within the cytoplasm creates a cleavage furrow which progresses to split the cell into two distinct daughter cells. The cell membrane develops around the two new cells, each containing identical genetic information. The completion of cytokinesis occurs after the completion of telophase.

DIFFERENCES IN PLANTS

In plant cells, cell walls prevent formation of the cleavage furrow. Instead, vesicles from the Golgi apparatus, carrying components for a new cell wall, move toward the midline of the cell. There, they coalesce forming the cell plate, and a new cell wall is formed. The two daughter cells grow largely by uptake of water, whereas animal cells increase in size by producing more cytoplasm.

CONTROL OF CELL DIVISION

Contact inhibition is one method of regulation, where physical contact with neighboring cells signals a halt to reproduction. Mitogens also regulate cell replication; these chemicals, produced by the body, can stimulate or inhibit cell division. Cancer is a disease in which uncontrolled or abnormal cell replication occurs.

Meiosis

There are two cell divisions in meiosis. The first cycle, meiosis I, is referred to as reduction division because the resultant daughter cells are haploid. The second cycle, meiosis II, is referred to as equatorial division, as haploid cells give rise to more

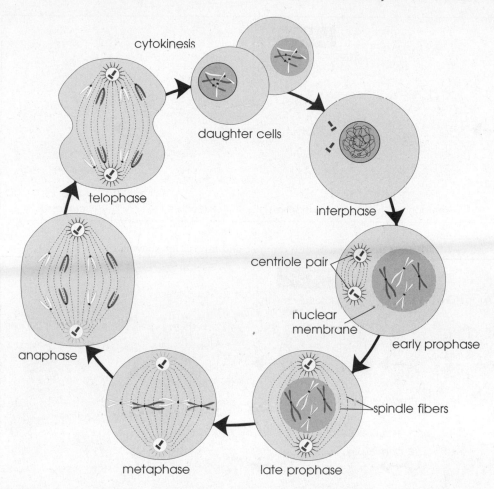

cytokinesis

daughter cells

telophase

interphase

centriole pair

nuclear membrane

early prophase

anaphase

spindle fibers

metaphase

late prophase

Mitosis in Animal Cells

haploid cells. Except for the gametes, each cell in our body receives half of its chromosomes from our mother and half from our father. A specific maternal chromosome, for example 15, is homologous to the paternal chromosome 15. In prophase I, the nuclear membrane disintegrates and homologous chromosomes find each other, forming tetrads. The chromosomes line up, gene by gene, oftentimes criss-crossing each other forming chiasmata. It is at this time that chromosomes may exchange portions of their genetic material with their homologues in a process called crossing over. Homologous chromosomes then line up at the metaphase plate, and are separated from each other during anaphase I. In some species, nuclear membranes re-form during telophase I, and cytokinesis completes the division, resulting in two haploid cells.

No DNA duplication occurs before meiosis II, but the replication that occurred before meiosis I leaves us with two sister chromatids for each chromosome. In prophase II, the nuclear membrane of each daughter cell disintegrates. Sister chromatids line up in metaphase II and are pulled apart in anaphase II. Nuclear membranes are re-formed in telophase II, and cytokinesis completes the formation of four haploid cells.

If the chromosomes do not separate properly, nondisjunction occurs. This produces one cell with too many copies of a particular chromosome (polyploidy) and another cell without any copies of that chromosome (aneuploidy). Down Syndrome is caused by nondisjunction, resulting in three copies of chromosome 21.

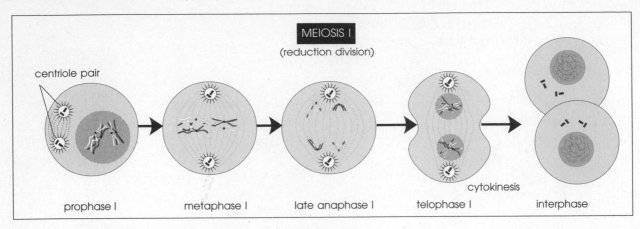

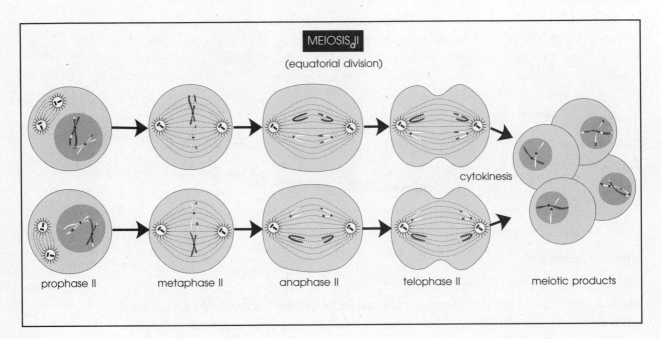

Meiosis in Animal Cells

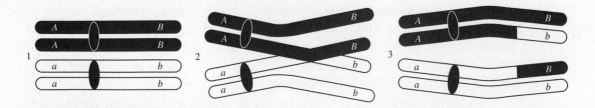

Schematic diagram of crossing over. (1) The two homologous doublestranded chromosomes, one bearing alleles *A* and *B* and the other alleles *a* and *b*, lie side by side. (2) A chiasma forms, causing corresponding breaks in one chromatid of each chromosome, and the fragments are exchanged. (3) After crossing over, one chromatid of the first chromosome bears alleles *A* and *b* and one chromatid of the second chromosome bears alleles *a* and *B*.

BIOLOGICAL ORGANIZATION AND RELATIONSHIP OF MAJOR TAXA

Taxa and Taxonomy

Taxonomy is the categorization of organisms based on similarities and differences. In order to make sense of the diverse array of living organisms, Carolus Linneaus (1707–1778) created a hierarchical classification system that we still use today. The categories, known as taxa, group similar species on different levels. The range of the Linneaus classification from largest to smallest is as follows: kingdom, phylum, class, order, family, genus, species. For instance, the full classification for humans is Animalia, Chordata, Mammalia, Primates, Homonidae, *Homo sapiens*.

The systems of classification help us to understand the world around us but are by no means definite. Many taxonomic debates are raging about such issues as which species belongs where and whether a so-called species is indeed one species or includes several species. Recently, scientists have debated the scientific validity of the current five-kingdom system and have thus created an even larger classification called the domain. Humans fall into the domain Eukarya.

TIP

Mnemonic:

Kings = **K**ingdom
Play = **P**hylum
Chess = **C**lass
On = **O**rder
Fine = **F**amily
Green = **G**enus
Silk = **S**pecies

Binomial Nomenclature

Linneaus also devised a system, based on the hierarchical classifications, to give each organism a unique scientific name. Binomial nomenclature, as it is called, gives each organism a name that is Latin and has two parts. The first part is the genus name, which denotes a group of similar life forms. For instance, all cats are in the genus *Felis*, and all dogs are in a different genus, *Canis*. The second part of the name is the species name, which is specific to a population of organisms that have similar characteristics, interbreed, and are reproductively isolated. In other words, a species can reproduce within its own species, but not with other species. The full names of the common house cat (*Felis domestica*) and Florida panther (*Felis concolor coryi*) indicate that both animals are cats but the two belong to different species.

Domains

The current classification includes three domains: Bacteria, Archaea, and Eukarya. This categorization actually splits the kingdom Monera, which contains all prokaryotes, into two separate groups: Bacteria and Archaea. It then combines all other kingdoms into the domain Eukarya.

Five-Kingdom Classification

As previously indicated, the five-kingdom classification is currently under scientific debate. It will be covered here because the DAT will test you on it. Because there are five kingdoms, the hierarchical system of naming is also known as the five-kingdom classification. The five kingdoms include: Monera, Protista, Fungi, Plantae, and Animalia.

Animals are multicellular heterotrophs that feed by ingestion. Some are sessile while others are mobile. They come in varying levels of complexity, from a sea sponge to a human. The more complex animals have specialized tissues, organs, and organ systems such as the digestive system, circulatory system, respiratory system, and musculoskeletal system. These organ systems vary from animal to animal, but the human organ systems will be reviewed in detail in a later section.

Animal cells grow by making more protein-rich cytoplasm; they then divide by mitosis. In mammals, meiosis produces haploid gametes, which cannot go on to produce viable organisms unless met and joined with another haploid gamete from the opposite sex. Most sea sponges, on the other hand, are hermaphrodites; that is, they have both male and female reproductive organs and are able to produce both types of gametes. Some animals undergo asexual reproduction, ranging from binary fission to budding to fragmentation. Some bee species have eggs that develop in a process called parthenogenesis, without ever being fertilized.

Animalia Phyla

Ninety-five percent of animals are invertebrates; that is, they do not have a backbone. Such animals are considered evolutionarily more primitive and are divided into several phyla. Vertebrates fall into the phyla Chordata. Every chordate has, in some stage of development, a notochord, a nerve chord, and pharyngeal slits. Some examples include humans and other mammals, fish, reptiles, birds, and sea squirts. Important invertebrate phyla are discussed in the next section.

LOWER INVERTEBRATES

Porifera

Porifera are sponges. Sponges are mostly marine, multicellular feeders, with a cellular level of design (no specialized tissues or organs). They exhibit radial symmetry; that is, they are organized like slices of a pie around a central mouth.

Cnidarians

Cnidarians are corals, sea anemones, and jellyfish. Cnidarians have a tissue level of design (no organs), are radially symmetrical, and are characterized by the presence of nematocysts (stinging cells).

Platyhelminthes

Platyhelminthes are flukes and tapeworms (parasitic, with complex life cycles) and flatworms (free-living and wormlike). Animals in this group exhibit cephalization, or the presence of a head and a tail region. They are also the first group to have bilateral symmetry, in which the right and left sides are identical (humans are bilaterally symmetrical).

Nematoda

Nematoda are roundworms. A simple and diverse group, the nematodes are among the most abundant animals on the earth today. Earthworms are *not* in this phylum.

HIGHER INVERTEBRATES

The higher invertebrates have a coelom at some stage of development. A coelom is a lined body cavity that aids in movement, nutrient transport, and gamete maturation.

GENERAL CHARACTERISTICS OF THE FIVE KINGDOMS

	Monera	Protista	Fungi	Plantae	Animalia
cell size	small ~1 - 10 μm	large ~10 - 100 μm	large ~10 - 100 μm	large ~10 - 100 μm	large ~10 - 100 μm
cell type	prokaryotic	eukaryotic	eukaryotic	eukaryotic	eukaryotic
nucleus	absent	present	present	present	present
chromosomal structure	nucleoid—single naked circle of DNA	chromosomes made of DNA, RNA, and protein	chromosomes made of DNA, RNA, and protein	chromosomes made of DNA, RNA, and protein	chromosomes made of DNA, RNA, and protein
mitochondria	absent	sometimes present	sometimes present	present	present
respiration	obligate anaerobes, facultative anaerobes, obligate aerobes	most obligate aerobes	most obligate aerobes	most obligate aerobes	most obligate aerobes
photo-synthesis	if present, enzymes bound to cell membrane, large variation in metabolic raw materials and end-products	if present, enzymes packaged into plastids, all generate oxygen	absent	generally present, enzymes packaged into chloroplasts, all generate oxygen	absent
metabolism	many variations	oxidative metabolism: glycolysis, Krebs cycle, electron transport	oxidative metabolism: glycolysis, Krebs cycle, electron transport	oxidative metabolism: glycolysis, Krebs cycle, electron transport	oxidative metabolism: glycolysis, Krebs cycle, electron transport
cell wall	polysaccharide-amino acid or peptidoglycans	some forms, various types	chitin	cellulose	absent
genetic recombi-nation	rare: conjugation transduction transformation	common: fertilization and meiosis	common: fertilization and meiosis	common: fertilization and meiosis	common: fertilization and meiosis
nutrition	autotrophic (photo- or chemosynthetic) and/or heterotrophic	autotrophic (photosynthetic) and/or heterotrophic	heterotrophic: absorption	autotrophic photosynthetic	heterotrophic: digestion
motility (single cell)	bacterial flagella composed of flagellin	9+2 undulipodia, ameboid	9+2 flagella only in zoospore gametes. All others nonmotile	9+2 undulipodia only in some gametes	9+2 undulipodia
cellularity	unicellular or colonial	unicellular, multicellular, or colonial	unicellular (yeast) or multicellular	multicellular	multicellular
cell division	mostly binary fission no centrioles, mitotic spindle or microtubules	mitosis/mitotic spindle/centrioles present	mitosis mitotic spindle centrioles absent	mitosis mitotic spindle centrioles absent	mitosis/mitotic spindle/centrioles present
development	N/A	varies	spores	multicellular embryo enclosed in maternal tissues	blastula

Mollusca

Mollusca are snails, clams, and squid. Mollusks are the earliest protostome phylum. Many are soft-bodied organisms with a hard outer covering.

Annelidae

Annelids are segmented worms (e.g., the common earthworm). Annelid bodies are made up of many identical segments.

Arthropoda

Arthropods include spiders, insects, and lobsters. The many species in this phylum are characterized by jointed appendages and an exoskeleton (external skeleton).

Echinodermata

Echinodermata are starfish, urchins, sand dollars, and sea cucumbers. One of two deuterostome phyla, echinoderms have pentaradial symmetry (five arms). Their larval stages are similar to those of chordates, suggesting that the phylum Chordata arose from the echinoderms.

Plantae

Without plants, humans could not exist. Not only do we rely on the photosynthetic organisms to produce oxygen and rid the air of excess carbon dioxide, but we also need plants for food, lumber, fuel, and medicine. Plants are multicellular organisms whose cells are surrounded by a cellulose cell wall. Like animals, each plant cell has identical DNA, but different combinations of genes are actively expressed in certain cells allowing for tissue and organ specialization. The roots absorb water and nutrients from the soil, the leaves engage in photosynthesis to make energy in the form of sugar, and the stem contains vascular tissue allowing for transport of these essentials from one part of the plant to the other. The xylem is the vascular tissue that transports water and minerals up to the leaves; phloem allows the sugars to "flow" down to the roots. The underside of leaves also have porelike structures called stomata, which are important for gas exchange with the environment. They are also important in transpiration, the evaporative loss of water from a plant. Stomata are regulated by guard cells. Water regulation in plants is an involved process. Plant cells with insufficient water shrivel, giving a limp or flaccid look to a plant. If this plant is then given an adequate water supply, each cell will take up the water, expanding its cell membrane against the cell wall, producing turgor pressure. Healthy plants are turgid.

Unlike an animal, a plant can continue to grow throughout its lifetime. This indeterminate growth occurs at the embryonic tissue called the meristem. Primary growth occurs in the vertical direction via apical meristems at the tip of the stem and root. Secondary growth gives the plant its girth by growth at the lateral meristems. The plane of cell division is determined in late interphase by microtubule arrangement. Cell growth in plants is largely due to uptake of water, stored in the central vacuole.

All plants are autotrophs. About 90% of plants have a mutualistic relationship with bacteria (e.g., nitrogen-fixing cyanobacteria) and/or fungi (forming micorrhizae). Even though they have the ability to produce their own nutrition, some plants, such as mistletoe, are parasites in their natural habitats, taking nutrition from oak trees. Others, like the venus flytrap, are carnivores, gaining extra minerals by trapping insects and other small animals and dissolving them with digestive enzymes.

The reproductive cycle of plants is called alternation of generations. In animals, the only haploid cells are gametes; in plants, an entire fully grown mature haploid organism is part of the life cycle. The haploid generation, called the gametophyte, undergoes mitosis-producing gametes, which fuse in fertilization, becoming a zygote. The zygote grows into a mature diploid plant, called the sporophyte. The sporophyte then undergoes meiosis-producing haploid gametes called spores. Spores develop into fully grown gametophytes without requiring the fusion of another gamete.

Flowering plants, called angiosperms, account for approximately 90% of plants and house their reproductive organs within the flower. The male reproductive organ is called the stamen, and the female reproductive organ is called the carpel. Pollination by animals, wind, or water brings the male gametes to the female gametes. Fertilization occurs; the ovule develops into a seed; and the ovary, into a fruit.

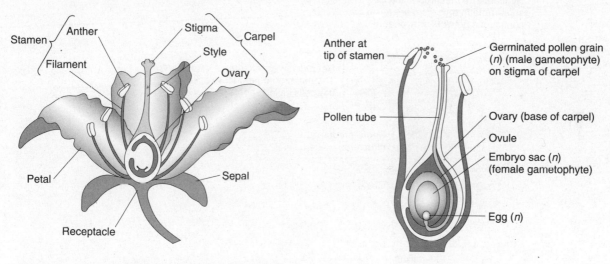

Typical structure and fertilization of flowering plants

Fungi

Humans often think of fungi as mold growing on rotting fruit or bread, ringworm, or athlete's foot. *Candida albicans* is the fungus responsible for yeast infections in the vagina and oral thrush in mouths of immunocompromised patients. But fungi are an integral part of the global ecosystem—they are the natural recyclers. They are necessary for the survival of many plant species, and therefore the production of oxygen in the atmosphere. Fungi, in a close symbiotic relationship with photosynthetic algae and cyanobacteria, form lichens. Lichens are integral in primary succession of ecosystems by decomposing remains and adding nutrients to the soil, preparing it for vegetation. It is also a fungus, *Penicillium*, that is the natural producer of the antibiotic penicillin.

Fungi are heterotrophs, but they do not ingest their food. Detriti decompose the organic remains and waste of plants and animals, recycling important nutrients in the environment. Others are parasites of plants and animals and feed directly off of host cells. Still others are micorrhizae. That is, they have a mutualistic symbiotic relationship with plant roots, with the plant providing nourishment for the fungi, while the fungi provides essential nutrients for the plant's growth. Ninety percent of plants have a fungi in a micorrhizal relationship with them. Fungi have cell walls made of chitin, the same material that comprises the cell walls of arthropods.

Unicellular fungi are called yeast. Multicellular are composed of hyphae, which form a large underground network called the mycelium. The mycelium may give rise to aboveground fruiting bodies, such as mushrooms. Hyphae can be composed of separated cells; cell walls that separate hyphae are called septa and have large pores through which cytoplasm and organelles can travel from cell to cell. Other hyphae have no septa and are one large syncytium of cytoplasm and nuclei; they undergo meiosis, but not cytokinesis. Some fungi have specialized hyphae that are able to penetrate cells walls of organisms with which they have a mutualistic or parasitic relationship. These specialized hyphae are called haustoria.

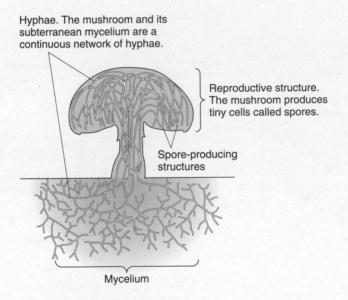

Structure of a multicellular fungus

Yeast reproduce by budding; they replicate their genetic material and then pinch off a portion of the membrane and cytoplasm forming a new cell. Multicellular fungi can often undergo asexual or sexual reproduction depending on environmental conditions. They spend the majority of their lives as haploid organisms. A generalized life cycle of fungi, including a sexual and asexual cycle, will be presented. Keep in mind that there are distinct variations among the life cycles and reproductive bodies in the five phyla of the Kingdom Fungi. The most primitive of these phyla, the chytrids, are the only fungi that have flagellated spores, called zoospores.

The sexual reproductive cycle begins when one fungi releases hormones. When the pheromone meets its match, the hyphae of the mating fungi grow toward each other until they fuse cytoplasm, called plasmogamy. They can remain in this phase of the cycle for days, months, or years. The nuclei then fuse in karyogamy, creating a diploid organism, followed by meiosis creating haploid spores, which then grow into mycelium of new organisms.

The asexual reproductive life cycle simply involves mitosis, forming clones in the form of spores. The spores can travel by air or water, or by flagella in the case of zoospores, and can then produce new organisms.

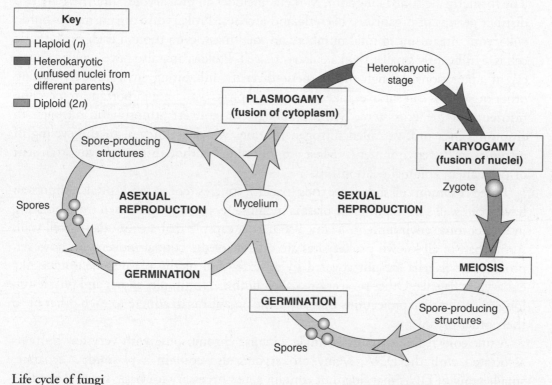

Life cycle of fungi

Protista

Recent advances in genetic comparison show that many protists are more closely related to plants, animals, or fungi than to each other. The formal Kingdom Protista has been abandoned, but scientists still used the term protist to refer to eukaryotic organisms that are not plants, animals, or fungi. Protists are extremely diverse; it is thought that endosymbiosis is responsible for much of this diversity. In endosymbiosis, a unicellular organism engulfs another unicellular organism without destroying it. It is thought that plastids, the pigment containing organelles, arose from endosymbiosis.

Most protists are unicellular organisms, but their single cells can often be quite complex with contractile vacuoles and specialized modes of locomotion. Nuclei of protists come in various numbers and sizes. Locomotion is accomplished by flagella, cilia, and pseudopodia in different species. Other protists are colonial or multicellular (e.g., algae). Nutritionally, some are photoautotrophs, others are heterotrophs that obtain nutrients either by ingestion or absorption, and some are mixotrophs, with the ability to be both autotrophic and heterotrophic. Most live in an aquatic or moist environment. Protists can be free-living (e.g., *Paramecium*), symbiotic (*e.g., Mixotricha paradoxa,* which live in the guts of termites, digesting the wood they eat), or parasitic (e.g., *Plasmodium,* the organism that causes malaria in humans).

Some protists adhere strictly to asexual reproduction, while others engage in some form of sexual reproduction. Algae, like terrestrial plants, have a life cycle involving alternation of generations.

Monera

The formerly identified kingdom, Monera, includes all prokaryotes, but there are two distinct groups of organisms: bacteria and archaea. Prokaryotic organisms far outdo eukaryotic organisms in total number and total mass, even though each prokaryotic cell is significantly smaller than a eukaryotic cell. Prokaryotes also have evolved a variety of adaptations through their genetic diversity, inhabiting environments that no other organisms can survive. Like fungi, many prokaryotes are important in recycling nutrients in the ecosystem. Some cyanobacteria convert atmospheric nitrogen to ammonia in a process called nitrogen fixation, which is integral to the cycling of nitrogen in the environment. Most are unicellular, although some have a transient or permanent colonial relationship.

Three common cell shapes are rods (bacilli), spheres (cocci), and spirals. Almost all have a cell wall surrounding the plasma membrane, preventing the cell from bursting in a hypotonic environment. Many also have a capsule that surrounds the cell wall. About half of all known prokaryotes are capable of directional movement; however, prokaryotic flagella are not covered by an extension of the plasma membrane like eukaryotic flagella. Other projections called fimbriae (multiple, short) and pili (fewer, longer) are hairlike projections that allow the organisms to adhere to each other or to their other organisms.

A nucleoid region contains a single, circular chromosome with very few proteins associated with the DNA. Many prokaryotes also contain a plasmid, a separate, smaller ring of DNA that does not contain genes necessary for basic survival but that can be utilized when the organism encounters an environmental threat. For example, certain bacteria have developed resistance to antibiotics through plasmids. Plasmids replicate independently of the cell's chromosome. Prokaryotic ribosomes are smaller than those found in eukaryotes.

Asexual reproduction occurs by way of binary fission. Horizontal gene transfer between organisms of the same or different species allows for added genetic diversity. Some prokaryotes may produce endospores, which are highly resistant, dormant forms of the organisms that may continue their life cycles when environmental conditions permit.

Prokaryotes may be obligate aerobes (requiring oxygen for survival), facultative anaerobes (using oxygen when available, but able to survive without it), and obligate anaerobes (that die in the presence of oxygen). The main forms of prokaryote nutrition are photoautotrophs, chemoautotrophs, and heterotrophs. They may be free-living, symbiotic, or parasitic.

A key difference between bacteria and archaea is the structure of their cell walls. Archaea cell walls contain a variety of polysaccharides and proteins, while bacteria cell walls contain peptidoglycans, which are sugar polymers cross-linked by peptide bonds. Within bacteria are two distinct types of cell walls. Most gram positive organisms have simple cell walls, while gram negative organisms have a more complex wall, which is then surrounded by an outer membrane.

Furthermore, many archaea, called extremophiles, have adapted to harsh environments where few other organisms can survive: too hot, too cold, too acidic, too salty. Some are even used as decomposers of human waste in sewage treatment plants, releasing methane as their own waste product.

STRUCTURE AND FUNCTION OF VERTEBRATE SYSTEMS

Integumentary System

The integumentary system, or skin, is divided into two sections: the epidermis and the dermis. The epidermis is the thin outer layer composed of stratified squamous epithelial cells, also called keratinocytes. It has no blood vessels or nerves. The epidermis itself has five layers, from outermost to innermost: stratum corneum, stratum lucidum, stratum granulosum, stratum spinosum, and stratum basale. Keratinocytes begin their epidermal fate at the innermost layer, the stratum basale. The cells undergo a progressive outward maturation through the layers, changing shape as they become filled with keratin. The outermost layer, the stratum corneum, is composed of flattened, dead cells, filled with keratin. These cells are continuously being lost and replaced. It is the structural protein, keratin, that toughens the skin, hair, and nails. The epidermis also contains melanocytes—cells responsible for brown pigment production—and specialized immune cells called Langerhans cells.

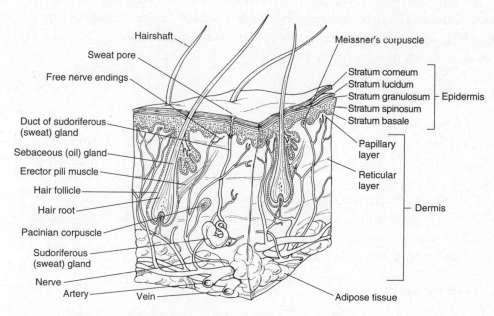

A general overview of the skin and the subcutaneous layer beneath it.

> **TIP**
>
> **Mnemonic**
> Epidermal Layers
> **Corn** = Corneum
> **Lovers** = Lucidum
> **Grow** = Granulosum
> **Several** = Spinosum
> **Barrels** = Basale

The dermis is the deep layer and is composed of connective tissue (including collagen and elastic fibers), sparse cells, and ground substance. Fibroblasts are the most abundant cell type in the dermis; however, there are also a number of immune cells scattered throughout. These cells include mast cells, lymphocytes, and macrophages. The dermis also contains blood vessels, hair follicles, sweat glands, sebaceous glands, and free and specialized nerve endings, including Pacinian and Meissner's corpuscles. The level beneath the dermis, called the subcutaneous layer, is filled with fatty deposits that help to store heat, as well as blood vessels, nerves, and lymphatics.

FUNCTIONS OF THE SKIN

The skin's major functions include protection and transmission of information from the environment to the brain. Nerves in the dermal layer of the skin can sense temperature, pressure, pain, and touch. One of the ways the body reacts to these external stimuli is thermoregulation, the process of keeping the body at a constant temperature. Most of the body's heat diffuses through the skin. The amount of heat lost can be changed by varying the blood supply to the small blood vessels in the skin. If the body temperature is too high, perhaps because of exercise or hot weather, the blood supply to the skin decreases and the capillaries close, thereby conserving heat. Also, high body temperature stimulates the sweat glands, to produce sweat, which evaporates and thus helps the body to cool. Sweat also contains metabolic wastes and therefore has an excretory function.

There are several ways in which the skin protects the body. First, the skin is a physical barrier against infection. Usually, disease-causing agents cannot enter the body where the skin is intact; entry occurs mostly through orifices or broken places in the skin. For this reason, burn victims have a very high risk of infection. The skin is also part of the immune system with its specialized immune cells that "sample" the environment. If these cells sense a threat, they relay a message to the extensive immune system, which responds appropriately. Finally, the skin's absorption of ultraviolet rays protects other layers of tissue from damage.

Skeletal System

The main functions of the skeletal system are support, protection, and, in conjunction with the muscular system, movement. Bones are also important for mineral storage and hemopoeisis (making blood cells). The human skeleton is divided into the axial skeleton, consisting of the skull, rib cage, sternum, and vertebral column, and the appendicular skeleton, consisting of the appendages and their attachments to the axial skeleton. Bone is mineralized connective tissue: a mix of cells, fibers, and minerals (calcium and phosphate). These materials are assembled in a way that makes bone rigid and strong, yet remarkably flexible.

TYPES OF BONES

There are five main types of bones in the body: long, flat, short, irregular, and sesamoid. Long bones are found in the arms, legs, toes, and fingers; they curve slightly to absorb shock and have large ends. The skull, ribs, hips, sternum, and scapula consist of broad plates of bone called flat bones. Short bones are present in the wrist and ankle. Irregular bones make up the vertebrae and parts of the face. Finally, sesamoid bones are embedded within tendons; one example is the kneecap.

BONE TISSUE

Bones come in two main densities: cancellous and compact. Cancellous bone is sometimes called spongy bone and consists of a network of supporting elements called trabeculae. Compact bone is composed of a dense matrix made up of structural units called osteons. Osteons are cylindrical sections; at the center of each is a Haversian canal, a tube that houses bundles of blood vessels and nerves. Surrounding the canals are concentric rings of bony tissue, which contain osteoblasts that lay down the bony matrix. The parallel osteons are connected by Volksmann's canals, which connect the Haversian canals to each other.

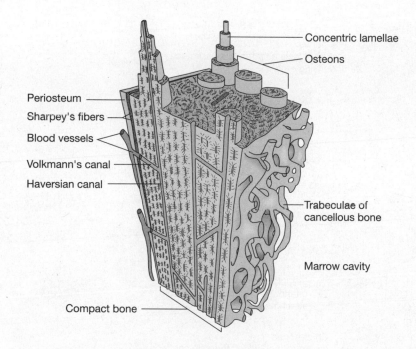

Compact bone is surrounded by the periosteum, attached by Sharpey's fibers. Compact bone is made up of osteons. Inside of compact bone is cancellous bone, with large trabeculae. In long bones, marrow space is the innermost compartment of bone.

The outer portion of any given human bone is made of compact bone. The inner portion is cancellous bone. At the center of long bones is the bone marrow, composed of fatty soft tissue and cells that produce red and white blood cells.

TIP	
Mnemonic	
osteo**B**lasts	**B**uild bone
osteo**C**lasts	**C**rush bone

CONNECTIVE TISSUES

Cartilage is a dense connective tissue essential to the skeletal system that does not contain blood vessels. It is more flexible than bone and functions well in absorbing shock, lubricating joints, and providing support. At birth, most of the skeleton is cartilage, later replaced by bone in a process called endochondral ossification. Bones that do not form from a cartilage template undergo intramembranous ossification. In adults, cartilage remains in the articulating surfaces of joints, the nose, ears, parts of the rib cage, and the rings of the trachea. Cartilage also remains at the ends of long bones in children and young adults. The junction of cartilage and bone in long bones is called the epiphyseal plate; this is where continued growth of long bones occurs.

Other connective tissues are the tendons, which attach muscle to bone, and the ligaments, which attach bones together at the joints.

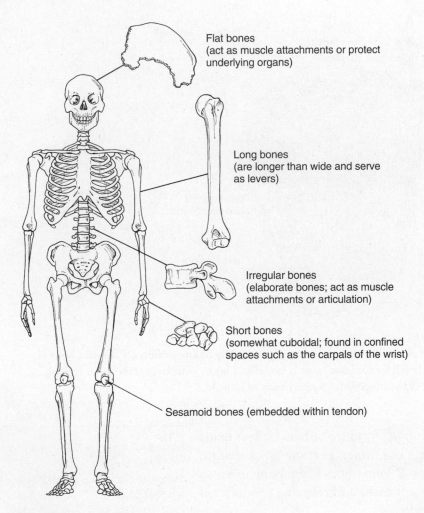

Flat bones
(act as muscle attachments or protect underlying organs)

Long bones
(are longer than wide and serve as levers)

Irregular bones
(elaborate bones; act as muscle attachments or articulation)

Short bones
(somewhat cuboidal; found in confined spaces such as the carpals of the wrist)

Sesamoid bones (embedded within tendon)

Five different types of bones and their locations.

JOINTS

Bones come together at joints. Immovable joints, like sutures between the skull bones, are called synarthroses. Cartilaginous and synovial joints (e.g., the knee) are movable. Cartilaginous joints are found throughout the axial skeleton, for example, between the vertebrae. These joints absorb shock and are termed amphiarthroses

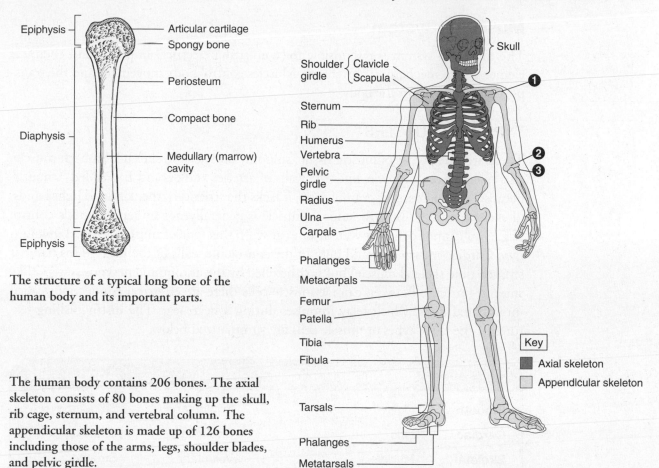

Epiphysis
Articular cartilage
Spongy bone
Periosteum
Diaphysis
Compact bone
Medullary (marrow) cavity
Epiphysis

The structure of a typical long bone of the human body and its important parts.

Skull
Shoulder girdle { Clavicle / Scapula
Sternum
Rib
Humerus
Vertebra
Pelvic girdle
Radius
Ulna
Carpals
Phalanges
Metacarpals
Femur
Patella
Tibia
Fibula
Tarsals
Phalanges
Metatarsals

❶
❷
❸

Key
■ Axial skeleton
☐ Appendicular skeleton

The human body contains 206 bones. The axial skeleton consists of 80 bones making up the skull, rib cage, sternum, and vertebral column. The appendicular skeleton is made up of 126 bones including those of the arms, legs, shoulder blades, and pelvic girdle.

because they allow for slight movement. Synovial joints are present in the appendicular skeleton and vary in form, depending on the location. Synovial joints are strong and have free movement; they are referred to as diarthroses. They are lubricated by synovial fluid, which reduces friction between tendons, ligaments, muscles, and bones. The knee and elbow are examples of synovial, diarthrotic joints.

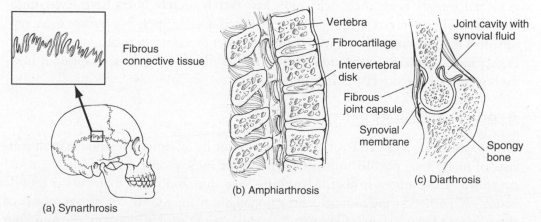

Fibrous connective tissue

(a) Synarthrosis

Vertebra
Fibrocartilage
Intervertebral disk
Fibrous joint capsule
Synovial membrane

(b) Amphiarthrosis

Joint cavity with synovial fluid
Spongy bone

(c) Diarthrosis

Three basic types of joints found in the human body. (a) An immovable joint such as found between bones of the skull. (b) A slightly movable joint such as found between vertebrae in the vertebral column. (c) A freely movable joint known as a synovial joint, such as found at the hip joint. Note the structural parts of the synovial joint.

Muscular System

The muscular system is responsible for converting electrical impulses and chemical elements into mechanical movement. Muscles control body movement and the transport of fluids within the body.

TYPES OF MUSCLES

There are three types of muscle tissue: smooth, cardiac, and skeletal. Smooth muscle, also called visceral muscle, lines the walls of arteries and organs. It is called "smooth" because, on microscopic examination, it lacks the striations, the dark and light bands, of skeletal muscle. Because smooth muscle is generally not under conscious control (e.g., you cannot constrict your arteries at will), this type of muscle is called involuntary. Cardiac muscle is found only in the contractile walls of the heart. This tissue is striated (like skeletal muscle) but is controlled by the autonomic nervous system (like smooth muscle). Between cardiac muscle cells there are electrical connections called intercalated discs, which relay impulses during a heartbeat. The distinguishing features of the three types of muscle cells are summarized below.

	#of Nuclei Per Cell	Action	Appearance
Smooth	One	Involuntary	Smooth
Cardiac	One	Involuntary	Striated
Skeletal	Multiple	Voluntary	Striated

Skeletal muscle is responsible for voluntary movement. If you lift this book, skeletal muscles are at work. Skeletal muscle is composed of two distinct fiber types: slow-twitch (red) and fast-twitch (white). Any given muscle can have a combination of these fiber types, and the proportion of fiber types can change with use of the muscle. Slow-twitch fibers contain many mitochondira, enabling the muscle to work for extended periods without fatigue. They also have an abundance of myoglobin, which gives red muscle fibers their rich color. Fast-twitch muscle fibers have fewer mitochondria. They contract with more force than red muscle fibers but fatigue more rapidly. In a long-distance runner who depends on her muscles not to fatigue, you would expect to have a large proportion of slow-twitch fibers in her legs. A sprinter, however, would have more fast-twitch fibers.

STRUCTURE OF SKELETAL MUSCLE

Skeletal muscle is attached to other muscle or bone by tendons. The muscle itself consists of many long parallel units called fibers, or muscle cells. Many closely packed myofibrils make up each fiber. Myofibrils have thin and thick filaments that slide across each other during muscle contraction. Thin filaments are composed mostly of three types of actin. Thick filaments are made of the protein myosin. Surrounding these filaments are two types of networks: sarcoplasmic reticulum, which stores calcium ions, and T-tubules, which help to conduct nerve impulses. Units of overlapping thin and thick filaments are called sarcomeres. Z-lines bind these units together.

Skeletal Muscle

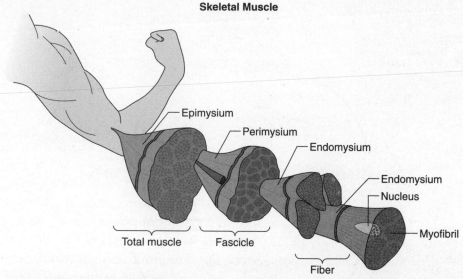

Composition of Skeletal Muscle

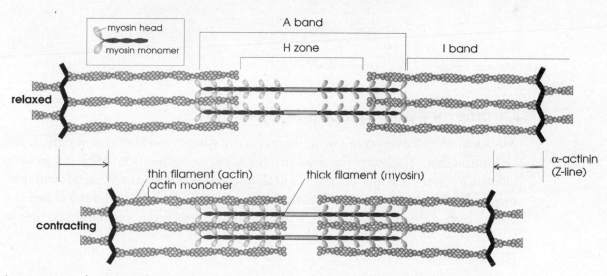

A sarcomere is the contractile unit of the muscle. A single sarcomere is defined from one Z-line to the next Z-line. During contraction, the H zone and I band shrink, but the A band stays constant.

SLIDING FILAMENT MODEL

Contraction of muscles begins with a nerve impulse, which triggers the release of stored calcium ions. What follows is best described by what is called the sliding filament model. The calcium ions expose binding sites in the actin filament. At these sites, a "head" of the myosin filament attaches and pulls the thinner actin filament inward. ATP in the muscle triggers the release of the myosin head, which now is free to attach again. The repeated attachment and release of many heads continue as long as there is stimulation or until the muscle fatigues.

Fatigue is defined as the muscle's inability to sustain contraction. Two factors lead to fatigue: depletion of ATP stores and the buildup of lactic acid. Lactic acid is produced when muscle cells are starved of oxygen and begin to function anaerobically.

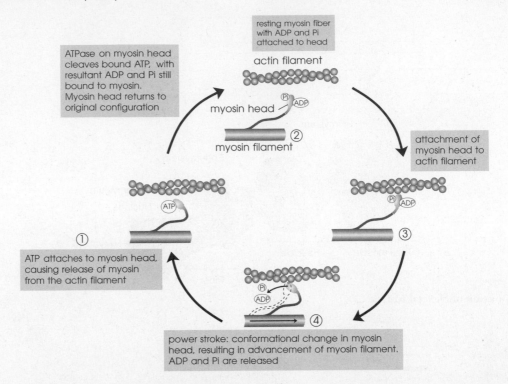

resting myosin fiber with ADP and Pi attached to head

actin filament

ATPase on myosin head cleaves bound ATP, with resultant ADP and Pi still bound to myosin. Myosin head returns to original configuration

myosin head

② myosin filament

attachment of myosin head to actin filament

③

ATP attaches to myosin head, causing release of myosin from the actin filament

①

power stroke: conformational change in myosin head, resulting in advancement of myosin filament. ADP and Pi are released

④

Molecular Basis of Muscle Contraction

Circulatory and Lymphatic Systems

The circulatory system transports vital nutrients, gases, wastes, chemical signals, and cells throughout the body. The fluid that houses these elements is the blood. In open circulatory systems, which are present in simpler animals such as arthropods and mollusks, blood bathes the organs directly. The human circulatory system is a closed system, meaning that the blood travels through blood vessels that form a closed loop.

BLOOD

Plasma, the fluid part of the blood, is 92% water. Plasma contains inorganic salts, proteins, hormones, nutrients, waste products, fats, and gases. The salts, called electrolytes, are important in maintaining osmotic balance. The plasma proteins function in clotting (fibrinogen and prothrombin), staving off infection (immunoglobulins), and regulating blood pressure (albumins).

Human blood contains many different types of cells. Almost half of the blood is made up of two types of blood cells: red blood cells, which carry oxygen, and white blood cells, which fight infection. Platelets are cell fragments that function in blood clotting. Red blood cells (erythrocytes) are shaped as biconcave discs; they produce hemoglobin, the oxygen-carrying protein. Some white blood cells (leukocytes) are phagocytic in that they engulf invading microbes. Other white blood cells, called lymphocytes, produce antibodies that either latch on to invading cells and help disable them (B-cells) or directly attack and destroy foreign cells (T-cells). Both white and red blood cells are formed in bone marrow. Platelets are not actually cells, but rather fragments of cells. These fragments attach to fibrin at the site of a cut; the result is a blood clot, which seals up the injury.

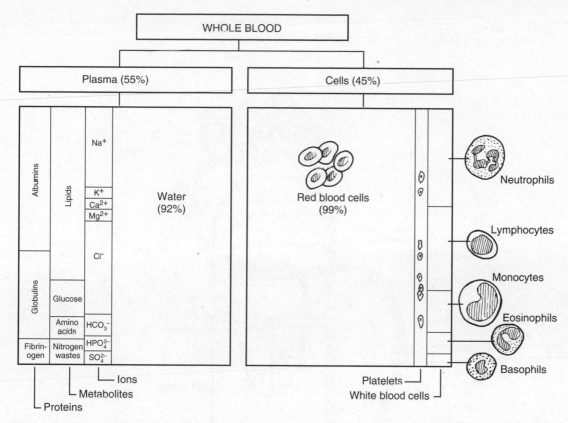

The composition of human blood. The two major components of whole blood are plasma and formed elements. The plasma contains water and numerous dissolved materials, including proteins, metabolites (nutrients and waste products), and ions. The great majority of formed elements are red blood cells.

ARTERIES AND VEINS

Blood travels through vessels called arteries and veins. Arteries carry blood away from the heart and have muscular walls that pulsate with every heartbeat. Systolic pressure is the maximum pressure attained during an arterial pulse, and diastolic pressure is the lowest. Arteries branch off into smaller vessels, the arterioles, and capillaries. Capillaries, the smallest vessels, are a single cell thick. Nutrients, gases, and other molecules in the blood diffuse through the thin capillary walls and surround the cell in a medium called interstitial fluid. Veins collect blood from the tissues and carry it back to the heart. Most veins have valves that prevent the blood from flowing backward. The vascular system is divided into two circuits: the pulmonary circuit and the

Arteries	Veins
Carry blood away from heart	Carry blood to heart
Systemic arteries carry oxygenated blood. Pulmonary arteries carry deoxygenated blood.	Systemic veins carry deoxygenated blood. Pulmonary veins carry oxygenated blood.
Muscular, elastic walls	Thin, inelastic walls
No valves	Valves to prevent backflow

systemic circuit. The coronary arteries are part of the systemic circuit and provide oxygenated blood so the heart itself can function.

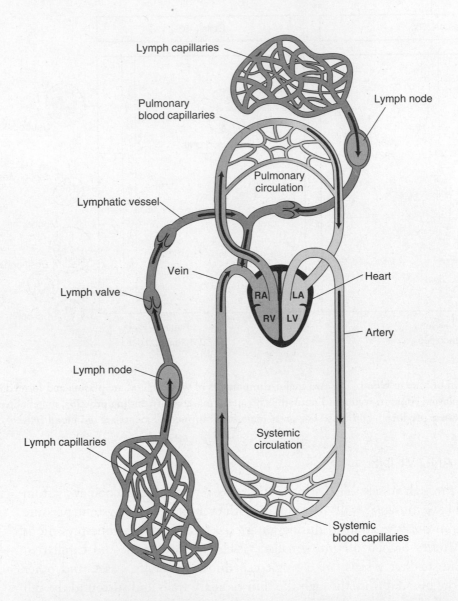

The two main cardiovascular circuits in the human body. In the pulmonary circuit, blood travels from the right ventricle to the lungs and returns to the left atrium. In the systemic circuit, blood travels from the left ventricle to the body and returns to the right atrium.

The lymphatic system as it relates to the circulatory system. Fluid seeps out of the circulatory system in the tissues and, while much of the fluid returns to the system, some fluid enters the lymph capillaries and returns to the circulation by this method. The lymphatic system is therefore a one-way system.

THE HEART

The heart is the center of both circuits of the circulatory system. Through several steps, called a heart cycle, the heart pumps blood into the lungs, where it is oxygenated; then it pumps the oxygenated blood back into the circulatory system. These are the events of a heartbeat:

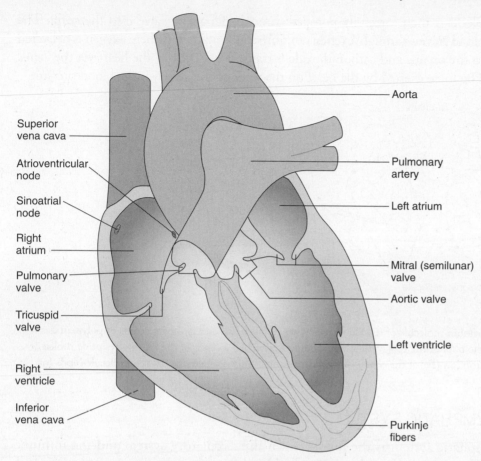

The heart. The contraction of both atria occurs simultaneously, as does the contraction of both ventricles. The sinoatrial (SA) node is the pacemaker of the heart and initiates the electrical impulse that causes the atria to contract, pushing blood into the ventricles. The impulse is then transmitted to the atrioventricular (AV) node, which subdivides into the Purkinje fibers. These fibers deliver an impulse to the ventricles, pushing blood from the right ventricle into the pulmonary arteries and from the left ventricle into the aorta.

Pulmonary Circuit

1. Deoxygenated venous blood enters the first chamber of the heart, the right atrium (RA), through the superior vena cava.
2. The tricuspid valve opens, allowing blood to flow to the right ventricle (RV).
3. Blood then passes through the pulmonary valve and into the pulmonary arteries, away from the heart.
4. Blood flows through the pulmonary arteries, arterioles, and finally reaches the capillaries, where carbon dioxide is unloaded and oxygen enters the blood. The oxygenated blood returns from the lungs via the pulmonary veins and enters the left atrium (LA).

Systemic Circuit

5. The heart pumps the blood through the mitral valve and into the left ventricle (LV).

6. Blood is then forcefully pumped through the aortic valve into the aorta. The blood travels through arteries, arterioles, and capillaries where oxygen is delivered to the organs and carbon dioxide is transported back to the heart via the veins. The force exerted by the heart on the walls of the vessels is the blood pressure.

The hemoglobin molecule of red blood cells. Two alpha chains and two beta chains of polypeptides make up the bulk of the molecule. A heme group is attached to each of the four polypeptide molecules. Note the iron ion (Fe) at the center of the heme group. This is where the oxygen molecule binds for transport.

THE LYMPHATIC SYSTEM

The lymphatic system is the link between the circulatory system and the immune system. As mentioned, molecules in the blood flow through the capillaries into the interstitial fluid. However, more fluid leaves the blood vessels and enters the body tissues than the reverse. What happens to the extra interstitial fluid? Unless collected, fluid would continue to build up in the tissues. Therefore, one of the functions of the lymphatic system is to absorb the excess fluid. Tiny tubes called lymph vessels collect the interstitial fluid, which passes through the lymph nodes and eventually cycles back into the circulatory system. The lymphatic system also plays a critical role in the body's defenses by producing lymphocytes and transporting white blood cells. Lymphatic vessels, like veins, have valves.

Respiratory System

The role of the respiratory system is to transport gases between the cells of the body and the environment. In humans, cellular respiration produces carbon dioxide, which is exchanged for oxygen, a necessary ingredient of respiration. Air (20% oxygen, 80% nitrogen) enters the body through the mouth and nose, moves through the pharynx to the trachea, and travels to the lungs. The lungs are made up of small passageways that end in air sacs called alveoli, where gas exchange occurs with the circulatory system. Alveoli have extremely thin walls and are surrounded by a network of pulmonary capillaries. Oxygen molecules diffuse across the thin walls and into the blood, while carbon dioxide diffuses into the air of the lungs. After gas exchange, the protein hemoglobin carries the oxygen in the blood, where it travels to the heart and the cells of the body. The deoxygenated air containing CO_2 waste is exhaled.

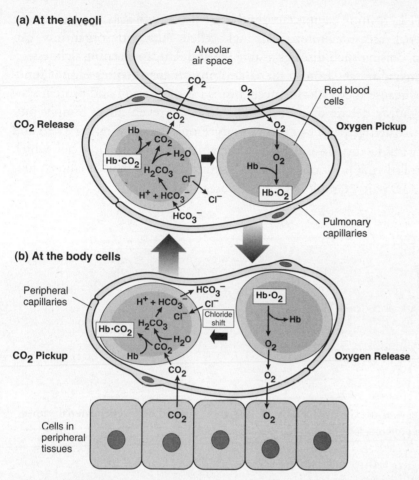

(a) At the alveoli

Alveolar air space

CO_2 O_2

Red blood cells

CO_2 Release

Hb CO_2

$Hb \cdot CO_2$ H_2O

H_2CO_3 Cl^-

$H^+ + HCO_3^-$ Cl^-

HCO_3^-

Oxygen Pickup

O_2

O_2

Hb

$Hb \cdot O_2$

Pulmonary capillaries

(b) At the body cells

Peripheral capillaries

$H^+ + HCO_3^-$ HCO_3^-

Cl^-

Cl^- Chloride shift

$Hb \cdot CO_2$ H_2CO_3

H_2O

CO_2

Hb

CO_2 Pickup

CO_2

$Hb \cdot O_2$

Hb

O_2

Oxygen Release

O_2

Cells in peripheral tissues

CO_2 O_2

A summary of transport and gas exchange mechanisms in the human body. (a) At the alveoli, CO_2 is released and oxygen is picked up. The gases pass across the membranes of the alveolus and the capillary. (b) At the body cells, the opposite occurs for the two gases. Note that oxygen is carried bound to the hemoglobin (Hb) of RBCs, while CO_2 is carried dissolved in plasma, bound to hemoglobin molecules, and as bicarbonate ions in sodium bicarbonate.

Immune System

The immune system protects the body against foreign invaders and from its own cells that have undergone cancerous changes. When a baby is born, it has not yet been exposed to pathogens, but it has innate immunity passed on by its mother. Innate immunity is transient and nonspecific but has a rapid response to a large variety of microbes. Acquired immunity occurs by exposure to pathogens throughout a lifetime. The response, via humoral and cell-mediated mechanisms, is slower and more specific, and the immunity is long-lasting.

PATHOGENS

The most common pathogens (microorganisms that invade the body and cause disease) are bacteria, viruses, and protozoans. Most types of these microorganisms are not harmful. In fact, our digestive tract is populated by billions of nonharmful bacteria. However, some species can cause serious diseases in humans by secreting toxins, attacking cells, or multiplying rapidly. Tuberculosis, syphilis, and leprosy are examples of bacterial diseases. Protozoans, single-celled eukaryotic organisms, can also be pathogenic, causing such diseases as malaria and African sleeping sickness.

Viruses are entirely different from bacteria and protozoans. Viruses cannot function on their own because they lack the mechanisms for respiration and protein synthesis. In fact, scientists debate as to whether viruses are even alive. Simply put, viruses are protein-coated genes. They can reproduce only by penetrating a cell and changing it into a virus factory. In the process, the virus destroys the host cell, which is why an uncontrolled viral invasion can be so harmful to an animal. Smallpox, herpes, measles, and AIDS are examples of viral diseases.

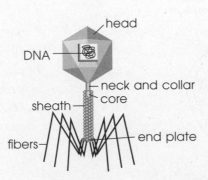

A T$_4$ **Bacteriophage: a virus that infects bacteria. Viruses are composed of genetic material, either DNA or RNA, and a protein coat.**

A virus enters the cell and changes its biochemistry to produce thousands of viral progeny. Generally, when viruses infect a cell, they use its resources to copy its DNA and produce viral RNA. Retroviruses, such as the AIDS virus, operate slightly differently. They have RNA gene material and can create an intermediate copy of DNA within the host. This DNA copy is then copied to form viral RNA. Viruses that infect bacteria are called bacteriophages.

HUMORAL VERSUS CELL-MEDIATED RESPONSE

The role of the immune system is to protect the body from foreign substances and damaged cells within the body, such as cancer cells. Foreign molecules in the body are called antigens. The body has two types of defense mechanisms to combat antigens: humoral immunity and cell-mediated immunity. Humoral immunity involves a diverse group of proteins called antibodies, or immunoglobulins, that recognize and bind to specific antigens, marking the antigen for destruction. Antibodies are Y-shaped proteins that have sequences that recognize a specific type of antigen. Humoral immunity occurs mostly in extracellular fluids. A cell-mediated response involves specialized cells that combat foreign cells. It is largely responsible for defending against infected and cancerous cells.

TIP

Vocabulary
AntiBODY—made by BODY to recognize foreign invaders. Also called immunoglobulins.
AntiGEN—foreign substances that are antibody-GENerating.

CELLS OF THE IMMUNE SYSTEM

The major cell type of the immune system is the lymphocyte. Lymphocytes originate in bone marrow and are found throughout the body. Large numbers are present in the lymph vessels and lymph nodes, spleen, thymus (in children and adolescents), and blood vessels. There are two types of lymphocytes: B-cells and T-cells. B-cells reside mostly in the bone marrow, are involved with humoral immunity, and can specialize into plasma cells that secrete antibodies. T-cells also originate in the bone marrow but then travel to the thymus to mature. They are involved in the cell-mediated response and come in three forms: helper T-cells, which stimulate the activity of other cells; killer T-cells (also cytotoxic cells), which destroy target cells directly; and suppressor T-cells, which decrease the activity of other B- and T-cells after infections are brought under control.

After encountering an antigen, the immune system "remembers" it by storing some of the lymphocytes that were mobilized for the attack. These cells are memory B- and T-cells, stored in the spleen and ready to react quickly should the antigen present itself again. When there is a large immune response, many memory cells remain. The result is permanent immunity, which occurs, for example, in the case of measles. After a mild response, there is a temporary immunity, such as is experienced after a bout with the flu.

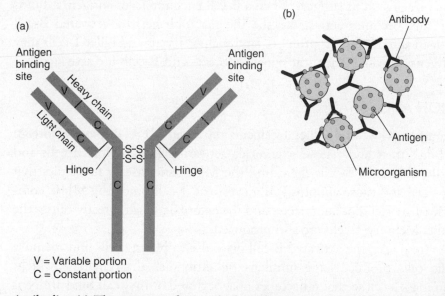

V = Variable portion
C = Constant portion

Antibodies. (a) The structure of an antibody molecule showing the four chains that make up the molecule. (b) The reaction between antibody molecules and antigens on the surface of a microorganism. Antibody molecules bind the microorganisms together and assist phagocytosis.

Other important cells in the immune system include phagocytic cells, which recognize the presence of an antigen, engulf it, and initiate a cell-mediated immune response. These phagocytic cells include macrophages, neutrophils, eosinophils, and dendritic cells. Natural killer cells, as opposed to B- and T-cells, are not very specific. They recognize harmful sequences in virus-infected and cancer cells, releasing chemicals that cause damaged cells to apoptose. Mast cells store histamine and activate an inflammatory response in response to physical injury or invasion by pathogens.

EVENTS OF AN IMMUNE RESPONSE

The following are the events of an immune response.

Self versus Nonself

The immune system must be able to distinguish between intruders and non-intruders. The proteins that identify the body's own cells are called major histocompatibility complexes (MHC). These proteins are unique to each individual and occur in every nucleated cell of the body. They help the body determine which cells belong to the body and which are foreign invaders or damaged. Autoimmune diseases occur when the body is unable to differentiate between self and nonself, and the immune system attacks its own cells. Phagocytic cells of the immune system that encounter foreign substances display MHC molecules on their membranes, activating an immune response.

Recognizing the Antigen

Macrophages and T-cells travel throughout the body searching for foreign MHC markers. If one is found by either type of cell, the cell will sound an "alarm" that the antigen has entered the body. The macrophage engulfs the antigen and displays pieces of the antigen's proteins on its surface. When a B-cell encounters an antigen, it binds to the antigen and becomes activated. Like the macrophage, the activated B-cell digests the antigen and displays its proteins. Both helper T-cells and killer T-cells may encounter antigens. Through chemical signals, more T- and B-cells are activated.

MOBILIZATION AND ATTACK

In a cell-mediated response, if a helper T-cell encounters an MHC displaying foreign substance, it binds to it and releases chemicals activating more helper T-cells and cytotoxic T-cells. Cytotoxic T-cells then bind the MHC and release molecules that enter the target cell and cause apoptosis. If a cytotoxic T-cell binds the MHC complex, the intermediate step does not occur, and the cytotoxic T-cell directly causes the target cell to die. Memory T-cells are also produced.

In a humoral response, the activated B-cell gives rise to plasma cells and memory B-cells. Plasma cells produce large numbers of antibodies that circulate widely. Antibodies can mark a cell so that it becomes phagocytosed or they can bind antigens in a way to inactivate them.

Halt

Suppressor T-cells send the message to plasma cells and T-cells to halt their replication and activity.

Memory

Some T- and B-cells become memory cells, stored in the spleen and ready for future encounters with the antigen.

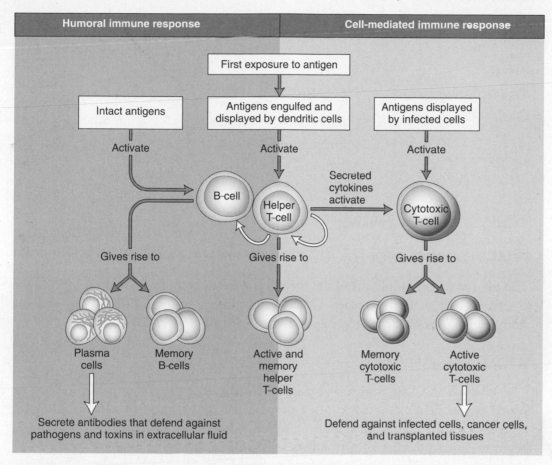

Humoral immune response	Cell-mediated immune response

A summary of humoral and cell-mediated immune responses

Digestive System

The roles of the digestive system are to convert material from food into nutrients that the body can use and to eliminate products that cannot be absorbed.

MOUTH

Digestion begins in the mouth, where the teeth are responsible for the mechanical breakdown of food into smaller particles. Humans have different types of teeth, with different shapes and functions. The incisors have sharp edges that cut food. The cuspids, also known as canines, and the bicuspids, also known as premolars, grasp and tear food. Molars, with large surfaces, grind the food.

Teeth are composed mostly of dentin, a calcium substance similar to bone. On the crown, the part of the tooth that is exposed, there is an outer thin coat of enamel, the hardest substance in the body. The innermost part of the tooth, called the pulp, is the living tissue, composed of nerves and blood vessels.

Salivary glands secrete saliva into the mouth. Saliva increases moisture and begins the chemical breakdown of carbohydrates via a digestive enzyme called salivary amylase. The tongue is a large muscle that tastes and manipulates food, and pushes the bolus of food to the pharynx to be swallowed.

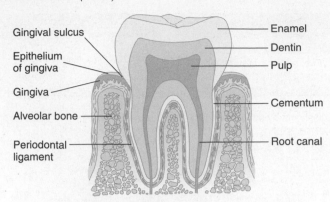

A tooth and its supporting structures

PHARYNX AND ESOPHAGUS

The pharynx, commonly called the throat, is a passageway that channels food to the esophagus and air to the trachea. Once in the esophagus, food is forced down to the stomach by a muscular contraction of the esophageal wall, called peristalsis.

STOMACH—CHYME

The stomach is a large muscular organ, where considerable amounts of food can be stored before being shunted to other parts of the digestive system. In the stomach, digestive enzymes and high concentrations of hydrochloric acid (HCl, pH of about 2) begin to digest proteins in the food, as well as break down the food into smaller and smaller particles. After a while, the food becomes a nutrient-rich acid broth known as chyme. This chyme is slowly released into the duodenum (the upper portion of the small intestine), where most of the breakdown of macromolecules occurs.

PANCREAS, LIVER, AND GALLBLADDER

Two glands, the pancreas and the liver, secrete substances into the duodenum that are crucial for digestion. The exocrine pancreas secretes molecules via ducts into the duodenum, as opposed to the endocrine pancreas, which secretes products (i.e., insulin) directly into the bloodstream. The exocrine pancreas delivers to the

The Characteristics of Several Components of Gastric Juice

Component	Source	Function
Pepsinogen	Chief cells of the gastric gland	Converts to pepsin
Pepsin	Formed from pepsinogen in the presence of hydrochloric acid	Protein-digesting enzyme capable of breaking down nearly all types of protein
Hydrochloric acid	Parietal cells of the gastric glands	Provides acidic environment; needed for converting pepsinogen into pepsin
Mucus	Goblet cells and mucus glands	Provides viscous, alkaline protective layer on the stomach wall
Intrinsic factor	Parietal cells of the gastric glands	Encourages the absorption of vitamin B_{12}

duodenum powerful hydrolytic enzymes that break down proteins, fats, and carbohydrates. It also delivers a strongly alkaline bicarbonate solution, which neutralizes the highly acidic chyme. The liver produces bile, a mixture that contains no digestive enzymes but does contain salts and lipids that aid in fat processing. Bile also has pigments, by-products of the liver's breakdown of red blood cells, that are removed from the body with the feces. The gallbladder, a small sac attached to the liver, stores the bile until it is needed.

SMALL INTESTINE

Food is broken down in the duodenum, but the nutrients of the food are absorbed in the other parts of the small intestine, the jejunum and the ileum. The lining of the lower small intestine has many folds and is covered with projections called microvilli, which maximize the surface area for the diffusion and active transport of molecules. The network of blood vessels surrounding the lower small intestine collects the nutrients and transports them to the liver, which regulates their release to the heart and the rest of the body.

LARGE INTESTINE—FECES

In the large intestine, or colon, water is reabsorbed from the chyme. Salts are actively transported from the large intestine, and water follows by osmosis, leaving dense feces. The feces, consisting mainly of undigested roughage, travel to the rectum, where they are stored before being eliminated via the anus.

Urinary System

The urinary system has two functions: (1) to remove metabolic wastes from the body and (2) to osmoregulate, or balance, the amounts of salts and water in the circulatory system. The kidneys, a pair of bean-shaped organs, are the sites of urinary function. Each kidney is made up of about one million functional units called nephrons. The nephrons perform three processes in controlling the salt and water concentrations of the blood. The kidney is a fascinating organ, but it can be overwhelming because of its intricate design.

FILTRATION, SECRETION, AND REABSORPTION

Blood enters the kidneys through the renal artery and travels through the arterioles into the capillaries. In the kidney, a ball of capillaries called the glomerulus is selectively porous, allowing water and small solutes such as amino acids, salts, and waste from the blood to be "filtered" out. Red blood cells and plasma proteins continue to circulate through the blood vessels, exiting the kidney via the renal vein. The filtrate enters a part of the nephron called Bowman's capsule. From there, it travels through the rest of the nephron: the proximal tubule, descending loop of Henle, ascending loop of Henle, distal tubule, and finally the collecting duct. Substances are either secreted (e.g., hydrogen ions to maintain pH) from the surrounding tissue into the filtrate, or reabsorbed (e.g., sugars, nutrients, amino acids) by the surrounding capillaries and returned to the bloodstream. Passive and active transport are involved in secretion and reabsorption. The collecting duct of each nephron opens into a larger opening, called a calyx. The calyces join to form the renal pelvis, leading into the ureter, connecting the kidney to the bladder. Through the collective action of the nephrons, the kidneys filter out waste products and water, forming a concentrated excretory fluid called urine. The bladder stores the urine, which eventually passes through the urethra and is eliminated from the body.

An important function of the urinary system is the removal of ammonia (NH_3), a nitrogenous by-product of cell metabolism that is highly toxic to the cells of the body. Because of its poisonous qualities, ammonia must be removed from the blood quickly or changed into a less toxic substance. In humans, the liver converts ammonia to a soluble form called urea. Urea can travel in the blood safely for longer periods than ammonia. The kidneys remove urea from the blood, where it becomes a major component of urine.

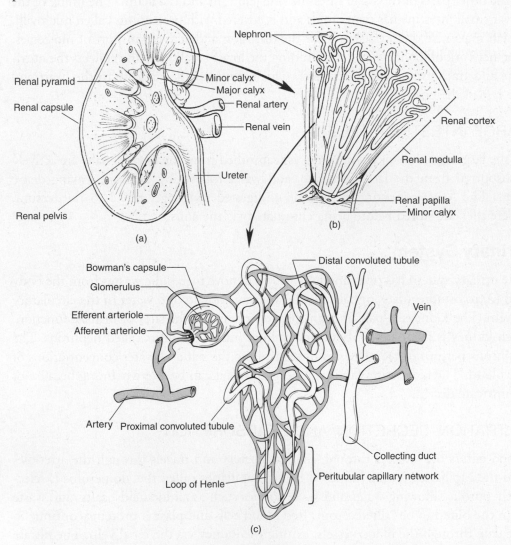

Structure of the kidney and its fine structures. (a) A sagittal section of the kidney showing the entry and exit of the renal artery and renal vein. The renal cortex is the outermost portion of the kidney, while the renal medulla is the inner portion. The urine collects in the calyces and renal pelvis before it is transported to the bladder, via the ureter. (b) The glomerulus, proximal tubule, and distal tubule are in the renal cortex. The Loop of Henle and collecting duct are in the renal medulla. (c) When the blood enters the kidney via the renal artery, it continues until it reaches the ball of capillaries called the glomerulus where it is filtered. The filtrate travels through the nephron, with substances being secreted into the filtrate or reabsorbed by the peritubular capillaries surrounding the nephron. Urine is concentrated in the collecting duct before emptying into the calyces.

Brain and Nervous System

The nervous system enables the body to receive and respond to stimuli from the environment. The primary cell of the nervous system is the neuron. Neurons process a stimulus and transmit it as an electric charge to other cells.

ANATOMY AND FUNCTION OF THE NEURON

A neuron consists of (1) a cell body (soma), which contains the nucleus and organelles; (2) dendrites, which are extensions of the cytoplasm that carry signals to the soma; and (3) the axon, which is a long nerve fiber that carries the electrochemical signal away from the soma and to other cells. The gap between two adjacent neurons or between a neuron and a target cell (i.e., muscle) is called a synapse. Most axons are covered with myelin sheaths, fatty insulating coats that speed up the conduction velocity of the axon. Myelin sheaths are made of Schwann cells, with gaps between them called Nodes of Ranvier. Schwann cells are examples of glial cells; that is, cells that are closely associated with neurons but do not transmit signals. Glial cells have very important supportive roles in the nervous system.

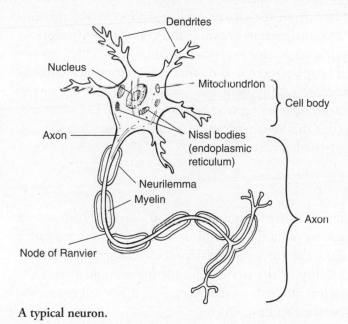

A typical neuron.

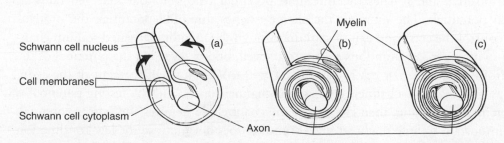

How the myelin sheath forms as the Schwann cell wraps itself around the axon in successive diagrams (a), (b), and (c). Myelin is the white, lipid-rich substance in the plasma membrane of the Schwann cell.

TYPES OF NEURONS

There are three types of neurons: sensory neurons (afferent), which interpret stimuli from the environment; interneurons, which relay the information to the brain where it is processed; and motor neurons (efferent), which control muscular movement. The axons and dendrites of these neurons are grouped together in bundles called nerves. For instance, a baseball player sees the ball coming toward him with sensory neurons in his eye. Interneurons relay the information to the brain where the speed and trajectory of the ball are processed, and an appropriate response is sent to the motor neurons of the baseball player's body, controlling the muscles so he can swing the bat.

TRANSMISSION OF INFORMATION

Several steps are involved in transmitting information through a nerve cell and to other cells.

Resting Potential

A neuron works because its membranes have electrical potential, or the force to move charged particles. When the neuron is not active, it is polarized, meaning that the electric charge inside the cell differs from the charge outside it. Specialized proteins in the membrane make up the sodium-potassium pump and create the difference in charge. Na^+ (sodium) ions are pumped outside the neural membrane, and K^+ (potassium) ions are pumped inside. The membrane is also selectively permeable, allowing K^+ ions to leak through much more readily than Na^+ ions. The result is that the inner surface of the nerve cell membrane is negatively charged relative to its outside. When the neuron is not firing, this difference in charge is called a resting potential. In many neurons, the resting potential is –70 mV.

Action Potential

Information in the nervous system is carried through electrical signals. These signals among nerve cells are sent as action potentials, or disturbances in the membrane's electrical potential that travels along the axon. An action potential begins with a stimulus, which changes the permeability of the nerve cell's membrane and upsets the normal balance of ions. Na^+ ions leak in, making the charge inside the cell more positive. Small changes in ion concentrations have no effect.

If, however, the stimulus is strong enough, the membrane potential becomes even more positive and reaches the threshold potential (the potential that generates an action potential). The moment the charge reaches threshold potential, the proteins that control the entry and exit of sodium through the membrane (gated sodium channels) swing open. Sodium ions rush into the cell, briefly reversing the potential of the cell from negative (−70 mV) to positive (+40 mV) in a small segment of the axon. Just as quickly, those channels close, other channels open, and the resting potential is restored. The opening, then closing, of the channels constitutes the action potential. It is important to note that a stronger stimulus does not increase the level or duration of the action potential; it only creates more frequent action potentials. After a segment of an axon is activated to produce an action potential, there is a period of time, called the refractory period, before this segment can be activated again.

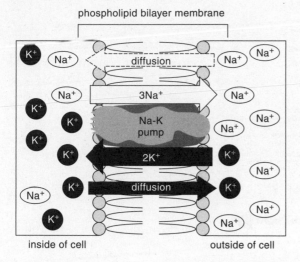

The Sodium-Potassium Pump

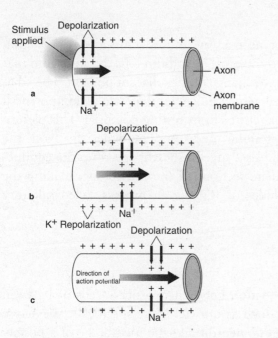

The action potential in a nerve cell. (a) A stimulus is applied to the membrane, and sodium ions (+) rush into the cell; the membrane loses its polarity, thereby generating an action potential. (b) The adjacent membrane area is depolarized by this action, and the action potential is propagated; meanwhile the original area undergoes repolarization with the accumulation of potassium ions (+) so it can "fire" again. (c) The action potential continues down the axon as successive areas undergo depolarization. Eventually, the action potential will pass into another nerve cell or a muscle cell.

An action potential is an example of an all-or-nothing response. If the stimulus is too low to cause critical changes in the permeability of the membrane, nothing will happen. If, however, the threshold potential is exceeded, an action potential is fired and is propagated along the axon and to other cells.

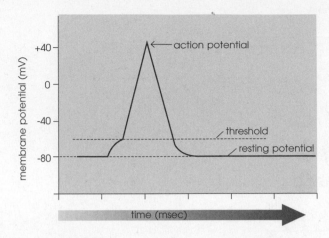

Action Potential

Propagation of the Impulse

Action potentials move along the membrane as a wave moves across a pool. An action potential fires only in a short portion of the axon. The sodium ions that rush into that portion also cause the electrical potential to change in the adjacent portion. The adjacent portion reaches a threshold potential, which quickly initiates an action potential in that area. Meanwhile, the original area returns to its resting potential. This pattern continues as the action potential moves along the axon. The wider the axon, the greater the speed of the action potential. Also, myelin sheaths speed up the conduction velocity of the impulse. They insulate sections of the membrane, making the impulse jump quickly between the Nodes of Ranvier (a process called saltatory conduction).

Transmission Between Cells

As stated previously, a synapse is the junction between two nerve cells or between a nerve cell and an effector membrane, such as muscle. More specifically, a synapse occurs between the axon of the presynaptic neuron and the membrane of a postsynaptic cell. There are two types of synapses: electric synapses, also called gap junctions, and chemical synapses. Gap junctions are protein channels that allow ions to flow freely from one cell to another, and thus to function as a unit. The transmission is virtually instantaneous, a feature that is important for some functions.

The more complex synapse is the chemical synapse, where a cell relays an impulse to another cell by converting the impulse into a chemical message. The chemical signals are called neurotransmitters. When an impulse travels to the synaptic knob of the presynaptic neuron and synaptic vesicles release the neurotransmitters into the synaptic cleft, the gap between the two cells lessens. The neurotransmitter binds to receptor sites on the postsynaptic membrane, thereby triggering a change in its permeability. The change either promotes or inhibits the propogation of the impulse. Very quickly, the neurotransmitter is eliminated from the synaptic cleft, and the system is ready for the next impulse.

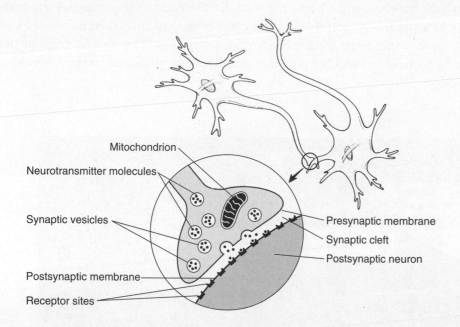

Mitochondrion

Neurotransmitter molecules

Synaptic vesicles

Postsynaptic membrane

Receptor sites

Presynaptic membrane

Synaptic cleft

Postsynaptic neuron

Activity at the synapse. When an action potential reaches the end of the axon, neurotransmitter molecules (such as acetylcholine) are released from synaptic vesicles by exocytosis at the presynaptic membranes. The molecules move across the synaptic cleft (space) and react with receptor sites on the surface of the postsynaptic membrane. This reaction generates an action potential in the postsynaptic neuron.

Processing Information

Nerve cells can receive impulses from thousands of axons. One impulse does not necessarily trigger the transmission of an action potential. Many excitatory impulses come together to make the cell fire, a process called summation. Remember that certain impulses can have an inhibitory effect so that impulses can also neutralize each other. The integration of the various sources by the nerve cell is the key to processing information.

CENTRAL AND PERIPHERAL NERVOUS SYSTEMS

The human nervous system is divided into two continuously interacting parts, the central nervous system and the peripheral nervous system.

The central nervous system, which processes information, consists of the brain and spinal cord. The spinal cord has two functions in the central nervous system: to relay information to and from the brain and to process simple stimuli. The spinal cord primarily integrates by way of a reflex, a connection of two or three neurons that unconsciously reacts to a simple stimulus. The knee jerk—the kicking response to a doctor tapping below the knee—is an example of a reflex.

The brain is the center of complex nerve integration. It is composed of three main parts: the cerebrum, the cerebellum, and the brainstem. The cerebrum is the largest part of the brain and it has various sections which control memory, thought sensation, and movement. The outer part of the cerebrum is composed of gray matter, a grouping of cell bodies. The interior consists of white matter, a network of axons. The cerebellum is largely responsible for the coordination and control of movement.

The brainstem has three main parts, the medulla oblongata, the pons, and the mid-brain. The brainstem is responsible for homeostasis and autonomic functions such as breathing, swallowing, heart muscle activity, and digestion. Two smaller parts of the brain, the hypothalamus and the pituitary gland, will be discussed in the Endocrine System section.

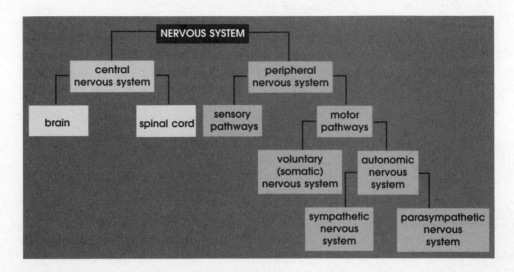

Organization of the Vertebrate Nervous System

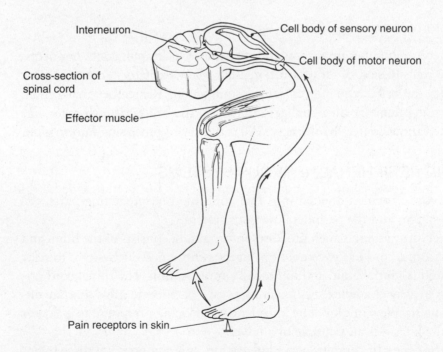

A typical reflex arc as shown by the withdrawal reflex. Impulses arise at the pain receptor and travel to the spinal cord by the sensory neuron. The interneuron interprets the impulse and dispatches a response via the motor neuron to the effector muscles that withdraw the foot from the pain. Note the position of the cell body of the sensory neuron outside the spinal cord in a ganglion and the cell body of the motor neuron within the cord. The brain is not involved in processing simple reflexes.

The peripheral nervous system collects and distributes information and is made up of sensory organs, motor (efferent) neurons, and sensory (afferent) neurons.

The motor division is divided into the somatic nervous system, which controls voluntary movements of skeletal muscles and the autonomic nervous system, which regulates smooth and cardiac muscles and organs of the digestive, cardiovascular, urinary, and endocrine system (involuntary actions).

The autonomic nervous system is further divided into the sympathetic and parasympathetic divisions. When there is danger, the sympathetic division is responsible for the "fight or flight response," including responses such as increased heart rate, hormone release, decreased digestion, and dilation of blood vessels to muscles. When no danger is perceived, the parasympathetic division controls responses that conserve energy—the "rest and digest response"—including decreased heart rate and increased digestion.

Endocrine System

The endocrine system is a network of internal communication, regulating the activities of various tissues of the body. Unlike the nervous system, which uses electrical impulses to trigger rapid response, the endocrine system relies on chemical signals called hormones to coordinate longer lasting activities, such as growth, reproduction, tissue repair, and nutrient balance in the blood.

HYPOTHALAMUS AND PITUITARY GLAND

The hypothalamus is a tiny brain region that connects the nervous system to the endocrine system. It receives information from nerves throughout the body and initiates an appropriate response, regulating body temperature, hunger, thirst, sexual desire, and pleasure. The hypothalamus is composed of neurosecretory cells that control the actions of the pituitary gland. The pituitary gland sits just under the hypothalamus and has two parts: the anterior pituitary gland (adenohypophysis) and the posterior pituitary gland (neurohypophysis). In the developing fetus, the anterior pituitary gland comes from tissues of the roof of the mouth. In the adult, various endocrine cells that make up the anterior pituitary gland produce and secrete a wide variety of hormones. The posterior pituitary is an extension of the brain tissue that makes the hypothalamus. It stores and secretes two hormones made by the hypothalamus.

HORMONES

Hormones are the chemical signals used by the endocrine system to regulate the body's activities. They are secreted by endocrine glands directly into the bloodstream and travel through the circulatory system to reach target organs and target cells. There, they bind to appropriate receptors and can cause dramatic changes in the cells' functioning. One hormone can have varied effects on different types of cells, as well as on several processes in one cell.

There are three main classes of hormones in the body: steroid, proteins and peptides, and amino acid derivatives. Steroid hormones, such as estrogen and testosterone, are lipids and can travel easily through cell membranes to bind with receptors inside the cell. Polypeptide and amino acid derivatives cannot traverse the membrane

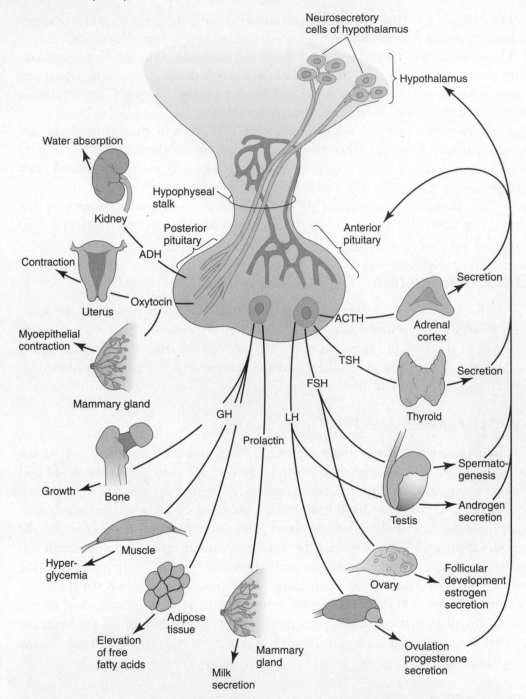

Endocrine glands secrete their hormones directly into the bloodstream. The posterior pituitary secretes ADH, which acts on the kidney, and oxytocin, which acts on the uterus and mammary glands. The anterior pituitary secretes GH, which acts primarily on bones, muscles, and adipose tissue; prolactin, which acts on the mammary gland; LH and FSH, which affect the gonads; TSH, stimulating the thyroid to release thyroxine; and ACTH, which acts on the adrenal cortex.

of their target cells but bind to receptors on the cell surface. Growth hormone is a peptide hormone.

For each hormone that successfully binds to a receptor, a number of second messengers are activated to take action in the target cell. These second messengers, in turn, activate multiple enzymes, which activate more enzymes, and so on, amplifying the effect of the hormone. This phenomenon is called the cascading effect and is one reason why very small amounts of a hormone in the blood can cause dramatic changes in physiology.

The main hormones made by the anterior pituitary are growth hormone (GH), adrenocorticotropic hormone (ACTH), follicle stimulating hormone (FSH), luteinizing hormone (LH), thyroid stimulating hormone (TSH), and prolactin. These hormones are secreted only when signaled by the secretion of thyroid releasing hormone (TRH) from the hypothalamus. Oxytocin and antidiuretic hormone (ADH) are made by the neurosecretory cells of the hypothalamus but are stored and secreted by the posterior pituitary gland.

Other important hormones that are not part of the hypothalamic-pituitary axis include insulin, glucagon, calcitonin, and parathyroid hormone (PTH). Insulin

TIP
Mnemonic
Hormones made and released by the *anterior* pituitary gland:
Follicle stimulating hormone
Luteinizing hormone
Adrenocorticotropic hormone
Thyroid stimulating hormone
Prolactin
I(gnore)
Growth hormone

is released by beta cells of the pancreas when blood sugar levels increase, facilitating the uptake of sugar by body cells and the liver. When blood sugar levels decrease, glucagon released by alpha cells of the pancreas stimulates the liver to break down stored glycogen into glucose that can be used by body cells. Blood sugar regulation is distorted in diabetes. Calcitonin and PTH are released by the parathyroid hormone in response to blood calcium level. If serum calcium is low, PTH stimulates release of calcium from bone as well as calcium reuptake by the kidney. If serum calcium is high, calcitonin stimulates calcium deposition in bones and reduces the amount of calcium reabsorbed by the kidneys.

REGULATION

Feedback loops involving positive and negative feedback regulate the endocrine system. Most responses in the body are regulated by negative feedback; that is, when a certain amount of a hormone builds up, it dampens the stimulus, thereby halting the production of more hormone. In positive feedback, the hormone acts to stimulate the original stimulus to produce even more hormone. Oxytocin is a common example of a hormone regulated by positive feedback.

Reproductive System

The reproductive systems of humans are designed to manufacture male and female germ cells, called gametes, and then provide a way for them to come together to form a zygote during sexual reproduction.

GAMETES

Gametes are germ cells produced by the gonads, with half the number of chromosomes (23) as the rest of the body's cells (46). Male gametes, called sperm, are small and motile; the predecessor cells of sperm, called spermatogonia, develop in the embryo. At puberty, the process of spermatogenesis occurs, creating haploid sperm. Female gametes, called eggs or ova, are large and nonmotile. Oogonia develop and begin the process of oogenesis in the embryo. At puberty, the process is reactivated.

There are three major differences between spermatogenesis and oogenesis. First, spermatogonia, the sperm cell progenitors, continue to divide mitotically throughout a mature adult male's lifetime. This allows for a male to produce up to 600 million sperm on a daily basis. Oogonia only divide mitotically in the embryo. Second, oogenesis has resting periods: meiosis begins in the embryo and is halted until puberty. Spermatogenesis starts at puberty and is a continuous process without major resting periods. Third, in oogenesis, cytokinesis is unequal, giving rise to only one viable gamete. Spermatogenesis involves equal cytokinesis and the production of four sperm. Lastly, in spermatogenesis, the daughter cells of the meiotic cycle are connected via cytoplasmic bridges until the last stage in development.

MALE REPRODUCTIVE SYSTEM

Male gonads, called testes, are composed of tightly wound seminiferous tubules. The specialized Sertoli cells of the seminiferous tubules are the site of spermatogenesis. Dispersed throughout the tubules of the testes are Leydig cells, which produce testosterone and other androgens. Testosterone has many functions, including regulation of sperm production.

The testes are housed outside the abdominal cavity in a skin pouch called the scrotum. The scrotum keeps the testes 2 degrees Celsius cooler than the rest of the body, allowing for healthy sperm production. Spermatogonia undergo two cycles of meiosis. After the first cycle, the germ cells are called primary spermatocytes and are still diploid. A second cycle produces haploid secondary spermatocytes, which continue to mature into spermatids. The spermatids then lose their cytoplasmic bridge connections, gain a flagellum tail, and become individual sperm cells. The sperm cell con-

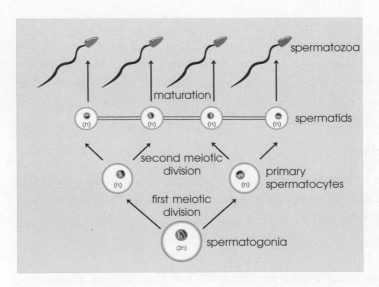

Spermatogenesis

tains many mitochondria, producing ATP to power the movement of the flagellum. The sperm, also called spermatozoa, then travel through the seminiferous tubules into the epididymis where they become motile. From there, they travel through the vas deferens, ejaculatory duct, urethra, and out the tip of the penis. Along the way, secretions from the bulbourethral gland, prostate gland, and seminal vesicles create semen.

> **TIP**
>
> **Mnemonic**
> Passage of sperm through male reproductive tract:
> **S**eminiferous tubules of the testes
> **E**pididymis
> **V**as deferens
> **E**jaculatory duct
> **N**(othing)
>
> **U**rethra
> **P**enis

FEMALE REPRODUCTIVE SYSTEM

Ovaries, the female gonads, are suspended within the abdominal cavity. They are composed of hundreds of thousands of follicles, each housing an egg. Females are born with approximately 400,000 follicles and do not produce any more after birth. From puberty until menopause, one mature follicle will release its egg during each menstrual cycle in a process called ovulation.

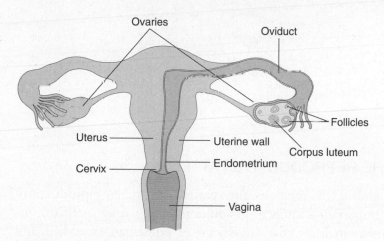

Female Reproductive Tract

Oogenesis begins in the embryo where oogonia in the ovaries begin the first cycle of meiosis, stopping at prophase I. These primary oocytes are reactivated by hormones at puberty. Follicle stimulating hormone encourages development of follicles, induces the completion of the first meiotic cycle, and begins meiosis II. The unequal division of cytoplasm results in one haploid secondary oocyte, which goes on to form an egg, and one polar body, which cannot form a viable gamete. Meiosis is again halted, this time at metaphase II. Each month from puberty until menopause, one follicle will mature and release its secondary oocyte from the ovary into the abdominal cavity in a process called ovulation. The follicle remains in the ovary, growing into the corpus luteum. The secondary oocyte is swept into the fallopian tubes by finger-like extensions and ciliated cells. If the oocyte is not fertilized, the corpus luteum disintegrates, the oocyte continues through the uterus, and menstruation occurs. A new follicle begins developing.

If the ovulated oocyte is successfully penetrated by a sperm, meiosis II is completed, resulting in a fertilized egg, called a zygote, and a second polar body.

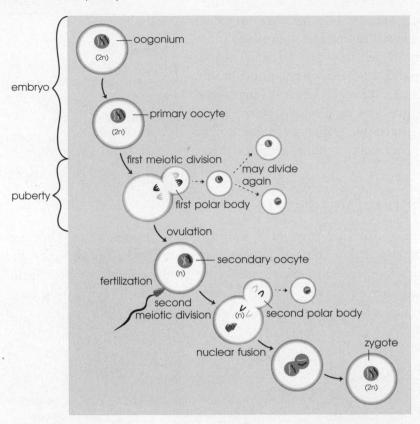

Oogenesis

HORMONES AND THE REPRODUCTIVE PATTERN

Sex hormones called androgens regulate the pattern in male reproduction. Testosterone is the most important androgen. In addition to regulating spermatogenesis, it accounts for secondary male sex characteristics (e.g., pubic hair, facial hair, and muscle growth) and determines certain sexual behaviors, such as sex drive and aggressiveness. Luteinizing hormone (LH) secreted by the anterior pituitary gland stimulates the Leydig cells of the testes to produce testosterone. Follicle stimulating hormone (FSH) acts with testosterone to continuously produce sperm. FSH and LH are gonadotropins, as they regulate functions of the gonads. The same gonadotropins play key roles in the female reproductive pattern, which is a 28-day cycle of egg release that differs greatly from the male's continuous gamete production. Changes in the blood levels of FSH and LH stimulate the ovaries to produce estrogen and progesterone, which in turn cause changes in the uterine wall. This process is called the menstrual cycle.

The menstrual cycle is divided into three main parts: the follicular phase, the luteal phase, and menstruation. At the beginning of the cycle, gonadotropin releasing hormone (GnRH) from the hypothalamus stimulates the anterior pituitary to release FSH and LH. These hormones trigger the growth of a follicle, which begins producing estrogen at low levels. Estrogen causes the endometrium to thicken. As the amount of estrogen rises, a feedback system causes a surge in LH and FSH. A day after the LH surge, ovulation occurs, ending the follicular phase. In the luteal phase,

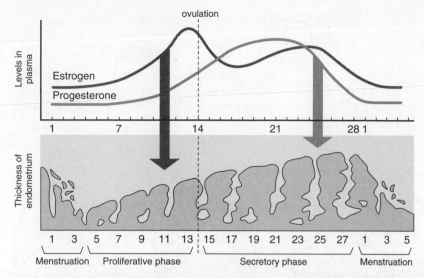

The menstrual cycle. Menstruation proceeds for several days. The follicular stage of the ovarian changes corresponds to the proliferative phase of the endometrium. After ovulation, the luteal phase in the ovary corresponds to the secretory phase of the uterine wall. The effects of estrogen and progesterone on the endometrium are illustrated by the vertical arrows.

LH stimulates the follicle to become the corpus luteum, which produces more estrogen and progesterone. The endometrial arteries enlarge and glands begin secreting nutrients. If the egg is not fertilized, the corpus luteum disintegrates, resulting in a drop in estrogen and progesterone. This causes spasm and rupture of the endometrial arteries, sloughing, and menstruation. The hormonal cycle then stimulates the next follicle to mature.

Conception is the point at which the egg becomes fertilized by a sperm cell. Fertilization occurs in the fallopian tubes, also called oviducts. The fertilized egg, or zygote, travels via the oviduct to the uterus, where it implants on the endometrium and develops into a fetus. The uterus, also called the womb, is a muscular organ with the ability to expand and accommodate the growing embryo and fetus.

DESCRIPTIVE EMBRYOLOGY AND DEVELOPMENTAL MECHANICS

Cleavage

About 24 hours after fertilization, the zygote develops by rapid mitotic cell divisions. The first divisions are called cleavages. In mammals and other animals along the deuterostome evolutionary line, cleavage is indeterminate, meaning that each cell can develop into a separate organism. For instance, indeterminate cleavage results in identical twins. Determinate cleavage occurs in the protostome evolutionary line (insects, crabs, and snails) in which cells specialize early in development. During the first three divisions, the cells continue to become smaller. Approximately the third day after fertilization, the fourth division occurs, creating a 16-cell mulberry-looking morula.

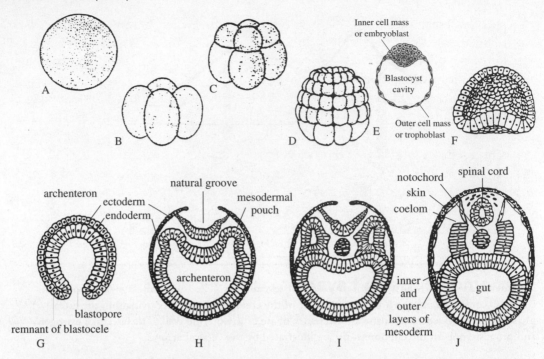

Early embryology of a primitive Chordate, amphioxus. (A) Zygote. (B–D) Early cleavage stages forming a morula (C) and then a blastula (D). (E) Longitudinal section through a blastula, showing the blastocele. (F–G) Longitudinal sections through an early and a late gastrula. Notice that the invagination is at the vegetal pole of the embryo, where the cells are largest. (H–I) Cross sections through an early and a late neurula. Invagination of the dorsal ectoderm is giving rise to the spinal cord, and pouches of the endoderm are giving rise to the mesoderm. (J) A later embryo in which both the spinal cord and the mesoderm are taking their definitive form. Notice that there is a cavity (the coelom) in the mesoderm.

From Morula to Gastrula

As the morula passes from the fallopian tubes into the uterine cavity, fluid penetrates the ball of cells and pushes them to the outer rim, with a small collection of cells at one end of the sphere. The inside of the ball becomes fluid-filled in a process called blastulation. At this stage, the embryo is called a blastula or blastocyst, and the fluid-filled center is called the blastocele. The blastula develops two specialized parts: the inner cell mass, which will later become the embryo, and the trophoblast, which will become the placenta. The embryo now becomes implanted into the uterine wall and continues to undergo mitotic cell divisions.

In a process called gastrulation, the cells of the blastula separate into three distinct layers. The outermost layer, the ectoderm, later becomes the epidermis of the skin, enamel of teeth, lens and cornea of the eyes, hair, nails, epithelial lining of the mouth and rectum, and the nervous system. The middle layer, the mesoderm, develops into the internal organs, the musculoskeletal, circulatory, lymphatic, and excretory systems, skeletal muscle, the lining of the body cavity, reproductive organs, dermis of the skin, and muscular layer of the digestive tract. The innermost layer, the endoderm, forms the lining of the digestive, respiratory, reproductive, and urinary tracts, the pancreas, liver, and thyroid. When the three layers have become apparent, the assemblage is called a gastrula. Gastrulation differs among different embryo types. In amphibians, the ball of cells invaginates like a racquetball being pushed in by a thumb. This creates an inner space, the archenteron, which becomes the digestive tract, and an opening called a blastopore, which becomes the anus. In mammals, the rapid inward migration of cells from the ectoderm forms the endoderm and the mesoderm, from which distinct structures arise.

At the end of gastrulation, the nervous system begins to develop in a process called neurulation. A hollow cord of cells in the mesoderm develops into the notochord, which later becomes part of the spinal column (every vertebrate has a notochord in some stage of development). Ectodermal cells above the notochord fuse to form the neural tube, which gives rise to the brain and spinal cord. Some ectodermal cells break off the neural tube and become neural crest cells. These cells move throughout the body and develop into many parts of the peripheral nervous system, such as sensory neurons and glial cells.

Mnemonic: Germ Layers

Ectoderm	Mesoderm	Endoderm
Sweat glands	**S**keletal system	**P**ancreas
Epidermis of the skin	**M**uscle	**E**pithelial lining of digestive tract
Eye—lens and cornea	**A**drenal cortex	**T**hyroid
Nervous system	**L**ining of the body cavity	
	Lymphatic system	**R**eproductive tract lining
Tooth enamel		**U**rinary tract lining
Hair	**R**eproductive organs	**L**iver
Epithelial lining of mouth/rectum	**E**xcretory system	**E**pithelial lining of respiratory tract
Nails	**D**ermis of the skin	
	Muscular layer of digestive tract	
	Circulatory system	

Development of the Fetus

After eight weeks of growth, the embryo is known as a fetus. In the first few weeks of development, the placenta and the umbilical cord form and become the specialized circulatory system between mother and fetus. This system provides the fetus with nourishment via oxygenated blood in the umbilical vein and removes metabolic wastes through the umbilical arteries. The umbilical cord develops from two embryonic sacs, the yolk sac (the site of early blood vessel development) and the allantois (an outpocketing of the gut that contains many blood vessels). The placenta is formed when part of the chorion fuses to the uterine walls. The chorion is a membrane that surrounds the amnion, which is the strong sac that houses the fetus and contains shock-absorbing fluid called amniotic fluid. In addition to supplying nutrients and removing wastes, the placenta prevents toxins and drugs from entering the fetus and functions as an endocrine gland, producing the essential hormones of pregnancy: progesterone, estrogen, and human chorionic gonadotropin (hCG).

CLASSICAL GENETICS
Genes

The traits passed from parent to offspring are carried by units of information called genes. Genes, studied in the field of genetics, are coded in fragments of DNA found in the chromosomes. Gregor Mendel (1822–1884) described several basic principles of inheritance of genetic information.

THE PRINCIPLE OF SEGREGATION
AND THE PRINCIPLE OF DOMINANCE

There are alternative forms, called alleles, of a single gene. For any inherited trait, an animal possesses an allele from each parent. The principle of segregation states that during meiosis, these alleles segregate from each other, resulting in gametes that carry one allele for each trait. For instance, if a white female cat mates with a black cat, their offspring will have two alleles for coat color, one white and the other black. When reproductive cells mature within the offspring, the alleles will separate, resulting in eggs or sperm that carry either the allele for white hair or the allele for black hair. The principle of dominance states that if the two alleles for a trait are different, one allele will be dominant (fully expressed in the individual) and the other will be recessive (will not show itself). Dominant alleles are written in capital letters; recessive alleles, in lowercase letters.

GENOTYPE VERSUS PHENOTYPE

Modern geneticists have contributed the concepts of the genotype, the genetic makeup of the organism, versus the phenotype, the actual physical characteristic of the organism. In other words, if a woman has brown eyes, that is her phenotype. However, her genotype is not as clear. She may possess either two alleles for brown eyes or a dominant allele for brown eyes and a recessive allele for blue eyes. An organism that possesses two matching copies of the same allele is said to be homozygous for that trait; those with two different alleles are called heterozygous. If a trait is known to be recessive but shows itself in an organism's phenotype, that organism is heterozygous recessive. That is, the organism has two copies of the recessive allele and no copies of the dominant allele. In the case of eye color, if *B* represents brown eye color and *b* represents blue eye color:

Genotype	Phenotype
BB or Bb	Brown eyes
bb	Blue eyes

To determine the genotype of an individual, Mendel devised the test cross, an experiment that mates a recessive homozygous individual with an individual of unknown genotype. Punnett squares like the following examples predict the frequencies of genotypes and phenotypes in the progeny of a cross. A brown-eyed parent of unknown genotype is crossed with a blue-eyed recessive homozygous individual.

Parent: *BB*   *Bb*

	B	*B*
b	*Bb*	*Bb*
b	*Bb*	*Bb*

	B	*b*
b	*Bb*	*bb*
b	*Bb*	*bb*

Offspring: Genotype: 100% *Bb*   Genotype: 50% *Bb*, 50% *bb*
             Phenotype: *Bb* = brown eyes   Phenotype: *Bb* = brown eyes
                                           bb = blue eyes

If all the offspring express the dominant phenotype, their eye color will be brown; the unknown phenotype is homozygous dominant. If the recessive phenotype appears in the offspring, the individual is heterozygous. If two heterozygous individuals are crossed, the Punnett square predicts that 50% of the offspring will be heterozygous (*Bb*), 25% will be homozygous dominant (*BB*), and 25% will be homozygous recessive (*bb*). In this case, the phenotype ratio would be three brown-eyed offspring to every one offspring with blue eyes.

The Punnett square for a cross of two heterozygous individuals is shown below:

Parent: *Bb* × *Bb*

	B	*b*
B	*BB*	*Bb*
b	*Bb*	*bb*

Offspring:

Genotype	Phenotype
25% BB	brown eyes
50% Bb	brown eyes
25% bb	blue eyes

The genotypic ratio of the offspring is 1:2:1 for *BB*:*Bb*:*bb*.

Independent Assortment

Mendel's third basic principle is the law of independent assortment, which states that unlinked traits separate independently of each other during meiosis. For instance, in pea plants, an allele for a wrinkled seed will have no effect on the color of the seed, that is, whether the seed will be green or yellow. With yellow and round seeds dominant, the following Punnett square predicts that a cross between a round, yellow seeded plant (*RRYY*) and a wrinkled, green seeded plant (*rryy*) will yield a 9:3:3:1 ratio in the second generation. This ratio is characteristic of crosses between individuals that are either homozygous recessive or homozygous dominant for two independently assorting traits.

RRYY* × *rryy

First Generation (F$_1$):

100% *RrYy*

RrYy* × *RrYy

Second Generation (F$_2$):

	RY	*Ry*	*rY*	*ry*
RY	*RRYY*	*RRYy*	*RrYY*	*RrYy*
Ry	*RRyY*	*RRyy*	*RyYy*	*Rryy*
rY	*rRYY*	*rRYy*	*rrYY*	*rrYy*
ry	*rRyY*	*rRyy*	*rryY*	*rryy*

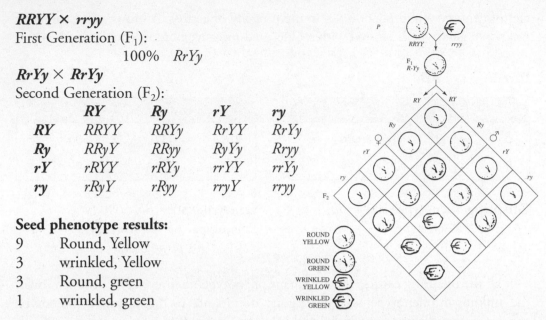

Punnett Square-Pea Dihybrid Cross

Seed phenotype results:

9 Round, Yellow

3 wrinkled, Yellow

3 Round, green

1 wrinkled, green

Degrees of Dominance

Some traits are inherited in a more complicated manner than can be explained by Mendelian genetics. For instance, two alleles do not always determine a trait. Some traits, such as coat color in rabbits, are polymorphic; multiple alleles with varying degrees of dominance determine the resulting coat color. Other traits, determined by an additive effect of two or more *genes,* are called polygenic. Genes that affect more than one phenotypic characteristic arc called pleiotropic.

Also, not all alleles can be categorized as simply dominant or recessive. Incomplete dominance is a situation in which one allele does not completely block the expression of another, and the alleles blend to form the phenotype. Petal color in snapdragon flowers is an example of incomplete dominance. If red (*RR*) and white (*rr*) flowering plants are crossed, the progeny will have pink flowers.

If a heterozygous phenotype expresses both alleles equally, the inheritance is codominant. A standard example of codominance is the inheritance of blood type. Blood types are determined by the alleles I^A, I^B, and i, corresponding to different types of antigens in the blood. An individual who is homozygous for I^A or I^B has an A or B phenotype and type A or B blood. If an individual is heterozygous ($I^A I^B$), however, the alleles are codominant and the phenotype is AB; this individual has type AB blood.

CHROMOSOMAL GENETICS

Chromosomes

Mendelian genetics is based on the behavior of chromosomes, the DNA and protein structures that contain the genetic information of an organism. Diploid (2*n*) species have two sets of chromosomes, one from each parent. Chromosome pairs, also called homologues, have an allele for a trait on each chromosome. Gametes have half the chromosome number and are referred to as haploid (*n*). In humans, the full complement of genetic material includes 22 chromosome pairs, called autosomes, which do not differ between the sexes, and an additional pair of sex chromosomes.

Sex Chromosomes

Sex chromosomes determine the sex of the individual; human males are heterologous, XY, and human females are homologous, XX. Sex chromosomes segregate like autosomes during meiosis, with each gamete receiving either an X or a Y chromosome from their father. The offspring will receive one of the two X chromosomes from the mother. If the sperm that fertilizes the egg has a Y chromosome, then the offspring will be male. If it has an X, the offspring will be female.

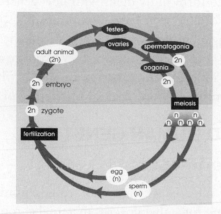

Generalized Animal Life Cycle

ASEXUAL AND SEXUAL REPRODUCTION

Asexual Reproduction

Many unicellular and some multicellular organisms produce new individuals through asexual reproduction. This process results in offspring that are genetically identical to the parent. There are three types of asexual reproduction. In binary fission, which occurs in some single-celled organisms such as bacteria, the genetic material is replicated while the cell elongates. The DNA has been duplicated, and the cell divides in half, producing two identical daughter cells. This process is similar to mitosis, but mitosis involves nuclear disintegration, and guidance of chromosomes by microtubules. In budding, small bud cells are pinched off the parent by cell division (yeast cells). In fragmentation, an organism may break or become fragmented into multiple pieces. Some or all of these fragments may grow into complete adults. A common example is the earthworm. Another example is a plant from which a cut branch can grow into a complete organism with its own root system.

Mutations can give rise to genetic diversity within a rapidly reproducing population of organisms, such as bacteria. Other forms of gene transfer and genetic recombination in prokaryotic organisms include transformation, transduction, and conjugation. In transformation, naked DNA from the environment is taken up by the prokaryotic cell and incorporated into its chromosome. In transduction, bacteriophages (viruses that infect bacteria) carry pieces of DNA from one bacteria to another. Conjugation is sometimes called bacterial sex and involves direct one-way transfer of genetic material from one organism to the other. The donor extends a sex pilus to the recipient, pulling the recipient closer. A cytoplasmic bridge then forms between the two cells. A single strand of DNA from the donor's bacterial chromosome or plasmid is transferred to the recipient. The bridge then breaks and the transferred DNA is taken up by the recipient's bacterial chromosome or plasmid.

Sexual Reproduction

Sexual reproduction combines genetic material from two sources to create offspring. During sexual reproduction, specialized cells, called germ cells, undergo meiotic division and come together to form individuals with new genetic combinations. Unlike mitosis, which produces diploid cells (paired chromosomes, $2N$), meiosis produces haploid gamete cells (single chromosomes, $1N$). When the single chromosomes of the gametes meet during sexual reproduction, they produce a diploid organism with a unique genotype. Even more genetic variation can occur when genes are exchanged between chromosomes during crossing over in prophase I of meiosis.

MOLECULAR AND HUMAN GENETICS

Independent Assortment

During metaphase I of meiosis when homologous chromosomes line up at the metaphase plate, there is no force that governs maternal chromosomes to orient themselves toward one pole and paternal chromosomes toward the other. For each homologous pair, there is a 50% chance that the maternal chromosome will situate itself toward one pole and a 50% chance it will go toward the other pole. Chromosome 1 has no effect on the positioning of the homologous pair of chromosome 7. Without considering crossing over, the number of combinations of a daughter cell formed by meiosis of a parent cell with two homologous pairs of chromosomes is four.

Linkage

If purple flowers usually produce long seeds and red flowers usually produce round seeds, it is reasonable to assume that flower color and seed shape are inherited together. This means that genes for these traits are linked on the same chromosome and will not follow Mendelian laws for independent assortment. Genes that are close to each other on a chromosome are more likely to be inherited together. On the other hand, genes that are farther apart have a higher probability of crossing over and exchange. The rate at which two linked genes become unlinked is called the recombination frequency. By establishing recombination frequencies, it is possible to make genetic maps that show the locations of the various alleles on the chromosome.

SEX-LINKAGE

Sex-linked genes are located on sex chromosomes. The X chromosome is much larger than the Y chromosome and carries the sex-linked genes. Because females have two X chromosomes, the dominant sex-linked allele is expressed and the recessive allele is not. In males, however, any allele on the one X chromosome is expressed. Inheritance

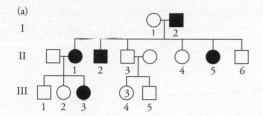

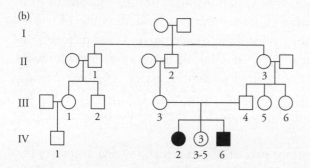

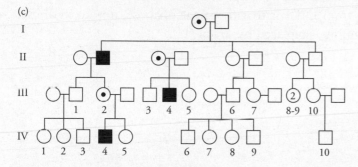

Pedigrees Can Track Patterns of Inheritance
Roman numerals identify generations; the numbers identify individuals within each generation.
(a) Inheritance of an autosomal dominant trait. Individual I-2 is a male heterozygous for the trait;
if he were homozygous, all of the progeny in generation II would show the trait. None of the
affected individuals in generations II or III can be homozygotes, because each has received a normal recessive allele from one parent. (b) Inheritance of an autosomal recessive trait. If the trait were
dominant rather than recessive, then either III-3 or III-4 would have to show the trait in order for
IV-2 and IV-6 to have inherited it. III-3 and III-4 are first cousins—their mating is represented by
the double horizontal line. There is no indication of sex linkage. (c) Inheritance of a sex-linked
recessive trait. The affected individuals II-1, III-4, and IV-4 are all males. The carriers are all
females. This is the pattern of inheritance for hemophilia.

of sex-linked genes is quite complicated. For example, a woman can be heterozygous
for a recessive sex-linked disease, such as hemophilia or color blindness, and act as a
carrier. She is not affected, but half of her sons will suffer from the disease. Also, the
male X chromosome is passed only to the female offspring. Therefore, an affected
male cannot pass on a sex-linked disease to his sons but can pass the gene on to his
daughters. If a daughter is homozygous for a recessive disease, she will be affected; if
she is heterozygous, she will act as a carrier.

   Over several generations, it is possible to track the inheritance of genes by means
of a pedigree. A pedigree depicts the pattern of inheritance of a particular trait in a
family and thus helps geneticists to understand the mechanism of gene transfer. In a
pedigree, a female is represented by a circle and a male by a square. A solid-colored

shape indicates that individual has the disease or trait being tracked. A dot or partially shaded shape indicates that the individual is a carrier but is not affected by the disease. A line through the shape indicates death.

Gene Structure

Genetic information is carried in strands of DNA (deoxyribonucleic acid). DNA is a nucleic acid, made up of the sugar deoxyribose, a phosphate group, and one of four nitrogenous bases: adenine (A), cytosine (C), guanine (G), and thymine (T). The combination of one sugar molecule, one phosphate molecule, and one nitrogenous base makes a nucleotide. The structure of DNA is a double helix, a coiled ladder with a sugar-phosphate backbone and rungs of paired nucleotide bases. The base-pairing rule is that the purines (A, G), pair up with the pyrimidines (T, C): A-T and G-C. Two hydrogen bonds hold adenine and thymine together, while three hydrogen bonds link guanine and cytosine.

Ribonucleic acid (RNA) is an important part of ribosomes and is also necessary for gene transcription and translation. It can be single-stranded or double-stranded. The difference in its composition from DNA is that the sugar is ribose, not deoxyribose, and the nitrogenous base thymine is replaced by uracil (U).

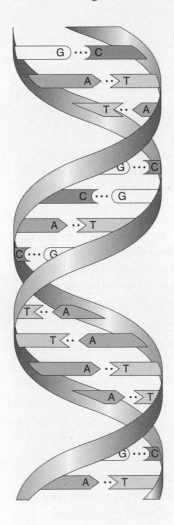

Nucleic Acid Base Structure

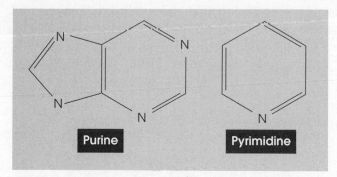

Nucleic Acid Base Structure

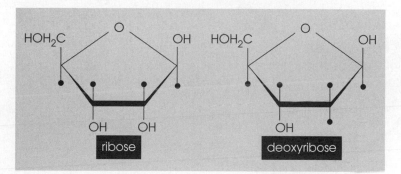

Pentose Sugars

DNA REPLICATION

The fundamental significance of DNA is that it is a replicable blueprint for life that can be passed on to future generations. It carries in it the instructions for a skin cell to become a skin cell, for stomach cells to specialize into stomach cells and then work together with the other organs of the digestive tract. The two strands of a DNA helix are antiparallel to each other; that is, one is in the 5' to 3' direction, and the other is in the 3' to 5' direction. During replication, bases are only added on the 3' end, making the overall direction of replication 5' to 3'. Because the strands are antiparallel, and because only a portion of the DNA is unwound at a time, only one strand will allow for the 5' to 3' directional addition. But both strands of the DNA double helix serve as a template to form a new DNA strand. The leading strand is the replicated DNA that is able to move in the 5' to 3' direction in a continuous fashion. The lagging strand makes short pieces of replicated DNA, called Okazaki fragments, in the 5' to 3' direction, which are then joined together. All living organisms—plants, animals, fungi, bacteria, protists—must replicate their DNA, whether they reproduce asexually or sexually. Please refer to the figure on the next page for a detailed illustration and explanation of the steps involved in DNA replication.

DNA Transcription and Translation

DNA encodes directions for the synthesis of proteins. Proteins, in turn, synthesize the molecules that make up the organism and make the organism function. In a process known as transcription, the portion of the DNA that encodes the specific protein is base-paired with RNA nucleotides creating a complementary strand of RNA called the messenger RNA (mRNA). The strand of DNA that is used as the template is the one that allows the RNA to grow in a 5′ to 3′ direction and is called the sense strand. The strand that is not used as a template for transcription is called the antisense strand. A complementary copy is not a duplicate, but rather a base-pair inverse of the original. For example, if a DNA base-pair sequence is ATGTCC, the RNA complement will be UACAGG.

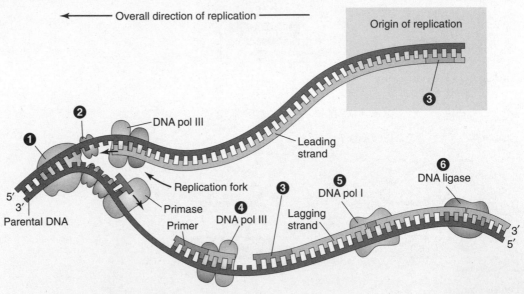

The Steps of DNA Replication

One or many origins of replication are identified. (1) DNA helicase unwinds the two strands of DNA, separating them from each other. (2) Single-strand binding protein helps stabilize the unwound DNA strands. (3) A small piece of RNA acts as a primer, which is necessary to begin the replication process. One primer is used for the entire leading strand. Multiple primers are used for the lagging strand. (4) DNA polymerase III adds nucleotides to the 3′ end of the primer, following the base-pairing rule of nucleotides. If an incorrect base pairing occurs, DNA polymerase III will correct it. (5) DNA polymerase I replaces the RNA primer with DNA nucleotides. (6) DNA ligase joins the Okazaki fragments of the lagging strand, as well as the DNA that replaced the RNA primer in the leading strand. After DNA replication is complete, each new helix is composed of one parent strand and one newly replicated strand.

Transcription has three main phases. Initiation begins when a promoter protein binds to the DNA at the starting point of transcription, unwinding the DNA. Elongation occurs when RNA polymerase adds RNA nucleotides, again following the base-pairing rule. Termination is different in prokaryotes and eukaryotes. In eukaryotes, a specific sequence of nucleotides indicates that the end of transcription is near. RNA polymerase continues to add 10 to 35 more base pairs before cutting the mRNA free. The mRNA then receives a 5′ cap of modified guanine, and a tail of 50 to 250 adenine nucleotides. Exons, the coding portions of the mRNA, are spliced together while the introns, the noncoding portions, are excised. The modified mRNA now exits the nucleus and enters the cytoplasm where the message will be translated into a protein.

The bases on a strand of mRNA code for different amino acids, which assemble to form proteins in a process called translation. Translation involves several steps. Different codons, or combinations of three base pairs, correspond to each of the 20 amino acids commonly used in proteins. GUU, for instance, is the three-letter code for valine, and UGG is the code for tryptophan. The mRNA is now used as a template, and a different kind of RNA, called transfer RNA (tRNA), is responsible

TIP

Mnemonic
Exons **Ex**it the nucleus.

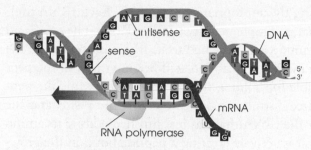

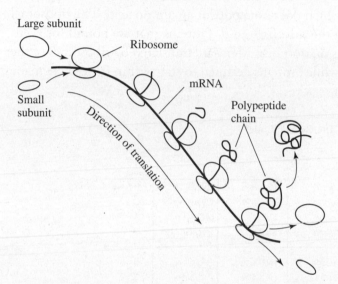

Elongation of mRNA During Transcription

Translation

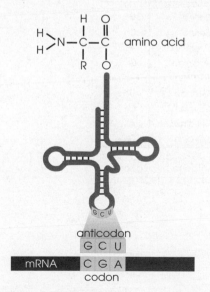

Structure of a tRNA

for decoding the message and adding the appropriate amino acids. Each tRNA molecule has an anticodon sequence that is complementary to the mRNA. The other end of a tRNA molecule has a specific amino acid attached to it. If the anticodon on the tRNA matches the message on the mRNA, the amino acid becomes part of the peptide chain. Ribosomes are responsible for holding the tRNA in place while the peptide bond is taking place. It has three distinct regions: the E site, the P site, and the A site. The E site is the exit site for the tRNA that has just finished adding its amino acid. The P site is for the tRNA that is actively creating a peptide bond in the growing polypeptide chain. The A site is for the tRNA that is bringing the amino acid, to be added after the amino acid from the tRNA in the P site. The ribosome moves along the mRNA strand. Protein synthesis ends when a tRNA reaches a stop codon on the mRNA, such as UGA, which does not code for an amino acid. The ribosomal subunits then disassociate from the mRNA strand. Proteins that are bound for eventual extracellular release, such as neurotransmitters, are translated by ribosomes of the rough endoplasmic reticulum, while proteins destined to stay within the cell are made with the help of free ribosomes.

The Genetic Code*

First Letter	Second Letter				Third Letter
	U	**C**	**A**	**G**	
U	Phenylalanine	Serine	Tyrosine	Cysteine	U
	Phenylalanine	Serine	Tyrosine	Cysteine	C
	Leucine	Serine	STOP	STOP	A
	Leucine	Serine	STOP	Tryptophan	G
C	Leucine	Proline	Histidine	Arginine	U
	Leucine	Proline	Histidine	Arginine	C
	Leucine	Proline	Glutamine	Arginine	A
	Leucine	Proline	Glutamine	Arginine	G
A	Isoleucine	Threonine	Asparagine	Serine	U
	Isoleucine	Threonine	Asparagine	Serine	C
	Isoleucine	Threonine	Lysine	Arginine	A
	Methionine (Start)	Threonine	Lysine	Arginine	G
G	Valine	Alanine	Aspartate	Glycine	U
	Valine	Alanine	Aspartate	Glycine	C
	Valine	Alanine	Glutamate	Glycine	A
	Valine	Alanine	Glutamate	Glycine	G

* The amino acids encoded by mRNA triplets (codons). Although the code depicted above is used by most organisms, subcellular organelles and some ciliate protists show minor variations. The code is also said to be degenerate because more than one triplet may code for a single amino acid.

EVOLUTION

Natural Selection

Evolution is the process by which the genetic makeup of populations changes over time. Charles Darwin's *The Origin of Species,* published in 1859, outlines several key concepts in the study of evolution: fitness, adaptation, and natural selection. Fitness is often confused with the ability of an organism to survive in an environment. However, this is not the criterion; an organism's fitness is determined by the ability to produce viable offspring. A healthy female tiger may be the strongest and fastest in the region, but her fitness is zero if she never mates. On the other hand, a male elephant seal that mates with many females has high fitness. Adaptation is a change over time in the genetic makeup of a population that increases its fitness. An individual with high fitness is more likely to produce more offspring than a less fit individual. Natural selection tends to select for characteristics of an organism that make it better adapted to its environment. For example, in early giraffe populations, natural selection favored individuals with long necks that could reach the leaves of trees. The result over time was a population shift toward individuals with very long necks that were better suited to life in the African savanna. Another example is bacterial resistance to antibiotics. Bacteria that have evolved to resist the effects of an antibiotic will flourish, while those that are susceptible to the effects of the antibiotic will struggle to survive. As new strains of antibiotic-resistant bacteria evolve, pharmaceutical companies must continue developing medications to fight diseases that are no longer curable with traditional antibiotics.

Cladistics

Cladistics is the study of groupings of organisms. An ancestor and all of its descendants are grouped into a clade. Phylogenetics uses similar-appearing diagrams; however, the length of the branch indicates the number of genetic changes that have occurred since a common evolutionary ancestor. Therefore, phylograms give information about evolution, while cladograms give information on groupings of organisms.

Analagous and Homologous Evolution

Over generations of evolution, certain species will come to have similar features. For example, a bird and a bat both have wings. But do they have a common ancestor? No. Evolution of similar structures that occur independently in separate lineages is called analogous, or convergent, evolution. Homologous, or divergent, evolution gives rise to similar structures from a common ancestral structure. For example, human and cat forelimbs arise from a common ancestral forelimb with bones.

POPULATION GENETICS

Hardy-Weinberg Equilibrium

Natural selection acts on individuals, but evolution acts on populations. Genetically speaking, evolution is defined as changes in allele frequencies of a population. The Hardy-Weinberg law is a hypothetical model that examines circumstances that cause evolution. In simple terms, if random sexual selection is the only factor affecting allele frequencies, then no evolution will occur—a situation known as Hardy-Weinberg equilibrium. However, if there are mutations, chance events, or unequal reproductive successes among genotypes in the population, the allele frequencies will not match those for Hardy-Weinberg equilibrium, and evolution will occur. The Hardy-Weinberg equilibrium is represented by the equation $p^2 + 2pq + q^2 = 1$, where p is the frequency of the dominant allele and q is the frequency of the recessive allele in a given population. The following example illustrates this principle with regard to scale color in fish. In this population, the known frequency for the dominant allele is 0.8 and that of the recessive allele is 0.2.

Hardy-Weinberg Equilibrium

$$p^2 + 2pq + q^2 = 1$$
$$A = p = 0.8$$
$$a = q = 0.2$$

Blue scales	$AA = p^2 = 0.8 \times 0.8 = 0.64$	
Blue scales	$Aa = 2pq = 2(0.8 \times 0.2) = 2(0.16) = 0.32$	
White scales	$aa = q^2 = 0.2 \times 0.2 = 0.04$	

$$0.64 + 0.32 + 0.04 = 1$$

This population is in Hardy-Weinberg equilibrium. If no changes occur in this population and mating continues to be random, the next generation of offspring will maintain these allele frequencies.

Mutations or Random Events

Mutations or random events can, by chance, quickly change the genetic makeup of a small population, a concept called genetic drift. If a nonlethal mutation in an individual greatly increases its fitness, that mutation will be passed on to many offspring. After only a few generations, the new gene will become common in the population. Lethal mutations kill the carrier, thereby preventing any chance to pass it on. In the same way, a gene can disappear from a population if a random event kills individuals with a certain genotype.

Reproductive Isolation

An extreme case of genetic drift is the founder effect, where a small number of individuals branch off the main population and colonize a new habitat. As the "colonists" are reproductively isolated from the larger population, the genetic makeup of their population can change drastically. For example, imagine that a country of people with varying eye color sends a group of homozygous brown-eyed colonizers to a distant island. The new island community will have only brown eyes, representing a dramatic shift in the allele frequency for that population.

When a population becomes reproductively isolated, the "colonizing" group becomes the "founder" of a new species. There are several mechanisms that bring about reproductive isolation.

ALLOPATRIC SPECIATION

Allopatric speciation arises from the separation of populations by a geographic barrier, such as a river or a mountain. The barrier prevents gene flow between the populations, and natural selection acts on each population separately. Allopatric speciation, for example, describes the genetic divergence of an animal on an island from the same animal on the mainland (e.g., Darwin's finches of the Galapagos islands).

PARAPATRIC SPECIATION

Parapatric speciation occurs when a small part of a larger population branches off in the absence of geographic speciation, separating itself without the presence of a geographic barrier. This can happen if selective pressures, such as temperature, predation, and food availability on a fringe of a population's range differ from those affecting the large range.

SYMPATRIC SPECIATION

In sympatric speciation, a new species originates within a larger population, usually by a genetic mutation. Sympatric speciation occurs frequently in plants, when chromosomal doubling results in unique genotypes that can reproduce only with each other.

POPULATION AND COMMUNITY ECOLOGY

The interactions between species and within each species in the community are studied in the field of ecology. Ecology seeks to answer such questions as these: Why does a species choose a certain environment to make its habitat? What factors affect the abundance of a species or group of species? What allows these organisms to coexist?

Populations

A population is a group of organisms from the same species that lives in the same niche. Populations are highly dynamic and can increase dramatically in number when times are good, and crash quickly if times are bad. The study of population dynamics is called population ecology. This field, for instance, predicts for fishermen whether a population of fish will decrease or increase on a given coastline.

Carrying capacity (K) is the limit to the number of individuals in a species. The limit is based on the concept that a niche has a finite amount of resources, such as food, water, and space, to support a population. The population, therefore, cannot grow indefinitely. Eventually it will reach the carrying capacity and the numbers of individuals will stabilize.

Different species have different strategies to maximize the growth of their populations. K-selected species are those that produce few offspring, invest heavily in parental care, and thus have offspring with a good chance of surviving to reproductive age. Humans are examples of a K-selected species. On the other hand, an r selected species has a large number of offspring and provides little parental investment, with the result that only a select few offspring survive to reproduce. Flies and most fish are examples of r-selected species. In stable environments, there tend to be more K-selected species, while in variable environments, r-selected species are common.

Communities

Populations of different species are assembled in nature as a community. For instance, different types of coral, fish, mollusks, arthropods, and microscopic species together form the community of a coral reef.

SUCCESSION

Communities are not permanent. In a gradual process called succession, the species composition in an area can change, and one community gives way to another. A barren field, for example, will first be populated by lichen, eventually being replaced by a grassy meadow, and can then become overgrown with trees and become a forest community.

NICHE

The sum of all the resources that a species uses in a community is called its niche. A niche first refers to an organism's habitat, that is, where it physically lives in the community. A niche is also defined by the conditions under which an organism can live, and the way in which an organism utilizes the resources in its environment. Temperature range, moisture level, food preferences, and feeding time are examples of factors that shape an organism's niche. The competitive exclusion principle states that no two species can occupy the same niche in the same place and time. For this reason, organisms are likely to exploit different resources and develop varying niches. For instance, different northeastern warbler species consistently forage in different zones of a tree. One species feeds on the bottom seeds, another on the top, and a third feeds in the middle, thereby avoiding competition for the limited resources in a single zone. It is important to note that all the warblers are physically able to feed on seeds from the entire tree. Therefore, they theoretically could exploit greater resources and have a much larger niche than they actually occupy. The fundamental niche encompasses the habitat and conditions in which a species *can* theoretically exist. However, many factors in nature often limit the fundamental niche to a smaller realized niche, where a species *actually* exists.

Interspecific Interactions Within a Community

Interspecific interactions are a set of relationships that can occur between different species in a community. They can have a positive (+) or negative (−) effect on each of the species involved.

COMPETITION (−/−)

When a specific resource is needed by two different species but is in limited supply, those two species compete for the resource. For example, lions and cheetahs prey on the same animals for food. Competition can lead to competitive exclusion, with local extinction of one of the species or niche differentiation, with one of the species redefining its ecological niche so that it will not be competing anymore. Competition is a negative interaction for both species involved.

If competition occurs within a species, for example male giraffes competing to mate with a female giraffe, it is called intraspecific competition.

PREDATION—PREDATOR-PREY OSCILLATIONS (+/−)

Predation is another major community interaction in which the predator kills and eats the prey. Organisms invest heavily in ways to avoid predation, resulting in such characteristics as camouflage, poisons, and protective coverings. An interesting defense against predators is mimicry. In Batesian mimicry, a harmless species resembles a dangerous species; in Mullerian mimicry, two poisonous snakes look alike. Predators have also developed specialized skills and body structures to help them successfully capture prey.

SYMBIOSIS

A close association between two species in direct contact in a community is called a symbiotic relationship. Parasitism (+/−) is a symbiotic relationship wherein one organism, the parasite, benefits and the other, the host, is harmed. Parasites rarely kill their hosts because they rely on them for nourishment. A helminth is a parasitic worm that can live in the intestines of humans, absorbing its host's nutrients for its own survival.

In mutualism (+/+), both organisms benefit from the interaction. Many corals, for example, benefit from the metabolic products of the single-celled algae called zooxanthellae, which in turn derive essential nutrients from the coral. Commensalism (+/0) is a relationship in which one organism benefits, while the other is neither helped nor harmed. A hermit crab, for example, uses an empty seashell from a deceased gastropod to protect its soft body. The gastropod is already dead and no longer needs its shell.

The tapeworm is a commonly known parasite that lives in the guts of humans, absorbing its host's nutrients. Hummingbirds have a mutualistic relationship with the flowers; they feed on the nectar, and in the process they cross pollinate the plants. Many animals serve as food for other animals. Sea sponges have been found to produce a compound that can support penicillin-resistant bacteria. Some leeches are parasites; others are used for medicinal purposes.

Ecosystems

An ecosystem is comprised of all the living and nonliving parts of a community. This includes the animals, plants, fungi, bacteria, as well as the rocks under which certain insects take shelter, the air, and the water source. Ecosystem ecology studies the flow of energy and nutrients in an ecosystem.

All organisms, at every level of the ecosystem, require energy and nutrients to function. In general, organisms are grouped as either producers or consumers. Primary producers, namely plants, are self-feeding (autotrophs), capturing energy from inorganic nutrients. All other organisms, including animals, fungi, and bacteria, cannot make their own food (heterotrophs) and obtain nutrients by eating producers or other heterotrophs. Primary consumers are herbivores and directly eat the primary producers. Carnivores that eat primary consumers are called secondary consumers, and carnivores that eat secondary consumers are called tertiary consumers.

The flow of food through an ecosystem is described by simplified diagrams called food webs. Each step in a food web is referred to as a trophic level. The 10% rule estimates that only 10% of energy transfers from a lower trophic level to a higher one. Primary producers are the first trophic level, primary consumers (herbivores) are the second, followed by secondary and tertiary consumers. When carnivores (or organisms at any other level) die, the decomposers (mostly fungi and bacteria) occupy the trophic level that returns the energy to the producers. Decomposers are also called detrivores.

Ecosystems have limited amounts of nutrients and water, so they are continuously recycled. Scientists have tracked and identified cycles for phosphorus, potassium, cal-

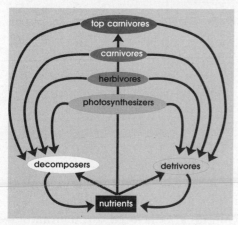

Generalized Food Web

cium, carbon, oxygen, sulfur, nitrogen, and water. All of these cycles have reservoirs of the particular chemical. The reservoirs are organic and inorganic and may contain the nutrient in immediately available forms, or forms that may become usable over time. A simplified example of the carbon and nitrogen cycles are illustrated.

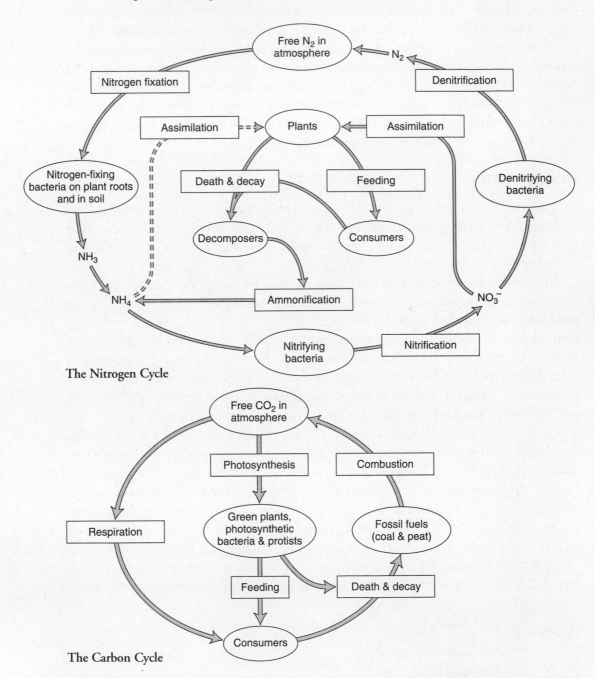

The Nitrogen Cycle

The Carbon Cycle

ANIMAL BEHAVIOR

Ethology

Behavioral science, or ethology, explores the way in which animals respond to their environment. Ethologists ask how and why an animal reacts to a stimulus in a certain way, and why a particular behavior was evolutionarily favored through natural selection. Some behaviors, called fixed action patterns (FAPs) are inherited. They are neither learned nor changeable and are hard-wired into the neural circuitry of the organism. An FAP occurs when a stimulus in the environment consistently triggers a programmed response sequence. A hatchling bird opening its mouth for food, an insect building a nest, and a baby suckling at a mother's breast are all examples of FAPs.

The spectrum of behaviors ranges from fully inherited to having a strong inherited component with some environmental factors, to shared components of inheritance and learning, to behaviors that are fully learned. Innate behaviors have a strong genetic influence. The direction and distance of flight for birds in migration is pre-programmed; however, some environmental cues are also necessary. Imprinting is a type of learning that combines inherited and learned behaviors. It happens during a critical period in an animal's development, when an innate behavior is customized to environmental information. A goose following its mother is displaying an imprinted behavior. If the mother is replaced by a human during the first few hours of life, the goose will follow that person as its "mother" for the rest of its life. Habituation is a simple form of learning in which an animal stops reacting to unimportant stimuli over a period of time. This allows animals to filter the "noise" and pay attention only to stimuli that have significance for them. Imagine moving near a fire station. The noise of the sirens might, at first, alarm you and wake you from your sleep. After the first few nights, your body learns to ignore the sound as an unimportant stimulus, allowing you to rest peacefully.

Associative learning involves the association of one thing in the environment with another thing in the environment. The two types of associative learning are classical and operant conditioning. In classical conditioning, an animal associates a neutral stimulus with another non-neutral stimulus. In Pavlov's defining experiment, he rang a bell, which normally has no salivary response in a dog, and then presented the dog with meat, which normally does cause a salivary response. After repeated rounds of this, the dog began to associate the sound of the bell with the meat, and therefore the sound of the bell alone was sufficient to produce a salivary response. In operant conditioning, an animal associates a behavior with a reward or punishment. For example, if you get sick from eating a certain food, you learn not to eat it anymore because of the negative consequence associated with it. Finally, insight learning takes place when an animal applies previous experience to a new situation; in other words, the animal is "thinking."

Social Behavior and Kin Selection

Social behavior is a vital part of life for many species. There are many complex behaviors associated with societies of animals such as competition for hierarchy, communication, parental investment in offspring, and courtship behavior. Sometimes, an animal will put itself in harm's way in order to benefit the other members of the society. An example is a ground squirrel that gives an alarm call. By giving the call, the individual warns others of danger but puts itself in peril by not immediately running away. This act, called altruistic behavior, is selected for evolutionarily because it increases the fitness of closely related individuals, a concept called kin selection.

GENERAL CHEMISTRY REVIEW OUTLINE (SNS Q41–Q70)

I. OVERVIEW
    A. A Method of Attack
    B. Problem Solving
    C. Scope of Examination
    D. General Concepts

II. ATOMIC AND MOLECULAR STRUCTURES
    A. Basic Concepts
    B. Electron Configuration, Orbital Types, and Quantum Numbers
        1. Lewis Dot Diagrams
        2. Atomic Theory
        3. Quantum Numbers
            a. Principal Quantum Number (n)
            b. Azimuthal Quantum Number (l)
            c. Magnetic Quantum Number (m_l)
            d. Spin Quantum Number (m_s)
        4. Order of Orbital Sequencing
    C. Molecular Geometry and Bond Types
        1. Molecular Geometry
        2. Bond Types
            a. Ionic
            b. Metallic
            c. Covalent
            d. Molecular

III. PERIODIC PROPERTIES
    A. Reading the Periodic Table
    B. Periodic Trends
        1. Atomic Radius
        2. Ionization Energy
        3. Electronegativity
        4. Electron Affinity
        5. Melting and Boiling Points
    C. Group Characteristics

IV. STOICHIOMETRY
    A. Percent of Composition
        1. Mole and Molar Mass
        2. Empirical Formulas
        3. Molecular Formulas

    B. Types of Reactions and Balancing Equations
        1. Types of Reactions
            a. Combination Reactions
            b. Decomposition Reactions
            c. Single-Replacement Reactions
            d. Double-Replacement Reactions
            e. Combustion Reactions
            f. Oxidation-Reduction Reactions (Half-Reactions)
            g. Neutralization Reactions (Hydrolysis Reactions)
        2. Balancing Equations
            a. Steps in Balancing Coefficients
            b. Calculations from Balanced Equations

V. GASES
    A. General Concepts—Standard Temperature and Pressure (STP)
    B. Kinetic Molecular Theory of Gases
    C. Graham's Law of Effusion
    D. Dalton's Law of Partial Pressures
    E. Boyle's Law and Charles's Law
    F. Ideal Gas Law
        1. Density = Grams per Liter
        2. Molar Mass

VI. LIQUIDS AND SOLIDS
    A. Graphical Analysis
        1. Heterogeneous Reactions versus Homogenous Reactions
        2. Energy Changes Accompanying Changes of State
    B. Summary of Characteristics of States of Matter
    C. Phase Diagrams

VII. SOLUTIONS
    A. Basic Definitions
    B. Concentration Calculations
        1. Conventional Concentration Units
        2. Mole Fraction
    C. Types of Problems
        1. Weight/Weight Calculation
        2. Weight/Volume Calculation
        3. Density Problems
        4. Dilution Problems
    D. Colligative Properties
        1. Lowering the Vapor Pressure
        2. Lowering the Freezing Point
        3. Boiling Point Elevation
        4. Osmotic Pressure

XII. CHEMICAL KINETICS
  A. Rate Laws
  B. Reaction Orders
  C. Activation Energy and Enthalpy
  D. Half-Life

XIII. NUCLEAR REACTIONS
  A. Radioactive Decay
  B. Alpha, Beta, and Gamma Decay

OVERVIEW
A Method of Attack

The general chemistry section is the second part of the Survey of the Natural Sciences. Remember that there will be no formal divisions between the three science sections that comprise the Survey of the Natural Sciences. Question 41 will begin the general chemistry section.

The general chemistry section is not only important in its own right. Because you will need a solid foundation in general chemistry to answer many of the organic chemistry questions, your score in organic chemistry will also be affected by your knowledge of general chemistry. For this reason, it would be prudent to place emphasis on the review of general chemistry prior to your review of organic chemistry.

For the biology section you are required to memorize and understand concepts; the general chemistry section requires that you problem-solve as well. This actually works to your advantage. How so?

Problem Solving

With a thorough review of the topics outlined in the scope of examination, you will have seen all of the possible types of questions that can be asked of you. There is virtually no chance that you will be asked to solve a problem that you can't work; understanding the basic concepts will get you far. Armed with the periodic table and a firm grasp of how to solve the common types of problems, you should do well on this section.

This review has been constructed to work through examples step by step, with an explanation of terminology preceding most of the problems presented. Remember that you will be given no formulas on the DAT, and calculators are not permitted. You will have a periodic table that you can display on your screen by clicking on the

"Exhibit" button in the lower right-hand corner. Do not forget that the periodic table is there—you will undoubtedly need it to correctly answer several questions! And, most certainly, do not waste time now trying to memorize parts of the table—that time can be utilized in better ways. Limit your review to the major topics, and master them. You should be able to talk out the steps in solving the problems. The ADA test constructors will most likely switch the given information around and ask you to solve for a variable that you are not used to or will change the problem in some other fashion.

The following is presented as a guide to attacking the problems on the exam. Although you may not need to follow the guide step by step on easier problems, it should help on difficult problems for which you cannot immediately see the path to the answer.

- **Identify the given facts**. What do you know from the question?

- **Identify what you are solving for or what is being asked**. Look at the answer choices.

- **Sketch a diagram or chart**. If you are asked to balance an equation or calculate the number of moles of a compound, a diagram or chart will help you think through the question.

- **Solve the problem**. The three methods for solving a problem given below are listed in order from most desirable to least desirable.

  1. Knowledge-based approach: You have prior knowledge of what is being asked, and the information you possess leads you to the right solution.

  2. Simplification: This involves breaking a complex problem down into simpler tasks. Then you can see more clearly how to solve these tasks individually and then solve the larger problem.

  3. Backward induction: Here, you look at the answers, and then narrow the choices by eliminating the incorrect or unlikely ones. This method uses trial and error to solve for the answers given.

- **Check the logic**. Does your answer make sense?

If you know the material and follow the problem-solving steps given above, regardless of what is asked you should be able to work the problem out. Think of the general chemistry section as a series of problems that can be solved by using knowledge and logic.

Scope of Examination

The area of chemistry encompasses more than any student could be expected to review, so the test constructors at the ADA have narrowed the field to a limited number of testable topics. *The best method of preparation is to achieve a superior level of knowledge of the topics outlined in the scope of the examination.* This review assumes that you have been exposed to the majority of terms and concepts. It is recommended that you refer to a general chemistry textbook to review any areas on which you feel a more thorough review is needed. Checking off the topics as you review them will ensure that you cover all the topics before exam day. The following is the scope of examination as defined by the ADA Department of Testing Services:

- Stoichiometry and General Concepts (percent composition, empirical formulae, balancing equations, moles and molecular formulas, molar mass, density, and calculations from balanced equations)

- Gases (kinetic molecular theory of gases, Dalton's, Boyle's, Charles's, and ideal gas laws)

- Liquids and Solids (intermolecular forces, phase changes, vapor pressure, structures, polarity, and properties)

- Solutions (polarity, properties (colligative, non-colligative), forces, and concentration calculations)

- Acids and Bases (pH, strength, Brönsted-Lowry reactions, and calculations)

- Chemical Equilibria (molecular, acid/base, precipitation, calculations, and Le Chatelier's principle)

- Thermodynamics and Thermochemistry (laws of thermodynamics, Hess's law, spontaneity, enthalpies and entropies, and heat transfer)

- Chemical Kinetics (rate laws, activation energy, and half life)

- Oxidation-Reduction Reactions (balancing equations, determination of oxidation numbers, electrochemical calculations, and electrochemical concepts and terminology)

- Atomic and Molecular Structure (electron configuration, orbital types, Lewis dot diagrams, atomic theory, quantum theory, molecular geometry, bond types, and sub-atomic particles)

- Periodic Properties (representative elements, transition elements, periodic trends, and descriptive chemistry)

- Nuclear Reactions (balancing equations, binding energy, decay processes, particles, and terminology)

- Laboratory (basic techniques, equipment, error analysis, safety, and data analysis)

General Concepts

The following basic concepts are not reviewed in this section because it is assumed that you have knowledge of them. Only a brief mention is given here; refer to a text, if necessary, for further information on these general concepts of chemistry.

- Matter is anything that occupies space and has mass.

- Weight is related to mass and gravitational force, weight can vary, but mass does not. Inertia is resistance to a change in direction.

- Density is mass divided by volume ($D = M/V$).

- Matter exists in three states: solid, liquid, and gas.

- Solids have definite size and shape.

- Liquids have size but not shape.

- Gases have neither shape nor size.

- If a substance consists of just one type of atom, it is an element.

- Combinations of elements in definite groupings are compounds.

- Mixtures can vary in composition.

- Energy exists in many forms and is either kinetic or potential.

- Reactions can be classified as exothermic ($\Delta H < 0$) or endothermic ($\Delta H > 0$), according to the equation $\Delta H = H_{products} - H_{reactants}$.

- Heat is measured by three common temperature scales: Celsius, Fahrenheit, and Kelvin. (See the appendix for formulas and relationships.)

- The International System (Système International, SI) of units is used in chemistry. (Common SI units are listed in the appendix.)

- Exponential notation is used in chemistry. Remember that exponents of 10 are added in multiplication and subtracted in division.

- The factor-label method of conversion is used to convert from one form of dimensional analysis to another. (In this commonly used system, units are crossed out in most chemical calculations.)

- Precision is concerned with the reliability or reproducibility of a measurement.

- Accuracy is concerned with the closeness of a measurement to an accepted value.

- Uncertainty is related to significant figures. (You need to know which digits are significant in a given measurement.)

ATOMIC AND MOLECULAR STRUCTURES

Basic Concepts

The *atom* is the smallest representative particle of an element. The atom is composed of smaller subunits:

- *proton:* a positively charged subatomic particle found in the nucleus

- *neutron:* an electrically neutral subatomic particle found in the nucleus and having approximately the same mass as the proton

- *electron:* a negatively charged subatomic particle found *outside* the nucleus; its mass is $\frac{1}{1836}$ the mass of a proton

Each principal energy level within an atom contains one or more sublevels. (Note that in the older terminology, the terms *shell* and *subshell* were used; the newer terminology has replaced *shell* with *principal energy level* and *subshell* with *sublevel.*)

The *valence principal energy level* refers to the electron population of the outer principal energy level. This number is important because these electrons come into contact with other atoms when forming compounds. In the periodic table the elements in each column have the same number of valence electrons.

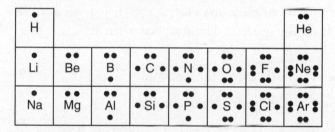

Representation of valence electrons as dots around the atomic symbol.

Electron Configuration, Orbital Types, and Quantum Numbers

The term *electron configuration* refers to the arrangement of electrons in an atom. In the most stable configuration of an atom the electrons are in their lowest possible energy state (ground state). As mentioned before, electrons are located in orbitals outside the nucleus and are in states of rapid motion.

LEWIS DOT DIAGRAMS

A Lewis dot diagram shows an element surrounded by a series of dots, which represent the valence electrons of the element.

Elements normally represented with Lewis electron-dot symbols.

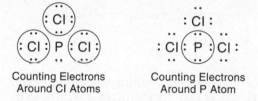

Counting Electrons
Around Cl Atoms

Counting Electrons
Around P Atom

Diagram illustrating how to count electrons around each atom by drawing a circle that includes all nonbonding electrons and all bonding electrons for that atom.

The *octet rule* states that atoms lose, gain, or share electrons until they are surrounded by eight valence electrons. The *noble gases* (except helium) have eight valence electrons and are therefore quite stable.

ATOMIC THEORY

John Dalton (1766–1844) created the atomic theory that explained the *law of conservation of mass*, the *law of definite compositions*, and *the law of multiple proportions*. His postulates were as follows:

• Matter is made up of small particles known as atoms.

- All atoms of a given element are identical.

- A chemical compound is composed of elements that are present in a definite, fixed numerical ratio.

- A compound is formed when atoms of more than one element combine.

- Atoms of different elements have different properties.

- In chemical reactions, atoms merely reshuffle from one combination to another; the atoms themselves do not change.

The *law of constant composition* states that the elemental composition of a pure compound is always the same. The *law of conservation of mass* (law of conservation of matter) states that matter is neither created nor destroyed in chemical reactions. The *law of multiple proportions* states that, when two elements combine to form more than one compound, in each case the masses of the elements that combine are ratios of small whole numbers.

Each atomic orbital has no more than two electrons of opposite spin.

QUANTUM NUMBERS

Principal Quantum Number (n)

The principal quantum number tells us an electron's *energy level*. It is related to the average distance of the electron from the nucleus. The number n can have any positive integer value (1, 2, 3, …). The larger the value of n:

- the farther the distance between the nucleus and the electron,

- the larger the average energy of the levels belonging to the shell,

- the less the difference in energy between adjacent shells: the difference between $n = 5$ and $n = 6$ is less than that between $n = 2$ and $n = 3$.

Note: The maximum number of electrons in energy level n is expressed as $2n^2$.

Azimuthal Quantum Number (l)

The azimuthal quantum number tells us the *angular momentum magnitude*. Each shell is made up of one or more subshells, designated as l. The number of subshells for a shell is equal to the value of n. The value of l may be 0 to $n - 1$.

EXAMPLE
If a shell has three subshells, what are the l values?
If the subshell n is 3, the l values are 0, 1, and 2. We associate letters with l values as follows: 0 = s, 1 = p, 2 = d.

Magnetic Quantum Number (m_l)

This number tells us the *angular momentum orientation*. It is the orientation of an orbital in space. The values for m_l are all integers from -1 to $+1$.

Principal Quantum Number, n (Shell)	Angular Momentum Quantum Number, l (Subshell)	Subshell Label	Magnetic Quantum Number (m_l)	Number of Orbitals in Subshell
1	0	1s	0	1
2	0	2s	0	1
	1	2p	−1, 0, +1	3
3	0	3s	0	1
	1	3p	−1, 0, +1	3
	2	3d	−2, −1, 0, +1, +2	5
4	0	4s	0	1
	1	4p	−1, 0, +1	3
	2	4d	−2, −1, 0, +1, +2	5
	3	4f	−3, −2, −1, 0, +1, +2, +3	7

Spin Quantum Number (m_s)

This number tells us the *electron spin direction*. Its values are $\pm\frac{1}{2}$. The significance of the spin is explained by the Pauli exclusion principle, which states that in a given atom no two electrons can have exactly the same quantum numbers. Each orbital can be filled by only two electrons, and the electrons can spin in only two directions: +spin and −spin.

Element	n	l	m_l	m_s
H	1	0	0	$\pm\frac{1}{2}$
He	2	0	0	$\pm\frac{1}{2}$
Li	2	0	0	$\pm\frac{1}{2}$
Be	2	0	0	$\pm\frac{1}{2}$
B	2	1	−1	$\pm\frac{1}{2}$
C	2	1	0	$\pm\frac{1}{2}$
N	2	1	+1	$\pm\frac{1}{2}$
O	2	1	−1	$\pm\frac{1}{2}$

Element	n	l	m_l	m_s
F	2	1	0	$\pm\frac{1}{2}$
Ne	2	1	+1	$\pm\frac{1}{2}$
Na	3	0	0	$\pm\frac{1}{2}$
Mg	3	0	0	$\pm\frac{1}{2}$
Al	3	1	−1	$\pm\frac{1}{2}$
Si	3	1	0	$\pm\frac{1}{2}$
P	3	1	+1	$\pm\frac{1}{2}$
S	3	1	−1	$\pm\frac{1}{2}$
Cl	3	1	0	$\pm\frac{1}{2}$
Ar	3	1	+1	$\pm\frac{1}{2}$
K	4	0	0	$\pm\frac{1}{2}$
Ca	4	0	0	$\pm\frac{1}{2}$

EXAMPLE

Which of the following quantum numbers are possible, and which are not possible, according to the rules for assigning quantum numbers?

1. $1, 0, 0, \frac{1}{2}$ Possible   **4.** $1, 3, 0, \frac{1}{2}$ Not possible

2. $3, 2, 2, -\frac{1}{2}$ Possible   **5.** $2, 0, 1, -\frac{1}{2}$ Not possible

3. $3, 1, 2, -\frac{1}{2}$ Not possible   **6.** $5, 0, 0, \frac{1}{2}$ Possible

ORDER OF ORBITAL SEQUENCING

Electrons fill sublevels starting with the lowest energy level first, then the next higher energy level, and so on, following the order below:

$$1s\ 2s\ 2p\ 3s\ 3p\ 4s\ 3d\ 4p\ 5s\ 4d\ 5p\ 6s\ 4f\ 5d\ 6p\ 7s\ 5f\ 6d$$

This sequence is much easier to remember if you understand the logic. The following figure illustrates that, if you start at the upper left and read the periodic table as you would text, the filling sequence makes sense. The maximum number of electrons in the *s* sublevel is 2 (one orbital); the *p* sublevel can hold 6 (three orbitals); the *d* holds 10 (five orbitals); and the *f* holds 14 (seven orbitals).

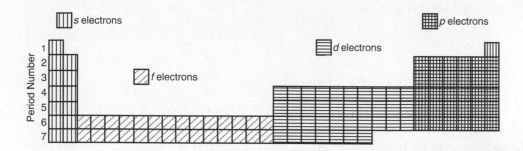

Periodic table divided to show the regions where *s, p, d,* and *f* electrons are the highest energy electrons in each atom.

Often chemists use an abbreviated version to simplify the electronic configuration. Inner electrons are represented by a noble gas, and valence electrons are written in electronic configuration. For example:

$$Fe = 1s^2 2s^2 2p^6 3s^2 3p^6 4s^2 3d^6$$

$$Fe = [Ar]: 4s^2 3d^6$$

When writing an electron configuration, keep *Hund's rule* in mind. This rule states that, for degenerate orbitals, the lowest energy is achieved when the number of electrons with the same spin is maximized. An orbital diagram is used to demonstrate this concept.

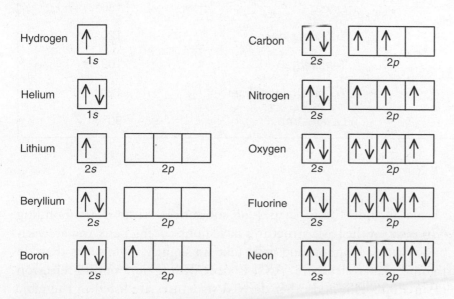

Orbital diagrams for the first 10 elements, showing only the valence electrons.

EXAMPLE

Write the orbital diagrams for hydrogen, helium, and nitrogen.

H has 1 electron in the ground state and is depicted as $\uparrow$ ($1s^1$).

He has 2 electrons with opposite spins and is shown as $\uparrow\downarrow$ ($1s^2$).

N has 7 electrons and is shown as $\underset{1s}{\uparrow\downarrow}$ $\underset{2s}{\uparrow\downarrow}$ $\underset{2p}{\uparrow\ \uparrow\ \uparrow}$ ($1s^2 2s^2 2p^3$).

A very common type of question asks you to write the electron configuration of a given element. An element such as scandium (Sc) would probably be chosen to test your awareness to go from $4s^2$ to $3d^1$. If you understand the sequencing of the periodic table, you will be able to write the electron configuration of any element.

Molecular Geometry and Bond Types

MOLECULAR GEOMETRY

Molecular geometry is the shape of the molecule that can be predicted by using the Lewis dot diagram. The *valence-shell electron-pair repulsion (VSEPR) theory* states that the geometry of the electrons around an atom will be an arrangement such that the electron pairs are as far away from each other as possible.

Notation	Shape	Angle(s)
AX	Linear	180°
AX_2	Linear	180°
AX_3	Trigonal planar	120°
AX_4	Tetrahedral	109.5°
AX_5	Trigonal bipyramidal	120°, 90°
AX_6	Octahedral	90°

The above table includes basic shapes of substances without nonbonding pairs. *Derived structures* of the basic structures have nonbonding pairs and are variations of the basic shapes. Nonbonding pairs take up slightly more space than do atoms. The trigonal planar structure, AX_3, is *bent* with a nonbonding electron pair in place of an atom. This and other derived structures are listed in the table on the following page.

Basic Structure	Derived Structure	Shape	Angle(s)
AX	AE	Single atom	None
AX_2	AXE	Linear diatomic	180°
AX_3	AX_2E	Bent	120°
AX_4	AX_3E	Triangular pyramidal	109.5°
AX_4	AX_2E_2	Bent	109.5°
AX_5	AX_4E	Seesaw	120°, 90°
AX_5	AX_3E_2	T-shaped	90°
AX_5	AX_2E_3	Linear	180°
AX_6	AX_5E	Square pyramidal	90°
AX_6	AX_4E_2	Square planar	90°

Commonly asked questions on the DAT refer to the following shapes:

- Bent (H_2O, SO_2)
- Linear (CO_2, $BeCl_2$)
- Trigonal pyramidal (NH_3)
- Trigonal planar (BF_3, BH_3)
- Tetrahedral (CH_4, CCl_4)

BOND TYPES

A chemical bond results from the concurrent sharing of electrons to two nuclei.

Type of Bond	Characteristics
a. Ionic	Solids *Atoms held together via electrostatic forces called ionic bonds* • transfer of electrons from metals to nonmetals • hard, brittle • high melting points • poor conductors of electricity
b. Metallic	Solids *Metallic bonds (positively charged ions in sea of electrons)* • variable hardness • variable melting points • good conductors of electricity • ductile and malleable with high deformity

Type of Bond	Characteristics
c. Covalent	Solids, Liquids, Gases *covalent bonds* • poor conductors of electricity and heat *polar covalent bonds* • unequal sharing of bonding electron pair • electronegativity difference of 0.4–0.7 • dipole moment *non-polar covalent bonds* • equal sharing of bonding electron pair • same electronegativity • diatomic molecules (H_2, Cl_2, O_2)
d. Molecular	*van der Waals forces (London dispersion) hydrogen bonds* • low melting points • poor conductors of electricity • high boiling points

PERIODIC PROPERTIES

Reading the Periodic Table

In the periodic table the elements are listed by increasing *atomic number,* from 1 to 115. In this example, the *atomic number* is above the symbol, and the atomic mass is below.

11
Na
22.98976

The atomic number indicates the total number of protons, which also equals the total number of electrons in a neutral atom.

The mass number is *number of neutrons + number of protons,* or *atomic number + number of neutrons.* This works out because electrons have practically no mass, and protons and neutrons have masses of about 1. Atomic numbers will always be whole numbers, and mass numbers will have several digits past the decimal point.

Isotopes are atoms with the same number of protons, but different numbers of neutrons. Therefore, isotopes have the same atomic number but different atomic masses. The term *isoelectric* refers to the fact that, when an atom loses or gains an electron, it becomes equivalent, in number of electrons, to the atom corresponding to its new charge.

EXAMPLE

1. Cl^- is isoelectric to Ar.

2. Si^{2-} is isoelectric to S.

The elements are organized in the periodic table in periods (rows) and groups (columns). As mentioned previously, atoms in the same column have the same valence orbitals and are more similar to each other than atoms in the same row. Each row corresponds to the principal quantum number.

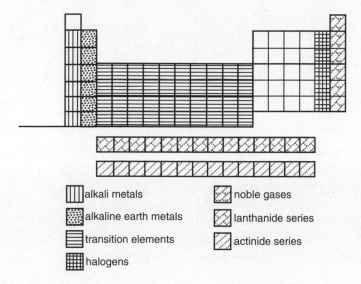

alkali metals

alkaline earth metals

transition elements

halogens

noble gases

lanthanide series

actinide series

Common form of the periodic table, showing groups of related elements.

Periodic Trends

ATOMIC RADIUS

Atomic radii increase on the periodic table as you move down and to the left. Within a group, the radius increases downward because each period has an additional outer principal energy level of electrons and is larger than the preceding principal energy level. The radius decreases as you move to the right of a row because the additional protons in the nucleus create a stronger positive charge that is able to draw electrons to the nucleus. With a stronger nucleus acting on electrons at the same distance, the electrons are drawn closer and a smaller radius results.

As an example, Mg^{2+} has a smaller radius than Mg because of loss of electrons. There is less electron-electron repulsion, and the electrons move closer to the nucleus. *Cations are always smaller* than neutral atoms of the same element, whereas *anions are always larger.*

IONIZATION ENERGY

Ionization energy is the energy that is needed to remove an electron from an atom. Remember that helium has the highest ionization energy; *ionization energy increases on the periodic table as you move up and to the right.*

ELECTRONEGATIVITY

Electronegativity is a measure of the ability of an atom to acquire an additional electron. *Electronegativity increases as you move up and to the right* on the periodic table. Remember that fluorine has the highest electronegativity.

H 2.1																	
Li 1.0	Be 1.5											B 2.0	C 2.5	N 3.1	O 3.5	F 4.0	
Na 1.0	Mg 1.3											Al 1.5	Si 1.8	P 2.1	S 2.4	Cl 2.9	
K 0.8	Ca 1.1	Sc 1.2	Ti 1.3	V 1.5	Cr 1.6	Mn 1.6	Fe 1.7	Co 1.7	Ni 1.8	Cu 1.8	Zn 1.7	Ga 1.8	Ge 2.0	As 2.2	Se 2.5	Br 2.8	
Rb 0.8	Sr 1.0	Y 1.1	Zr 1.2	Nb 1.3	Mo 1.3	Tc 1.4	Ru 1.4	Rh 1.5	Pd 1.4	Ag 1.4	Cd 1.5	In 1.5	Sn 1.7	Sb 1.8	Te 2.0	I 2.5	
Cs 0.7	Ba 0.9	La 1.1	Hf 1.2	Ta 1.4	W 1.4	Re 1.5	Os 1.5	Ir 1.6	Pt 1.5	Au 1.4	Hg 1.5	Tl 1.5	Pb 1.6	Bi 1.7	Po 1.8	At 2.2	
Fr 0.7	Ra 0.9	Ac 1.0															

Periodic table showing the electronegativities of the elements.

ELECTRON AFFINITY

Electron affinity is the energy required to add an electron to an atom. Fluorine has the highest electron affinity. Electron affinity increases on the periodic table as you move up and to the right. This concept is closely related to electronegativity.

MELTING AND BOILING POINTS

Melting and boiling points tend to decrease from the top to the bottom of a group for metals. Nonmetals show an increase from top to bottom.

Group Characteristics

Group IA (Alkali metals)

- Metallic character increases as you go down the group.
- React easily with nonmetals (one electron in outer principal energy level).

Group IIA (Alkaline earth metals)

- Two electrons in outer principal energy level.

Groups IIIB–VIIIA and IB–IIB (Transitional elements)

- Most have metallic character.
- Good electrical conductors.

Transitional elements have unusual characteristics. If you are questioned about a characteristic that is unfamiliar, the element involved is most likely transitional.

Group VIIA (Halogens)

- Seven electrons in outer shell.
- Fluorine has highest electronegativity.

Group 0 (Noble gases)

- Nonreactive because of full outermost principal energy level.
- Have no electronegativity.

STOICHIOMETRY

The term *stoichiometry* refers to the quantitative relationships among compounds in a chemical reaction. Knowing these relationships among reactants and products enables chemists to produce the desired amount of products with just the right amount of reactants. Stoichiometry involves the factor-label (or the "crossing-out-units") method of conversion. It is important to form the habit of writing the units because they are as important as the numbers that are associated with them. Showing units will also help you see what you have been given and what you are looking for in a problem. Be sure to cancel the units as you work out stoichiometry problems.

Percent of Composition

It is important to understand the *law of constant composition.* The elemental composition of a pure compound is always the same. For example:

- ^{12}C has 12.00 atomic mass units per atom.

- 12 amu ^{12}C has 6.02×10^{23} atoms.

  Avogadro's number $= 6.02 \times 10^{23} = 1$ mole.

MOLE AND MOLAR MASS

A *mole* (mol) is the amount of any substance that contains as many units as the number of atoms in 12 grams of ^{12}C. It is the central unit of measurement in chemistry.

The percentage of a given element in a compound is given by the following formula:

$$\text{Percent of element} = \frac{(\text{atoms of element}) (\text{atomic mass})}{\text{formula mass of compound}} \times 100$$

EXAMPLES

1. What percentage of oxygen is present in $KClO_3$?

   $\% \, O = \dfrac{(3) \, (16 \, g)}{122.6 \, g} \times 100 = 39.2\%$

2. Given a 60-gram sample of $KClO_3$, how many grams of oxygen are present?

   $(0.392)(60) = 23.520 \, g$

EMPIRICAL FORMULAS

An *empirical formula* gives the simplest whole-number ratio of elements in a particular compound. You may be asked to find the empirical formula from a given percent composition.

EXAMPLE

The percent composition of a compound is as follows: 12.1% C, 16.2% O, and 71.7% Cl. What is the empirical formula of this compound?

1. Assume that there are 100 g of sample. Therefore, there are 12.1 g of C, 16.2 g of O, and 71.7 g of Cl.

2. Convert grams to moles for each element. Obtain the molar masses (g/mol) of the elements from the periodic table.

$$\text{moles C} = (12.1 \text{ g}) \times (1 \text{ mol C}/12.0 \text{ g}) = 1.01 \text{ mol C}$$

$$\text{moles O} = (16.2 \text{ g}) \times (1 \text{ mol O}/16.0 \text{ g}) = 1.01 \text{ mol O}$$

$$\text{moles Cl} = (71.7 \text{ g}) \times (1 \text{ mol Cl}/35.5 \text{ g}) = 2.02 \text{ mol Cl}$$

3. Divide by the smallest number of moles calculated (1.01 mol O) to get a ratio. The ratio of C:O:Cl is 1:1:2. Therefore, the empirical formula is $COCl_2$.

MOLECULAR FORMULAS

The *molecular formula* gives the actual number of atoms of each element in a particular compound.

You may be asked to find the molecular formula from the empirical formula. The molecular formula of the molecule will be a multiple of the ratio found in determining the empirical formula. In the example above, the empirical formula for $COCl_2$ had the ratio 1:1:2, so the ratio of the molecular formula must be

1	$\times$	1:1:2	=	1:1:2 or $COCl_2$
2	$\times$	1:1:2	=	2:2:4 or $C_2O_2Cl_4$
3	$\times$	1:1:2	=	3:3:6 or $C_3O_3Cl_6$
4	$\times$	1:1:2	=	4:4:8 or $C_4O_4Cl_8$

The molecular mass must be supplied in the question to determine which formula is correct.

EXAMPLE

Given the empirical formula $COCl_2$, what is the molecular formula if the mass of the compound is 294 grams?

The mass of $COCl_2$ is about 99 grams; $\frac{294}{99}$ = approximately 3. Therefore, 3 times the empirical formula gives the molecular formula $C_3O_3Cl_6$.

Types of Reactions and Balancing Equations

TYPES OF REACTIONS

There are often questions on the DAT asking you to identify a given reaction as to type. There are four major types of reactions: combination, decomposition, single-replacement, and double-replacement. Three other common reactions are included here as well. To understand why reactions take place, you need first to understand several basic concepts: *heat of formation, solubility, entropy, enthalpy,* and *limiting reactants.*

Combination Reactions

Combination reactions involve the formation of one product by two or more substrates. These reactions are also called synthesis reactions. If the heat of formation is negative, the reaction proceeds spontaneously and is exothermic. A reaction will occur spontaneously to achieve a lower energy state. With large negative values of heat the reaction proceeds rapidly, whereas with small negative values the reaction proceeds at a barely noticeable rate. In the following reaction, 1 mole of zinc and 1 mole of sulfur combine to form 1 mole of zinc sulfide:

$$Zn + S \rightarrow ZnS \quad (\emptyset H + -48.5 \text{ kcal})$$

Decomposition Reactions

Decomposition reactions involve the formation of two or more products by one substrate. A very high positive value for the heat of formation indicates that a reaction will decompose explosively. Conversely, a very high negative value for the heat of formation indicates that the reaction is highly exothermic and will be difficult to decompose. In the following example, a low negative value for the heat of formation results in the decomposition of 2 moles of mercuric oxide:

$$2HgO \rightarrow 2Hg + O_2 \quad (\emptyset H = -21.7 \text{ kcal/mol})$$

Single-Replacement Reactions

In a single-replacement reaction a single element reacts with a compound to produce a different element and a new compound:

$$2AgNO_3 + Zn \rightarrow 2Ag + Zn(NO_3)_2$$

In this single-replacement reaction the element zinc replaces silver, producing a new single element and a new compound.

Double-Replacement Reactions

Double-replacement reactions involve two compounds. The cations for each compound switch places.

$$MgSO_4 + BaCl_2 \rightarrow MgCl_2 + BaSO_4$$

In this reaction the two cations replaced each other, thus the term *double-replacement reaction.*

Combustion Reactions

Combustion reactions start by combining an organic (carbon-containing) substance with oxygen and then continue to form carbon dioxide and water:

$$C_5H_{12} + 8O_2 \rightarrow 5CO_2 + 6H_2O$$

If the original organic compound contains an element other than carbon, hydrogen, and oxygen, these elements must be in their elemental states in the product.

Oxidation-Reduction Reactions (Half-Reactions)

Oxidation-reduction reactions involve the transfer of electrons by a compound or an ion. If electrons are on the right (product) side, an oxidation reaction has occurred. If the electrons are on the left side, a reduction reaction occurred. These reactions are usually broken down into two half-reactions to help keep track of the electrons.

$$Fe^{2+} \rightarrow Fe^{3+} + e^-$$ oxidation half-reaction
$$I_2 + 2e^- \rightarrow 2I^-$$ reduction half-reaction

As long as the electrons cancel, the half-reactions can be combined to form a complete oxidation-reduction reaction.

$$I_2 + 2Fe^{2+} \rightarrow 2Fe^{3+} + 2I^-$$

> **TIP**
>
> **Remember:** *Subscripts are never changed when balancing equations. Coefficients in front of a compound are changed.* Therefore, the amount, not the identity, of a substance changes. Balancing equations is done largely by trial and error. The process is best accomplished by balancing the most complex molecule first.

Neutralization Reactions (Hydrolysis Reactions)

This is a form of a double-replacement reaction using an acid and a base to form salt and water. It is also referred to as a neutralization reaction because the acid and base are neutralized.

$$HCl + NaOH \rightarrow NaCl + H_2O$$

BALANCING EQUATIONS

Since atoms are neither created nor destroyed in any reaction, equal numbers of atoms of each element must be maintained on both sides of the equation.

Steps in Balancing Coefficients

EXAMPLE

Balance the following equation:

$$C_4H_{10} \text{ (l)} + O_2 \text{ (g)} \rightarrow CO_2 \text{ (g)} + H_2O \text{ (l)}$$

First, balance the carbons:

$$C_4H_{10} + O_2 \rightarrow 4CO_2 + H_2O$$

Next the hydrogens:

$$C_4H_{10} + O_2 \rightarrow 4CO_2 + 5H_2O$$

Then the oxygens:

$$C_4H_{10} + \frac{13}{2} O_2 \rightarrow 4CO_2 + 5H_2O$$

Equations can contain only whole numbers, so multiply everything by 2:

$$2C_4H_{10} + 13O_2 \rightarrow 8CO_2 + 10H_2O$$

Look over the equation to make sure everything checks out. The coefficients indicate the numbers of molecules and the numbers of moles involved in the reaction.

$2C_4H_{10}$	$+$	$13O_2$	$\rightarrow$	$8CO_2$	$+$	$10H_2O$
2 molecules		13 molecules		8 molecules		10 molecules
$2(6.02 \times 10^{23}$ molecules)		$13(6.02 \times 10^{23}$ molecules)		$8(6.02 \times 10^{23}$ moleclues)		$10(6.02 \times 10^{23}$ molecules)
2 mol		13 mol		8 mol		10 mol

Calculations from Balanced Equations

A common type of problem that may be asked requires calculations from your balanced equation. Use the above reaction to solve the following problem:

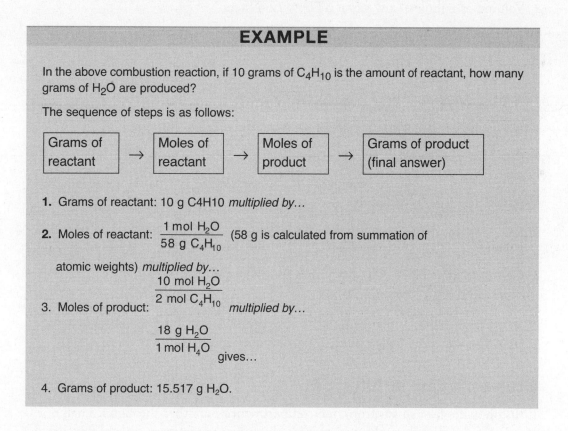

EXAMPLE

In the above combustion reaction, if 10 grams of C_4H_{10} is the amount of reactant, how many grams of H_2O are produced?

The sequence of steps is as follows:

Grams of reactant	$\rightarrow$	Moles of reactant	$\rightarrow$	Moles of product	$\rightarrow$	Grams of product (final answer)

1. Grams of reactant: 10 g C4H10 *multiplied by...*

2. Moles of reactant: $\dfrac{1 \text{ mol } H_2O}{58 \text{ g } C_4H_{10}}$ (58 g is calculated from summation of atomic weights) *multiplied by...*

3. Moles of product: $\dfrac{10 \text{ mol } H_2O}{2 \text{ mol } C_4H_{10}}$ *multiplied by...*

   $\dfrac{18 \text{ g } H_2O}{1 \text{ mol } H_4O}$ gives...

4. Grams of product: 15.517 g H_2O.

Other related problems are *weight/weight problems, weight/volume problems,* and *density problems.* These types of problems involve solute/solution reactions.

GASES

General Concepts—Standard Temperature and Pressure (STP)

When dealing with gases, we consider them to be in a hypothetical "ideal" state. We assume that they have nonexistent intermolecular forces and occupy no volume.

Volumes of gases change extensively with changes in pressure and temperature. Gases as a whole have distinct properties, making them unique from solids and liquids.

- Gases expand to fill their containers (gas volume = volume of container); volumes of solids and liquids are not determined by container.

- Gases are quite compressible under high pressure (pressure = force/area); solids and liquids are not as compressible.

- Gases form homogenous mixtures with each other regardless of their identities; with liquids this is not always the case.

Standard temperature and pressure (STP) of the gas laws:

- Temperature = 0.0°C (273.15 K)

- Pressure = 1 atmosphere

- Volume of 1 mole of any gas at STP = 22.4 liters

All gases show similar physical characteristics and behaviors. To understand the gas laws, it is important to understand the kinetic molecular theory of gases.

Kinetic Molecular Theory of Gases

The *kinetic molecular theory of gases* may be summarized as follows:

- Attractive and repulsive forces between gas molecules are negligible.

- The volume of all the molecules of the gas is negligible compared to the volume in which the gas is contained.

- Collisions between gas molecules are elastic; henceforth there is no gain or loss of energy.

- Gas molecules collide with each other and the walls of their container in a random, continuous motion.

The average kinetic energy of gas particles is proportional to their absolute temperature and is the same for all gases at a given temperature.

Graham's Law of Effusion

Effusion is the flow of gas from one compartment to another through a small opening. Rates of effusion can be compared by keeping the temperature and pressure the same. *Graham's law* states that the rates of effusion are inversely proportional to the square roots of the densities of the gases:

$$\frac{\text{Rate of effusion of gas A}}{\text{Rate of effusion of gas B}} = \sqrt{\frac{\text{Density of B}}{\text{Density of A}}} = \sqrt{\frac{\text{Mm of B}}{\text{Mm of A}}}$$

where Mm is equal to molecular mass.

Lightweight gases effuse and diffuse more rapidly than gases of larger molecular weight.

Dalton's Law of Partial Pressures

Dalton's law states that the total pressure of a mixture of gases is equal to the sum of the individual pressures exerted by all the gases.

$$P_{total} = P_1 + P_2 + P_3 + \cdots$$

This relationship allows us to write the following equation:

$$P_{total} = \frac{RT}{V}(n_1 + n_2 + n_3 + \cdots)$$

where $R = 0.0821$ L-atm/K-mol, $T =$ Kelvin temperature, and $n =$ number of moles.

EXAMPLE

What pressure, in atmospheres, is exerted by a mixture of 3.00 grams of H_2 and 8.00 grams of N_2 at 273 K in a 10.0-liter vessel?

$$n_{H_2} = 3.00 \text{ g } H_2 \times \frac{1 \text{ mol } H_2}{2.02 \text{ g } H_2} = 1.49 \text{ mol } H_2$$

$$n_{H_2} = 8.00 \text{ g } N_2 \times \frac{1 \text{ mol } H_2}{28.0 \text{ g } H_2} = 0.286 \text{ mol } N_2$$

Now that we have the numbers of moles, we can move on.

$$P_{total} = \frac{RT}{V}(n_1 + n_2 + n_3 + \cdots)$$

$$= \frac{(0.0821 \text{ L-atm/K-mol})(273 \text{ K})}{10.0 \text{ L}} \times (1.49 \text{ mol} + 0.286 \text{ mol})$$

$$= 3.98 \text{ atm}$$

Another simplified formula that may come in handy is

$$P_{partial} = P_{total} \times \text{mole fraction}$$

Boyle's Law and Charles's Law

With *Boyle's law,* pressure and volume are inversely proportional to one another and temperature is constant; therefore, ignore the denominator in the combined gas law formula given below. With *Charles's law,* volume and absolute temperature are directly proportional and pressure is constant; therefore, ignore P in the numerator of the formula:

$$\frac{P_1 V_1}{T_1} = \frac{P_2 V_2}{T_2}$$

There are no direct questions on the DAT on the combined gas law; but if you can remember the relationships it states, you will find it easier to memorize Boyle's and Charles's laws.

Ideal Gas Law

The *ideal gas law* combines the principles of Boyle's law, Charles's law, and Avagadro's principle:

$$PV = nRT$$

The ideal gas law assumes that each gas occupies the entire volume of the vessel with its own partial pressure. We can use this relationship to find the density and molar mass of the gas.

DENSITY = GRAMS PER LITER

• Obtain the number of grams from *n*(grams/molecular weight).

• Obtain the number of liters by solving the ideal gas law equation for *V*.

MOLAR MASS

• Divide the weight by the volume.

• Multiply this number (grams/liter) by 22.4 liters/mole.

LIQUIDS AND SOLIDS

Graphical Analysis

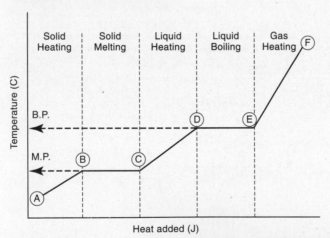

Typical heating curve, bringing a sample from the solid state on the left to the gaseous state on the right.

On the above figure, M.P. = melting point and B.P. = boiling point.

ENERGY CHANGES ACCOMPANYING CHANGES OF STATE

The joule (J) is a unit of thermal energy and is the SI unit for quantity of heat. In past years, calories (1 calorie = 4.184 joules) were also used as measures of thermal energy.

A → B = specific heat (amount of heat needed to raise the temperature of 1 g of substance 1°K) of a solid (J/gm°K)

B → C = heat of fusion (J/gm); melting (reverse is freezing = crystallization)

C → D = specific heat of a liquid (J/gm°K)

D → E = heat of vaporization (J/gm); liquid → gas (reverse is condensation)

E → F = specific heat of a gas (J/gm°K)

Sublimation is the phase change from solid to gas without passing through the liquid phase.

HETEROGENEOUS REACTIONS VERSUS HOMOGENEOUS REACTIONS

Homogeneous reactions occur in one phase (Example: solid only). Heterogeneous reactions occur in two or more phases (Example: solid and liquid).

ENERGY CHANGES ACCOMPANYING CHANGES OF STATE

The calorie (cal) is a unit of thermal energy. One calorie is equal to 4.184 joules (J). The joule is the SI unit for quantity of heat.

EXAMPLE

Calculate the joules necessary to change 5 grams of ice at −10°C (263°K) to steam at 130°C (403°K).

Necessary constants:

Specific heat of ice = 2.108 J/gm°C (or gm°K) ΔH_{fusion} = 355 J/gm

Specific heat of water = 4.184 J/gm°C (or gm°K) $\Delta H_{vaporization}$ = 2260 J/gm

Specific heat of steam = 2.00 J/gm°C (or gm°K)

Approach this problem by breaking down the process into simple steps.

1. Change ice (solid) at −10°C to ice (solid) at 0°C.
   Joules = grams × specific heat × temperature change
      = 5 gm × 2.108 J/gm°C × 10°C
      = 105.4 J

2. Change ice (solid) at 0°C to water (liquid) at 0°C.
   Joules = grams × ΔH_{fusion}
      = 5 gm × 355 J/gm
      = 1775 J

3. Change water (liq) at 0°C to water (liq) at 100°C.
   Joules = grams × specific heat × temperature change
      = 5 gm × 4.184 J/gm°C × 100°C
      = 2092 J

4. Change water (liq) at 100°C to water (gas) at 100°C.
   Joules = grams × $\Delta H_{vaporization}$
      = 5 gm × 2260 J/gm
      = 11300 J

5. Change water (gas) at 100°C to water (gas) at 130°C.
   Joules = grams × specific heat × temperature change
      = 5 gm × 2.00 J/gm°C × 30°C
      = 300 J

Calculate the total joules by adding steps 1 through 5. In this case, 105.4 + 1775 + 2092 + 11300 + 300 = 15572.4 J = 15.5724 kilojoules.

Summary of Characteristics of States of Matter

In the following table, the states of matter are listed in decreasing order according to the four characteristics of density, expandability, diffusibility, and compressibility (e.g., solids are the most dense, whereas gases are the least dense).

Density	Expandability	Diffusibility	Compressibility
1. Solids	Gases	Gases	Gases
2. Liquids	Liquids	Liquids	Liquids
3. Gases	Solids	Solids	Solids

Phase Diagrams

Another popular series of questions on the DAT involves phase diagrams. A phase diagram is a graphical way to show the different states of matter under which equilibrium exists. Defining the areas on the graph has been the route the DAT has taken to test knowledge on this section.

The *critical point* is the point where the vapor pressure curve ends. Beyond this point the gas and liquid phases are indistinguishable. The *triple point* is the point where all three curves intersect. At this point all three phases are in equilibrium.

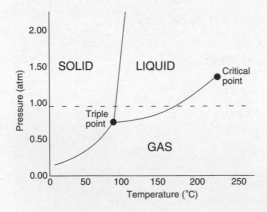

A typical phase diagram of the pressure-temperature regions where gas, liquid, and solid phases exist. Each line represents an equilibrium between two phases, and the triple point indicates the pressure and temperature at which all three phases are in equilibrium.

SOLUTIONS

Basic Definitions

Solute: substance that is dissolved in a solution.

Solvent: dissolving medium of a solution; usually the component present in greater amount.

Electrolyte:	solute that produces ions in solution (conducts electric current).
Non-electrolyte:	substance that does not ionize in water, thereby resulting in a nonconducting solution.
Saturated solution:	solution that has the maximum amount of solute that can be dissolved in the solvent at the particular temperature.
Unsaturated solution:	solution that has more capacity for solute to be dissolved.
Supersaturated solution:	solution containing more solute than a saturated solution.
Solvation:	clustering of solvent molecules around a solute particle.
Hydration:	water is the solvent that clusters around solute.
Miscible:	capable of mixing in all proportions.

Concentration Calculations

1. CONVENTIONAL CONCENTRATION UNITS

- Molarity (M) The number of moles of solute per liter of solution
- Molality (m) The number of moles of solute per kilogram of solvent
- Normality (N) The number of equivalents of solute per liter of solution (1 equivalent of reagent A will react with 1 equivalent of reagent B as in acid-base)

EXAMPLE

What is the normality of 2.5 M H_2SO_4?

2 H ions $\times$ 2.5 M = 5.0 N

MOLE FRACTION

The mole fraction is the ratio of the number of moles of a particular component to the total number of moles in a solution.

EXAMPLE

A solution contains 3.0 moles of water and 2.0 moles of methanol. What is the mole fraction of water?

3.0 mol/(3.0 mol + 2.0 mol) = 0.60

Types of Problems

WEIGHT/WEIGHT CALCULATION

These types of problems deal with the *weight fraction*.

$$\text{Weight fraction} = \frac{\text{grams of component}}{\text{total grams of solution}}$$

Multiplying the answer by 100 gives the *weight percent*.

WEIGHT/VOLUME CALCULATION

To find the weight/volume percent, use the following formula:

$$\text{Weight/volume precent} = \frac{\text{weight of solute (g)}}{\text{volume of solution (mL)}} \times 100$$

DENSITY PROBLEMS

Density, as you know, is equal to mass/volume. This value can be used to help calculate the weight percent. Density acts as a conversion factor to go from milliliters to grams in the denominator.

EXAMPLE

A solution has a molarity of 1.433M of Substance Z. Substance Z has a molecular weight of 42.37. The density of the solution is 1.012 grams per milliliter. Find the weight percent of Substance Z.

Since a molar solution of a solute is defined as a mole of solute per liter, there are 1.433 moles × 42.37 grams/mole = 60.72 grams of Substance Z in 1 liter or 1000 mL of solution. The solution density is 1.012 grams per milliliter, hence the total grams per 1000 mL is 1.012 grams per milliliter × 1000 mL = 1012 grams.

$$\text{Weight percent is equal to } \frac{\text{grams of component}}{\text{total grams of solution}} \times 100 = \frac{60.72 \text{ grams solute}}{1012 \text{ grams solution}} \times 100 = 6\%$$

DILUTION PROBLEMS

If a solution is diluted or concentrated, the number of moles *does not change,* but the volume of solution and the concentration *do change.* The formula is as follows:

$$M_1 \times V_1 = M_2 \times V_2$$

Colligative Properties

The colligative properties of the solvent depend on the *concentration* of solute particles present, not on the kind of solute particles. Typical problems involve vapor pressure lowering, freezing point lowering, boiling point elevation, and osmotic pressure.

LOWERING THE VAPOR PRESSURE

If a solute (A) is added to a pure solvent (B), the vapor pressure above the solvent decreases. The more particles dissolved in a solvent, the lower the vapor pressure. Raoult's law governs this relationship.

$$\Delta \text{ vapor pressure} = (\text{mole fraction}) \times \text{vapor pressure of pure solvent}$$

$$\text{mole fraction} = \frac{\text{moles of solute}}{(\text{moles of solute} + \text{moles of solvent})}$$

LOWERING THE FREEZING POINT

The more particles of solute added to a solution, the greater the reduction of temperature needed to allow the molecules to orient themselves in a crystalline structure.

$$\Delta \text{ freezing point depression} = K_f \times \text{molality}$$

where K_f is a constant for the solvent ($1.86°C/m^{-1}$ for water).

BOILING POINT ELEVATION

Boiling occurs when the vapor pressure is equal to the external pressure on the surface. Since adding solutes lowers the vapor pressure, a higher temperature is needed to raise the vapor pressure and cause the solution to boil.

$$\Delta_{\text{boiling point}} = K_b \times \text{molality}$$

where K_b is a constant depending on solvent.

OSMOTIC PRESSURE

Solvent moves across a semipermeable membrane if the solute concentrations on the two sides of the membrane are not the same (i.e., are either hypotonic or hypertonic), *not* isotonic.

$$\text{Osmotic pressure} = \text{molarity of solution} \times R \times T$$

where R is a constant and T is the temperature in kelvins.

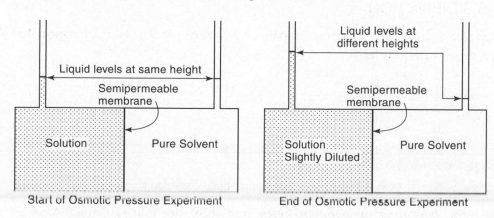

Start of an osmotic pressure experiment with equal pressures acting on both compartments. At the end of the experiment, the pressure developed is the osmotic pressure.

ACIDS AND BASES

Basic Information

An *acidic solution* is an aqueous solution that has a pH less than 7. It contains more H^+ ions than OH^- ions. A *basic solution* is an aqueous solution that has a pH greater than 7. It contains more OH^- ions than H^+ ions. Brönsted-Lowry, Arrhenius, and Lewis have provided different definitions of the same concept. Be sure that you can see that all three describe the same concept.

BRÖNSTED-LOWRY'S DEFINITION

An *acid* is a substance that donates a proton (H^+) to another substance. A *base* is a substance that accepts a proton (H^+) from another substance.

In a solution, when an acid donates a proton, the acid becomes a substance that can now accept a proton. This is the concept behind conjugate acid-base pairs.

$$AH \quad + \quad B \quad \leftrightarrow \quad BH^+ \quad\quad + \quad A$$

acid   base   conjugate acid   conjugate base

A conjugate acid forms when a proton is added to a base. A conjugate base forms when a proton is lost from an acid. The stronger the acid, the weaker the conjugate base; the opposite is true for a strong acid. This concept applies also to bases.

ARRHENIUS'S DEFINITION

An *acid* is a substance that, in the presence of an aqueous solution, donates a H^+ to that solution. A *base* is a substance that, in the presence of an aqueous solution, produces OH^-. The amount of dissociation defines the strength of the acid or base. A substance that dissociates completely is considered to be a strong acid or base (large K_a or K_b), and one that dissociates partially is considered to be weak (small K_a or K_b).

$$AH \xrightarrow{H_2O} A^- + H^+$$

$$K_a = \frac{[A][H]}{[HA]}$$

LEWIS'S DEFINITION

An *acid* is a substance that accepts a pair of electrons. A *base* is a substance that donates a pair of electrons.

```
    F              H                 F  H
    |              |                 |  |
F—B      +    :N—H       →      F—B—N—H
    |              |                 |  |
    F              H                 F  H

Lewis acid     Lewis base      Lewis acid-base compound
```

The term *amphoteric* (*amphiprotic*) refers to a substance that can function as an acid or a base, depending on its environment.

pH and pOH

EXPLANATION OF FORMULAS

pH (potential for Hydrogen) measures the hydrogen ion concentration $[H^+]$. The formula is as follows:

$$pH = -\log [H^+] = \log \frac{1}{[H^+]}$$

pOH measures the hydroxide ion concentration. Here is the formula:

$$pOH = -\log [OH^-] = \log \frac{1}{[OH^-]}$$

The equilibrium-constant expression for the autoionization of water is as follows:

$$K [H_2O] = K_w = [H^+][OH^-] = 1.0 \times 10^{-14}$$

THE pH AND pOH SCALES

pH	1	2	3	4	5	6	**7**	8	9	10	11	12	13	14

Strong acid ←————————— neutral —————————→ Strong base

pOH	14	13	12	11	10	9	8	**7**	6	5	4	3	2	1

CHEMICAL EQUILIBRIUM

Equilibrium Constant

At equilibrium, the rate of the forward reaction equals that of the reverse reaction. Rate will be discussed more fully later, but it is helpful to give this equation here:

$$\text{Rate} = k[A]^x [B]^y$$

We write this equation for both the forward and reverse reactions of a particular reaction at equilibrium. By setting them equal to each other and solving for k, we get the equilibrium constant.

EXAMPLE

What is the equation for the equilibrium constant of the following reaction?

$$2[A] + [B] \longleftrightarrow 3[C] + 2[D]$$

$$\text{Rate (forward)} = k[A]^2 [B]; \text{Rate (reverse)} = k[C]^3 [D]^2$$

$$k_{\text{forward}} [A]^2 [B] = k_{\text{reverse}} [C]^3 [D]^2$$

$$K_{eq} = \frac{[C]^3 [D]^2}{[A]^2 [B]}$$

TIP

Note: Pure solids and liquids are not in the equilibrium constant expression.

To determine the direction of the reaction (i.e., if products or reactants are favored in the given reaction), you must find the value of Q_c, the reaction quotient. This value, Q_c, is found with the same method as k_c. Rather than using the concentrations at equilibrium, Q_c utilizes the experimental set of concentrations.

By comparing Q_c to k_c, we can tell whether the given reaction will favor the formation of products or reactants, or whether the reaction is at equilibrium.

$Q_c = K_{eq}$ The reaction is at equilibrium.

$Q_c > K_{eq}$ The reaction favors the reactants.

$Q_c < K_{eq}$ The reaction favors the products.

$$aA + bB \longleftrightarrow cC + dD$$

$$Q_c = \frac{[C]^c [D]^d}{[A]^a [B]^b}$$

EXAMPLE

$$A + B \longleftrightarrow 2C$$

Given: $K_{eq} = 62$ at 500°C; $[A] = 7.69 \times 10^{-2}$; $[B] = 3.45 \times 10^{-4}$; $[C] = 5.21 \times 10^{-3}$ at 500°C.

Is this equation at equilibrium or will a reaction take place to reach equilibrium? If a reaction takes place to reach equilibrium, will it favor the formation of products or reactants?

1. Write the reaction quotient, Q_c:

$$Q_c = \frac{[C]^2}{[A][B]}$$

2. Substitute concentrations given in the question:

$$Q_c = \frac{(5.21 \times 10^{-3})^2}{(7.69 \times 10^{-2})(3.45 \times 10^{-4})} = 1.02$$

$$Q_c = 1.02 \text{ at } 500°C$$

$$k_{eq} = 62 \text{ at } 500°C$$

$Q_c < k_{eq}$, therefore a reaction will take place in order to reach equilibrium. It will favor the formation of products as it moves in a forward direction.

If a reaction is at equilibrium, any change in stress to the system will cause the reaction to move to the left or right to counterbalance that alteration. In these problems, either the reactants or the products will be favored. The following examples illustrate how changes in concentration, pressure/volume, and temperature will affect a reaction at equilibrium.

CHANGES IN REACTANT/PRODUCT CONCENTRATION

Increasing the concentration of a substance causes the reaction to use that substance, making more of the substances on the other side of the equation. Increasing concentration causes a shift to the other side.

CHANGES IN PRESSURE AND VOLUME

Increasing the pressure of a system at equilibrium will cause a shift to the side that reduces pressure. An increase in volume has the same effect as a decrease in pressure.

EXAMPLE

What will occur with an increase in pressure in the following reaction at equilibrium?

$$N_2 \text{ (g)} + 3H_2 \text{ (g)} \leftrightarrow 2NH_3 \text{ (g)}$$

There are 2 moles of gas on the right side of the equation and 4 moles on the left. An increase in pressure favors the formation of more NH_3. The reaction favors the side with fewer gas molecules.

CHANGES IN TEMPERATURE

We treat heat as a product in an exothermic reaction, and as a reactant in an endothermic reaction.

EXAMPLE

Add heat to the following endothermic reaction:

$$\text{Reactants} \longleftrightarrow \text{products}$$

When heat is added, the reaction will try to normalize by shifting to the right:

$$\text{Reactants} + \text{HEAT} \longleftrightarrow \text{products}$$

Acid/Base Calculations

Some acid/base calculations have already been addressed (pH, K_a, etc.) in other sections. Neutralization, buffers, and titration must be reviewed as well.

The formula for *neutralization* is

$$\text{Volume}_{acid} \times \text{Normality}_{acid} = \text{Volume}_{base} \times \text{Normality}_{base}$$

A *buffer* is a solution that undergoes a limited change in pH upon addition of a small amount of acid or base. *Buffering capacity* refers to the amount of acid or base the buffer can neutralize before the pH begins to change to an appreciable degree.

The *Henderson-Hasselbach equation* is used to estimate the pH of a buffer.

In a weak acid buffer solution:

$$pH = pK_a + \log \frac{[\text{base}]}{[\text{acid}]}$$

Note that when:

$$[\text{base}] = [\text{acid}], pH = pK_a$$

Titration is a method used to determine the pH of an unknown solution. A *standard solution* of known concentration is mixed with the unknown solution. The *equivalence point* is reached when the numbers of equivalents of the standard and unknown solutions are equal in the titration procedure. The *end point* is the point in the titration when the indicator changes color, showing that enough standard solution has been added to terminate the reaction. A *titration curve* is a graph of pH as a function of the volume of standard solution added.

Precipitation

K_{sp}

The *solubility product constant* (K_{sp}) is equal to the product of the molar concentrations of ions in a saturated solution, each raised to a power equal to its coefficient in the balanced equation.

$$\text{Dissolution: } A_x B_y \text{ (s)} \longleftrightarrow x A^{y+} \text{ (aq)} + y B^{x-} \text{ (aq)}$$

$$\text{Solubility product constant, } K_{sp} = [A^{y+}]^x \times [B^{x-}]^y$$

Often a reaction is written out and you are asked to formulate the expression for the K_{sp}; or the solubility data are given, and you are asked to find the K_{sp}.

EXAMPLE

The molar solubility in water of $Pb(IO_3)_2$ is 4.0×10^{-5} mole per liter. What is the value of K_{sp}?

$$Pb(IO_3)_2 \text{ (s)} \longleftrightarrow Pb^{2+} \text{ (aq)} + 2IO_3^- \text{ (aq)}$$

$$K_{sp} = [Pb^{2+}][IO_3^-]^2$$

Upon dissolution:

$$1 \text{ mol } [Pb^{2+}] \rightarrow 4.0 \times 10^{-5} \text{ mol/L}$$

$$2 \text{ mol } [IO_3^-] \rightarrow 4.0 \times 10^{-5} \text{ mol/L} \times 2$$

$$K_{sp} = (4.0 \times 10^{-5})(8.0 \times 10^{-5})^2$$

$$= 2.6 \times 10^{-13}$$

The *ion product* is the product of the concentrations of the dissolved ions, each raised to its stoichiometric coefficient.

Ion product $< K_{sp}$:   Unsaturated   No precipitate will form.

Ion product $= K_{sp}$:   Saturated   No precipitate will form.

Ion product $> K_{sp}$:   Unsaturated   Precipitation occurs.

OXIDATION-REDUCTION REACTIONS

Oxidation and Reduction Definitions

Oxidation is the loss of an electron by a substance. *Reduction* is the gain of an electron by a substance. An easy mnemonic to remember is "*LEO* the lion says *GER*" (lose e^- → oxidation; gain e^- → reduction). These two processes occur simultaneously in oxidation-reduction (redox) reactions, thereby conserving the original number of electrons. An *oxidizing agent* is *reduced* and causes the other atom to be oxidized. A *reducing agent* is *oxidized* and causes the other atom to be reduced.

Determination of Oxidation Numbers

Oxidation numbers are used to keep track of the changes that take place in a redox reaction. The rules for assigning numbers are as follows:

- A free element (Na, H_2, P_4, N_2) has the oxidation number 0.

- The oxidation number of any monatomic ion (an ion of only one atom) is equal to the charge on the ion (Na+ = +1; Al^{3+} = +3).

- The oxidation number of oxygen is -2 except in peroxides, where it is -1 (peroxides = H_2O_2; Na_2O_2).

- The oxidation number of hydrogen is $+1$ except when it occurs after a metal ion, when it is -1.

- The oxidation number of fluorine is -1.

- The oxidation numbers of Group IA elements are $+1$.

- The oxidation numbers of Group IIA elements are $+2$.

- The sum of all the oxidation numbers in a compound is 0, except for polyatomic ions, where the sum is equal to the charge of the ion.

Steps in Balancing Redox Reaction Equations

- Determine what substances are undergoing oxidation and what substances are undergoing reduction.

- Write the half-reaction for each process.

- Balance each half-reaction equation.
  Acidic solution: Use H_2O and H^+.
  Basic solution: Use H_2O and OH^-.

- Balance charges, using electrons.

- Multiply one or both half-reactions by a whole-number factor to get the electrons lost to equal the electrons gained.

- Add the two balanced half-reactions.

EXAMPLE

Balance the following equation, which involves an acidic solution:

$$Cr_2O_7^{2-} \text{ (aq)} + Cl^- \text{ (aq)} \rightarrow Cr^{3+} \text{ (aq)} + Cl_2 \text{ (g)}$$

Steps 1 and 2:

$$Cr_2O_7^{2-} \text{ (aq)} \rightarrow Cr^{3+} \text{ (aq)} \qquad\qquad Cl^- \text{ (aq)} \rightarrow Cl_2 \text{ (g)}$$

Step 3:

Since this is an acidic solution, use H_2O and H^+ to balance the half-reaction equations:

$$14 H^+ \text{ (aq)} + Cr_2O_7^{2-} \text{ (aq)} \rightarrow 2Cr^{3+} \text{ (aq)} + 7 H_2O \text{ (} l \text{)}$$

and

$$2Cl^- \text{ (aq)} \rightarrow Cl_2 \text{ (g)}$$

Step 4:

Equalize the total charge on both sides.

$$6e + 14 H^+ \text{ (aq)} + Cr_2O_7^{2-} \text{ (aq)} \rightarrow 2Cr^{3+} \text{ (aq)} + 7 H_2O \text{ (} l \text{)}$$

and

$$2Cl^- \text{ (aq)} \rightarrow Cl_2 \text{ (g)} + 2e^-$$

Step 5:

Multiply the second half-reaction equation by 3 to equalize the electrons on both sides.

$$6Cl^- \text{ (aq)} \rightarrow 3Cl_2 \text{(g)} + 6e^-$$

Step 6:

Finally, add the two balanced half-reactions.

$$14 H^+ \text{ (aq)} + Cr_2O_7^{2-} \text{ (aq)} + 6 Cl^- \rightarrow 2Cr^{3+} \text{ (aq)} + 7 H_2O \text{ (} l \text{)} + 3Cl_2 \text{ (g)}$$

Electrochemical Concepts and Calculations

ELECTROLYTIC CELL

An electrolytic cell has nonspontaneous reactions that are driven by an outside source of electrical energy (electrolysis). The oxidation-reduction reactions occur in the electrodes. The *positive electrode* (*anode*) is where *oxidation* takes place. The *negative electrode* (*cathode*) is where *reduction* takes place.

An electrolytic cell can be used to decompose molten sodium chloride:

$$2NaCl \text{ (} l \text{)} \rightarrow 2Na \text{ (} l \text{)} + Cl_2 \text{ (g)}$$

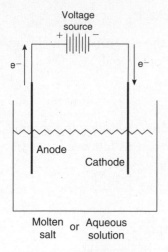

Setup of an electrolytic cell.

FARADAY'S LAW

Faraday's law states that the amount of oxidation-reduction reaction occurring in an electrolytic cell is proportional to the amount of current passing through. It relates the number of electrons to the amount of electric charge. The coulomb (C) is the unit of electric charge.

$$96,485 \text{ C} = 1 \text{ mole electrons} = 1 \text{ faraday (F)}$$

GALVANIC CELL

A galvanic cell produces an electric current as a spontaneous reaction occurring between the electrolytes of the cell, for example, a battery. The two half-cells must be separated from each other but connected by a salt bridge, which allows ions to be exchanged.

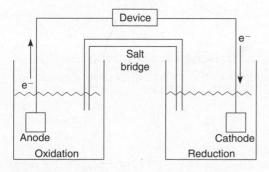

The galvanic cell.

a. Electromotive Force (emf)

Electromotive force (emf) is the driving force that pushes the electrons through the circuit. It is the potential difference between the electrodes of the cell.

b. Standard Electrode Potential (E°)

The value $E°$ is the emf measured under standard conditions, thus allowing a comparison between half-cell reactions. The standard conditions are as follows:

• The temperature is 25°C.

• The concentration of each ion is 1 M.

• The partial pressure of each gas in the reaction is 1 atmosphere.

• Metals are in their pure states.

When $E°$ values are compared, the *higher number is oxidized*, and the *lower number is reduced.*

$$\text{Emf of cell} = E_{\text{oxidation}} + E_{\text{reduction}}$$

> **TIP**
>
> **Note:** The half-cell potential for a reduction reaction is equal in magnitude but opposite in sign to the half-cell potential for an oxidation reaction.

A positive emf value indicates a spontaneous reaction, while a negative one indicates a nonspontaneous reaction.

THERMODYNAMICS AND THERMOCHEMISTRY

Laws of Thermodynamics

FIRST LAW

The total energy of a system and its surroundings is conserved. Energy is neither created nor destroyed.

$$\text{Change in internal energy } (\Delta E) = \text{heat added } (q) + \text{work done on system } (w)$$

SECOND LAW

In any spontaneous process the entropy of the universe increases. Processes that are spontaneous in one direction are not spontaneous in the reverse direction. *Entropy* (S) is a measure of the randomness of a system.

THIRD LAW

The entropy of a pure crystalline substance at absolute zero (0.0 K or −273°C) is zero.

Hess's Law

Hess's law states that, whether a reaction occurs in one step or in a series of steps, the change in enthalpy is an additive property. Change in enthalpy (ΔH) refers to the thermal energy gained or lost when a change takes place under constant pressure.

EXAMPLE

Using the given information, predict the ΔH for the reaction $SO_2 \rightarrow SO_3 + \frac{1}{2}O_2$

$$S + \frac{3}{2}O_2 \quad \rightarrow \quad SO_3 \quad \Delta H = -54.31 \text{ kcal/mol}$$

$$S + O_2 \quad \rightarrow \quad SO_2 \quad \Delta H = -32.92 \text{ kcal/mol}$$

Solve this problem by reversing the second equation. Change the sign of ΔH, and then subtract the terms on each side of the equation to get the final equation.

$$\begin{array}{lll} S + \frac{3}{2}O_2 & \rightarrow \quad SO_3 & \Delta H = -54.31 \text{ kcal/mol} \\ SO_2 & \rightarrow \quad S + O_2 & \Delta H = -32.92 \text{ kcal/mol} \\ \hline SO_2 & \rightarrow \quad SO_3 + \frac{1}{2}O_2 & \Delta H = -21.39 \text{ kcal/mol} \end{array}$$

Spontaneity Prediction

GIBBS FREE ENERGY

Gibbs free energy (G) is a thermodynamic state function that combines enthalpy and entropy. For a change occurring at a constant temperature and pressure, the formula is

$$\Delta G = \Delta H - T\Delta S$$

Entropy (S) is a measure of the randomness of a system. *Enthalpy* (H) is a measure of the amount of heat. If ΔG is negative, the reaction is spontaneous and forward. If ΔG is zero, the reaction is at equilibrium. If ΔG is positive, the reaction is nonspontaneous, but the reverse reaction is spontaneous.

STANDARD FREE-ENERGY CHANGE

The standard free-energy change for a reaction equals the sum of the standard free-energy values per mole of each product, each multiplied by the corresponding coefficient in the balanced equation, minus the corresponding sum for the reactants.

$$\Delta G° = \Sigma n\Delta G°_f(\text{products}) - \Sigma m\Delta G°_f(\text{reactants})$$

EXAMPLE

$$N_2 \text{ (g)} + 3H_2 \text{ (g)} \rightarrow 2\ NH_3 \text{ (g)}$$

For N_2(g): $\Delta G°_f = 0.0$

For H_2(g): $\Delta G°_f = 0.0$

For NH_3(g): $\Delta G°_f = -16.66$ kJ/mol

Set up the equation and plug in the numbers:

$$\Delta G = 2\Delta G°_f(NH_3) - [3\Delta G°_f(H_2) + \Delta G°_f(N_2)]$$

$$\Delta G = -33.32 \text{ kJ}$$

CHEMICAL KINETICS

Rate Laws

The rate of a reaction is the change in concentrations of the reactants divided by the time. The rate law for almost all reactions, $aA + bB \rightarrow cC + dD$, has a rate proportional to $[A]^a [B]^b$.

$$\text{Rate} = k [A]^a [B]^b$$

EXAMPLE

Find the rate law from the given information:

Trial	$[A]_{initial}$ (m)	$[B]_{initial}$ (m)	Initial rate (m/s)
1	0.100	0.100	2.0×10^{-5}
2	0.100	0.200	4.0×10^{-5}
3	0.200	0.200	16.0×10^{-5}

Look for the trials in which the concentrations are the same (i.e., trials 1 and 2). In trial 2, the concentration of B doubles while the concentration of A stays the same, and the rate increases by 2.

$$\text{Trial 1 rate:} \quad k [A]^x [B]^y = k(1.00)^x (1.00)^y$$

$$\text{Trial 2 rate:} \quad k (1.00)^x (2.00)^y$$

Now, divide rate 2 by rate 1:

$$\frac{\text{Rate 2}}{\text{Rate 1}} \quad \frac{4.0 \times 10^{-5}}{2.0 \times 10^{-5}} = \frac{\cancel{k}\,\cancel{(1.00)^x}(2.00)^y}{\cancel{k}\,\cancel{(1.00)^x}(1.00)^y} = (2.00)^y$$

$$2 = (2.00)^y$$
$$y = 1$$

Make the same comparison between trials 2 and 3, and find $x = 2$.

The overall *reaction order* is the sum of the two orders ($2 + 2 = 4$).

To find the rate law, solve for k using the data from any of the trials and the values for x and y:

$$\text{Rate} = k [A]^x [B]^y \rightarrow k = \frac{\text{rate}}{[A]^x [B]^y}$$

$$k = \frac{2.0 \times 10^{-5} \text{ M/s}}{(1)^2 (1)^2}$$

$$\text{Rate law} = 2.0 \times 10^{-5} \text{ M}^{-2} \text{ s}^{-1} [A]^2 [B]^2$$

Reaction Orders

- *Zero-order reactions* have a constant rate, and they occur independently of the concentrations of the reactants.

- *First-order reactions* have a rate $\propto [A]^x$, where $x = 1$. The rate is therefore proportional to the concentration of one reactant.

- *Second-order reactions* have a rate $\propto [A]^1[B]^1$, or a rate $\propto [A]^2$.

Chemical reactions are usually accelerated by

- increasing the concentrations of reactants,

- increasing the temperature of reaction,

- increasing the surface area of reaction,

- the presence of a catalyst.

A *homogenous catalyst* is a catalyst that is in the same state as the reactants. A *heterogeneous catalyst* is in a different phase than the reactants.

> **TIP**
>
> **Note:** Third-order and higher order reactions are also feasible, as well as mixed-order reactions (fractional order).

Activation Energy and Enthalpy

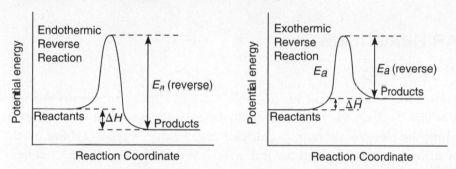

Reaction profiles illustrating the activation energy of reverse reactions and the fact that ΔH of the reverse reaction is opposite in sign to ΔH of the forward reaction.

In this reaction profile, E_a is the activation energy of the reaction. It is the difference in potential energy between the activated complex and the reactants and represents the energy of collision necessary to drive this reaction. The activation energy can be reduced by the addition of a catalyst. The catalyst works by increasing the frequency of collisions in the forward reaction (E_a) and similarly in the reverse reaction ($E_{a\ reverse}$). $E_{a\ reverse}$, the activation energy of the reverse reaction, is the difference between the potential energy of the transition state and the products.

ΔH represents the change in enthalpy. Enthalpy is equal to the potential energy of the products minus the potential energy of the reactants. If this number is negative, the reaction is exothermic (heat is released). If this number is positive, the reaction is endothermic (heat is absorbed).

The *transition state* (activated complex) is the arrangement of reactant and product molecules at the point of maximum energy in the rate-determining step of a reaction.

Collision theory states that reactant molecules must possess the correct orientation and enough energy to combine and form an activated complex.

Half-Life

The half-life ($t_{1/2}$) is the length of time required for the concentration of a reactant to decrease to one-half of the original amount.

For a first-order reaction:

$$t_{1/2} = \frac{0.693}{k}$$

For a second-order reaction:

$$t_{1/2} = \frac{1}{k\,[X]}$$

In these formulas, k = rate constant of reaction and X = initial concentration.

Here is an example of the most common type of question asked in this category: Given x grams, use the equation

$$\frac{x}{2^n} = \text{remaining amount}$$

where n = number of half-lives and x = number of grams.

This equation gives the final product remaining.

NUCLEAR REACTIONS

Radioactive Decay

Radioactivity occurs as a result of an unstable nucleus that spontaneously emits energy and/or small subatomic particles. Radioactive isotopes emit subatomic particles including the electron (beta particle), neutron, helium nucleus (alpha particle), and positron. As a result, the nuclear mass and/or nuclear charge changes, forming a radioisotope.

In the past, the questions for this section have taken one of two forms. You may be required to fill in the missing element, or simply identify the type of radioactive decay.

Alpha, Beta, and Gamma Decay

Type of Decay	Charge	Radiation	Penetrating Power
Alpha	+2	4_2He	1
Beta	−1	Electrons	100
Gamma	0	High-energy photons	1,000

Alpha decay is a form of radioactivity that involves the emission of helium nuclei, termed alpha (α) particles, $^4_2$He:

$$^{222}_{86}\text{Rn} \quad \rightarrow \quad ^{218}_{84}\text{Po} \quad + \quad ^4_2\text{He}$$

or

$$^{222}_{86}\text{Rn} \quad \rightarrow \quad ^{218}_{84}\text{Po} \quad + \quad \alpha$$

Beta decay involves the emission of electrons. Beta particles (β) have no mass and have a charge of -1, indicated as $_{-1}^{0}e$.

$$_{6}^{14}C \quad \rightarrow \quad _{7}^{14}N \quad + \quad _{-1}^{0}e$$

or

$$_{6}^{14}C \quad \rightarrow \quad _{7}^{14}N \quad + \quad \beta$$

Neutrons are emitted in nuclear reactions ($_{0}^{1}n$):

$$_{49}^{21}Sc \quad \rightarrow \quad _{50}^{20}Ca \quad + \quad _{0}^{1}n \quad + \quad _{-1}^{0}e$$

Positrons are the positive equivalents of beta particles. Positrons have no mass and a $+1$ charge.

$$_{6}^{11}C \quad \rightarrow \quad _{5}^{11}B \quad + \quad _{+1}^{0}\beta$$

Reactions involving positrons may also involve *electron capture,* a process whereby an electron combines with a proton to form a neutron:

$$_{6}^{11}C \quad + \quad _{-1}^{0}\beta \quad \rightarrow \quad _{5}^{11}B$$

Gamma rays are emitted when decay occurs, leaving the nucleus with excess energy. The loss of this excess energy is called gamma radiation. No change of charge or mass occurs with gamma radiation. *X rays* are similar to gamma rays; neither is incorporated into written equations, nor does either change the identity of the isotope.

ORGANIC CHEMISTRY REVIEW OUTLINE (SNS Q71-100)

I.   OVERVIEW
    A. A Method of Attack
    B. The Visual Thought Process
    C. Organic Models
    D. Scope of Examination
    E. General Concepts

II.   BONDING
    A. Three Types of Bonds
        1. Ionic
        2. Covalent
        3. Hydrogen
    B. Orbitals
        1. Atomic Orbitals
        2. Molecular Orbitals
            a. Sigma Bond
            b. Pi Bond
        3. Hybrid Orbitals
            a. sp^3
            b. sp^2
            c. sp
    C. Bond Rotation and Energy; Newman Projections
        1. Rotation and Energy
        2. Newman Projections
            a. Ethane
            b. Butane
        3. Energy Diagrams
    D. Other Related Concepts
        1. Ring Strain
        2. Cyclohexane
        3. Bond Cleavage

III.   NOMENCLATURE
    A. IUPAC Rules
    B. General Molecular Formulas
        1. Alkanes
            a. Alkyl Substituents
            b. Rings

    B. Alkanes, Alkenes, and Alkynes
        1. Alkanes
        2. Alkenes and Alkynes
    C. Alcohols, Ethers, and the Carbonyl Compounds
        1. Alcohols
        2. Ethers
        3. Aldehydes
        4. Ketones
        5. Carboxylic Acids
    D. Carbohydrates, Lipids, and Amines
        1. Carbohydrates
        2. Lipids
        3. Amines
    E. Optically Active Stereoisomers

VII. ACID-BASE CHEMISTRY
    A. General Information
        1. Relevance to Understanding Reactions
        2. Review of Definitions
            a. Brönsted-Lowry Acid and Base
            b. Lewis Acid and Base
        3. Strength and Stability of Acids and Bases
    B. Resonance
        1. Terms and Concepts
        2. Rules for Drawing Resonance Forms
        3. Effects of Resonance on Acidity
    C. Inductive Effects and Electronegativity

VIII. MECHANISMS AND REACTIONS OF THE MAJOR FUNCTIONAL GROUPS
    A. General Information
        1. A Brief Review
        2. Structure and Stability of Radicals
    B. Alkane Reactions
        1. Free-Radical Halogenation of Alkanes
        2. Nucleophilic Substitution and Elimination
             a. The Basics
            b. S_N1
            c. S_N2
            d. $E1$
            e. $E2$
    C. Alkene and Alkyne Reactions
        1. Markovnikov's Rule—HX Addition
        2. Anti-Markovnikov Reactions—Radical Halogenation

    E. Carboxylic Acids, Esters, and Ethers
        1. Carboxylic Acids
           a. Oxidation of Alkenes
           b. Grignard Reagent with Carbon Dioxide
           c. Oxidation of 1° Alcohols
           d. Saponification of Esters
        2. Esters—Acid and Alcohol
        3. Ethers
           a. Williamson Ether Synthesis
           b. Dehydration

X.   ORGANIC ANALYSIS
    A. General Concepts
    B. Some Simple Chemical Tests
    C. Infrared (IR) Spectroscopy
        1. Concept of Oscillation Frequencies
        2. Common IR Spectrums
    D. Nuclear Magnetic Resonance (NMR) Spectroscopy
        1. NMR and the Concept of Chemical Shift Values
        2. Spin-Spin Splitting
        3. Shielding and Deshielding
        4. Chemical Shift Values

OVERVIEW

A Method of Attack

The organic chemistry section is the third and last part of the Survey of the Natural Sciences. There will be only 30 questions on which to demonstrate your knowledge of organic chemistry. Students should realize that the American Dental Association does not expect dental school applicants to have a full mastery of the subject matter. Thankfully, the ADA realizes that practicing dentists do not need a Ph.D. in organic chemistry. However, *a solid foundation in the major concepts is expected. The goal of this review is to thoroughly cover the concepts that are outlined in the ADA's scope of examination.*

The approach you choose for your review of organic chemistry is important. This review should be different from your reviews of both biology and general chemistry. The biology review called for extensive memorization, and the general chemistry review emphasized analytic problem solving skills. *The organic chemistry review demands both.* The best method of studying organic chemistry is to *visualize* and *conceptualize* the interactions of the molecules involved and to understand why certain reactions occur. Too many students attempt to learn organic chemistry through memorization alone. Finding similarities and trends among reactions is much more useful than memorizing individual reactions. Taking the time to think through the concepts presented is vital to a successful outcome on the actual exam. Each topic included in the ADA scope of exam can be tested through an infinite number of questions, and the student who can apply general principles to a wide range of problems will be the most successful.

The Visual Thought Process

It has been stressed that the best method of preparation is to fully visualize the topic discussed. But how do you implement this method into your review for the DAT? The following example may be helpful. In the review of the chemical and physical properties of alkanes, the following statement is made: "Alkanes are *nonpolar hydrocarbons that are insoluble in water.*" You should visualize hydrogens bound to sp^3 hybridized carbons in the tetrahedral configuration and should realize that, because of the symmetry, no dipole is created. This explains why alkanes are *nonpolar hydrocarbons.* In addition, the structure of water should come to mind. You will recall that the H_2O molecule is in a bent formation with two lone pairs of electrons, creating a dipole. By realizing that polar and nonpolar molecules are not soluble with one another, you can see that the claim that alkanes are *insoluble in water* can be justified.

The visual thought process also identifies what information is known and what is not. For example, if you, the diligent student, were able to visualize the hydrocarbon configuration but could not link it to the solubility in water, you would refer to Section VI.A.2 on solubility and then make the link between polarity and solubility. It takes time to adopt this thought process, which is slow and tedious, but we believe that *it is the most efficient and effective method of learning organic chemistry.*

Organic Models

Model sets are an excellent aid in this visual type of learning. Since, however, model sets are not allowed in the actual exam, *they should only be used initially to understand the concepts presented.* The organic chemistry section intentionally tests the student's ability to visualize in three dimensions. The only way to improve this ability is through practice.

Scope of Examination

It is important to keep in mind that the goal of your review of organic chemistry is to score well on this section of the DAT. *Mastering the fundamental concepts outlined in the scope of examination is the best method of preparation for the DAT.* Following is the scope of examination, as defined by the ADA Department of Testing Services:

- Mechanisms Energetics, Structure, and Stability of Intermediates (S_N1, S_N2 elimination, addition, free radical, and substitution mechanisms)

- Chemical and Physical Properties of Molecules and Organic Analysis (inter- and intra-molecular forces, separation, introductory infrared spectroscopy, ^{1}HNMR spectroscopy, ^{13}CNMR, chemical identification, stability, solubility, and polarity)

- Stereochemistry (conformational analysis, geometric isomers, stereoisomers (enantiomers, diastereomers, meso compounds), optical activity (planes of symmetry))

- Nomenclature (IUPAC rules and functional groups in molecules)

- Individual Reactions of the Major Functional Groups and Combinations of Reactions to Synthesize Compounds (carbon-to-carbon bond formation, functional groups conversions, multistep synthesis, redox reactions, name reactions, Grignard, Wittig, Diels-Alder, Aldol reaction)

- Acid-Base Chemistry (resonance effects, inductive effects, and prediction of products and equilibria)

- Aromatics and Bonding (concept of aromaticity, resonance, atomic/molecular orbitals, hybridization, bond angles/lengths)

A one-year introductory course covering the major concepts of organic chemistry is required by most dental schools. This review assumes that you have been exposed to the majority of terms and concepts. It is recommended that you refer to an organic chemistry textbook to review areas for which you feel additional study is needed.

Check off each topic on the outline as you review the material. Doing so will ensure that, by the end of your review, you have covered all the topics outlined in the ADA's scope of examination.

General Concepts

Organic chemistry assumes a fundamental knowledge of general chemistry. *Review general chemistry before beginning this section.* Organic chemistry is the study of carbon-containing molecules. *Electrophiles* are electron loving (are themselves electron deficient), and *nucleophiles* are nucleus loving (are themselves electron rich). Bonds form between the two. Nature prefers lower states of energy, which are more stable. High-energy bonds are more reactive and less stable; low-energy bonds are less reactive and more stable. *Electronegativity* is the ability of an atom to attract electrons. Electronegativity increases on the periodic chart upward and to the right. The number of *valence electrons* determines the number of bonds an atom will form. *Atomic orbitals* are theoretic regions around the nucleus that have a high probability of containing electrons.

IIIIII······   into the plane of paper

◄━━━   out of the plane of paper

Valency, you recall, determines the number of bonds formed by an atom. Carbon has four electrons in its outer shell and forms four bonds to obtain an octet. Be sure to review *Lewis structures* and the *octet rule*.

BONDING

Understanding electronegativity, the octet rule, valency, and trends of the periodic table is essential to understanding bonding. Refer to the general chemistry section for a review of these concepts if you have not done so already.

Three Types of Bonds

IONIC

Ionic bonds form between atoms with different electronegativities. An atom with a high electron affinity will take electrons from an atom with a low ionization potential. Ionic bonds are strong bonds that have great intermolecular forces, resulting in high melting and boiling points.

COVALENT

In ionic bonding, electrons are transferred from atom to atom. The atoms of covalent bonds, however, have similar electronegativities and therefore share electrons. Covalent bonds are found in diatomic molecules and in most organic compounds. A difference in electronegativity of atoms in a covalently bonded molecule creates a polar covalent bond. In fact, most covalent bonds are polar, and the molecule creates a dipole. This simply means that the atom in the bond with less electronegativity takes on a slightly positive charge (+), and the atom with greater electronegativity takes on a slightly negative charge (−). Understanding this concept is key to understanding why organic reactions occur as they do.

HYDROGEN

Hydrogen bonds form a weak dipole interaction between a hydrogen atom and a negatively charged atom. Hydrogen bonding determines most of the physical properties of organic molecules.

1.

$$\ddot{O} = C = \ddot{O}$$

No Net
Dipole

2.

No Net
Dipole

3.

Net Dipole

4.

Net Dipole

Orbitals

ATOMIC ORBITALS

Atomic orbitals are theoretic areas around the nucleus where electrons of a given energy level can be found. These orbitals are often referred to *as electron clouds*. An *s* orbital takes on a *spherical cloud*, whereas a *p* orbital is more elongated and resembles a *dumbbell-shaped cloud*.

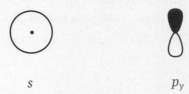

s p_y

MOLECULAR ORBITALS

The sharing of electrons in covalent bonds results in an overlap of two of the atomic orbitals, forming two *molecular orbitals*. One of these will be of *higher energy* and *antibonding*, while the other will be of *lower energy* and *bonding*. Electrons fill the bonding, lower energy level first.

Sigma Bond

End-on-end overlap of orbitals forms a sigma (σ) bond. The bonding of four hydrogen atoms to a carbon atom results in four sigma bonds. A sigma bond allows the two bonded atoms to *freely rotate*.

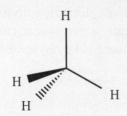

Methane with
4 σ bonds

Pi Bond

The pi (π) bond is formed from the *parallel overlap of p orbitals*. These parallel overlaps are above and below the plane of the sigma bond. *Pi bonds do not permit rotation.*

Single bonds are sigma bonds, double bonds contain one sigma and one pi bond, and triple bonds contain one sigma and two pi bonds.

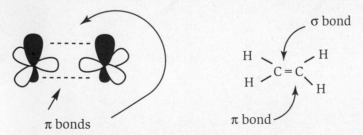

HYBRID ORBITALS

Hybridization of atomic orbitals occurs to achieve lower energy states and results in shapes more conducive to overlapping when atomic orbitals become molecular orbitals. This overlapping creates stronger bonds. It is important to remember that nature does not like high-energy states and that chemical reactions occur primarily to obtain lower energy states. Therefore, while paradoxical, the stronger the bond the less energy in the system. Strong bonds and low energy create very stable systems.

   Hybridization is the result of nature's creating a system to reduce the energy in the bond and thus achieve a more stable system. This desire to achieve stability results in a change of electron configuration. In the hybridization of carbon (6 electrons, electron configuration of $1s^2\ 2s^2\ 2p^2$), an electron from the $2s$ orbital moves into the vacant $2p_z$ orbital. Then each of the three $2p$ orbitals and the one $2s$ orbital has one electron. The mixing of these four orbitals (that is, the hybridization) results in four identical hybrids that are one part s and three parts p.

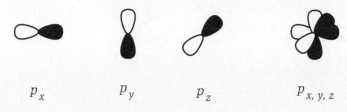

$$p_x \qquad p_y \qquad p_z \qquad p_{x,\,y,\,z}$$

sp^3

The sp^3 hybrid orbital consists of one s (spherical) and three p (dumbbell-shaped) orbitals that are mixed to form four new sp^3 orbitals. These four orbitals are arranged in a *tetrahedral* conformation, which maximizes the distance between the electron clouds. The angle between clouds created by sp^3 hybridization is 109.5°.

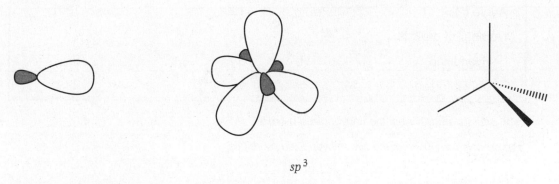

$$sp^3$$

sp^2

The sp^2 hybrid consists of one s orbital and two p orbitals that mix to form three sp^2 orbitals. The fourth p orbital remains unhybridized. This planar conformation creates an angle of 120° between the orbitals. The three sp^2 orbitals lie on the same plane, and the unhybridized dumbbell-shaped p orbital is perpendicular to this plane (the p orbital is 90° from the plane of the three sp^2 orbitals).

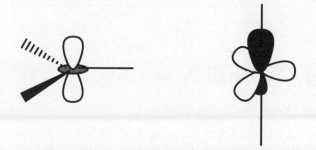

$$sp^2$$

sp

When one *s* and one *p* orbital form a hybrid, two *sp* orbitals are created and two *p* orbitals remain unhybridized. The two *sp* orbitals are 180° apart (linear), and the two unhybridized orbitals are perpendicular to each other and to the *sp* orbitals. The *lengths* and *strengths* of these hybridized orbitals are *inversely related*, with the *sp* bond being the shorter and stronger.

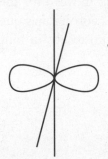

Two unhybridized *p* orbitals

Comparison of *sp*³, *sp*², and *sp* Orbitals

	*sp*³	*sp*²	*sp*
Conformation	Tetrahedral	Planar	Linear
Angle (°)	109.5	120*	180†
Number of orbitals	4	4	4
Hybridized	4	3	2
Unhybridized	0	1	2

*sp² orbitals are 90° from the unhybridized p orbital.

†sp orbitals are 90° from the two unhybridized p orbitals.

Type	Strength	Length	Sigma	Pi	Free Rotation
*sp*³	Weak	Long	1	0	Yes
*sp*²	⇓	⇓	1	1	No
sp	Strong	Short	1	2	No

Bond Rotation and Energy; Newman Projections

ROTATION AND ENERGY

The free rotation about a single bond creates a variety of arrangements of atomic structures, some more energetically desirable than others. For example, an ethane molecule has two carbons, each having three hydrogens and one sp^3 bond between the carbons. The ethane molecule can be illustrated with the dotted-line wedge, the sawhorse, or the *Newman projection*.

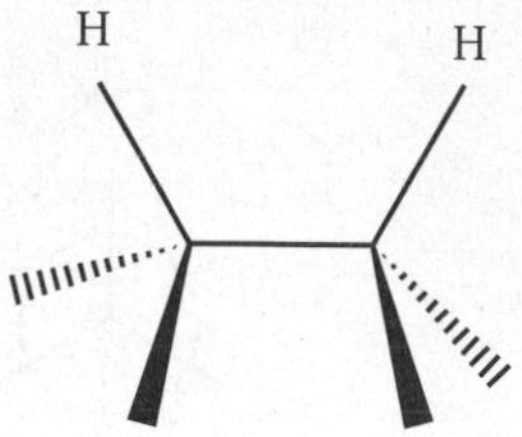

Dotted-Line
Wedge

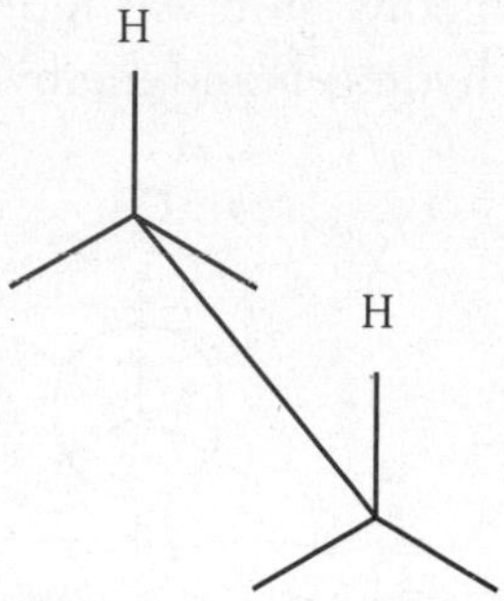

Sawhorse

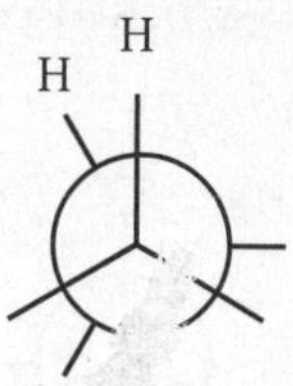

Newman Projection

NEWMAN PROJECTIONS

Newman projections are used to illustrate the energetically favorable and unfavorable positionings of atoms.

Ethane

The Newman projection of ethane helps to visualize the positioning of the hydrogens on the carbons. The projection is drawn looking down the axis of the carbon-carbon bond. In the case of ethane, the closer the hydrogens are to one another, the greater the energy and the less stable the molecule. The *anti* is the most favorable positioning, followed by the *gauche*. The *eclipsed* is the least favorable positioning. Rotating the back carbon 60° will change the positioning from anti to gauche, and with another turn the positioning goes from gauche to eclipsed. In ethane, the gauche and anti positionings are identical (sometimes referred to as *staggered*); however, with the addition of more carbons the anti position is indeed more energetically favorable.

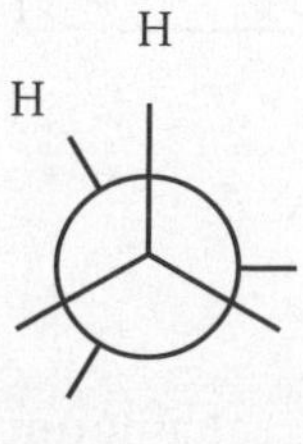

Eclipsed

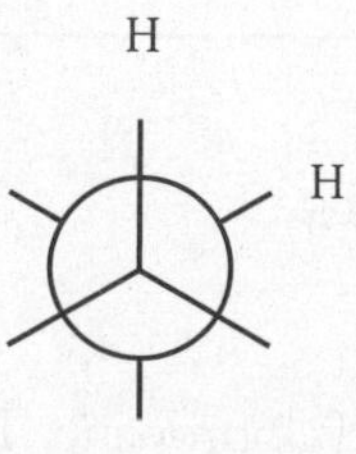

Gauche

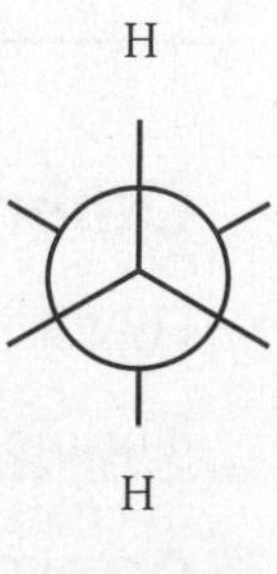

Staggered
or
Anti

Butane

The Newman projection of butane shows a slightly more complicated situation. In this projection, the axis that is rotated is between the second and third carbons. Rotating the third carbon (out of view) illustrates the various positions possible. The eclipsed position of two methyl groups is more energetically unfavorable than is an eclipsed conformation of hydrogen and methyl.

Eclipsed   Gauche   Anti

Energy Diagrams

As a rule of thumb, *a molecule attains the lowest possible energy by maximizing the distance between its atoms*. In most energetically unfavorable positions the larger groups are eclipsed, and in the most energetically favorable position the larger groups are anti to each other. The relative energy states of molecules are represented by energy diagrams.

Below is the *energy diagram* for butane.

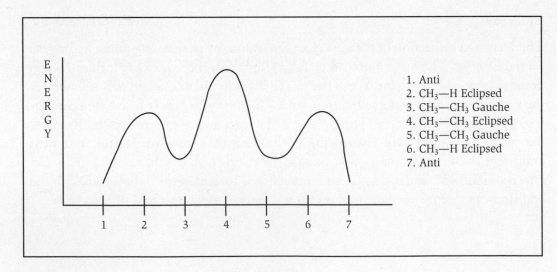

1. Anti
2. CH₃—H Eclipsed
3. CH₃—CH₃ Gauche
4. CH₃—CH₃ Eclipsed
5. CH₃—CH₃ Gauche
6. CH₃—H Eclipsed
7. Anti

Other Related Concepts

RING STRAIN

The most *ring strain* is found in cyclopropane. This molecule gives off a great amount of energy when the ring is broken because of its extreme divergence from the desired bond angle. Of all the cycloalkanes, the six-membered ring *cyclohexane* has the least strain created from bond angles stretching from their desired angle. The molecule benzene has no ring strain.

CYCLOHEXANE

Cyclohexane is a molecule that appears in two conformations, the *chair* and the *boat*. The molecule undergoes *ring flip*, switching between boat and chair conformations, to maximize the distance between substitutents. The chair conformation has *six axial* hydrogens (vertically oriented) and *six equatorial* hydrogens (horizontally oriented). Hydrogens in the same position (equatorial or axial) on adjacent carbons are trans to one another. Hydrogens in the axial position are cis to hydrogens in the equatorial position on adjacent carbons. The following illustration may help to clarify the positioning of hydrogens on the chair configuration of cyclohexane. Also, if an organic model set is available, building the cyclohexane and then inverting the ring between the chair and boat conformations will help to visualize this transformation.

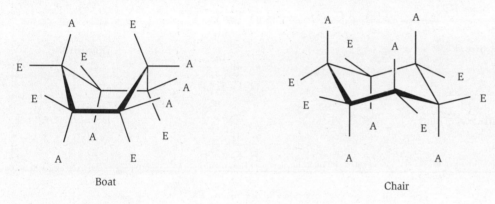

Boat   Chair

BOND CLEAVAGE

In *heterolytic cleavage* (*heterolytic* means "*different breaking*") both electrons are taken by one of the atoms in a molecule. This results in charged products. A simple example of heterolytic cleavage is the dissolution of water. In *homolytic cleavage* (*homolytic* means "*similar breaking*") each atom takes one electron. No charge results from homolytic cleavage; however, *radicals* are formed that are extremely reactive.

NOMENCLATURE

IUPAC Rules

1. Determine the longest continuous chain of carbon atoms and use this as the parent name. When a functional group is present, use the longest chain that includes the functional group. Drop the *-e* from the alkane name, and add the suffix of the corresponding functional group.

Functional Group(s)	Suffix	Generalized Structural Formula	Example
Alkane	-ane	R–H	pentane
Alkene	-ene	R=H	pentene
Alkyne	-yne	R H	pentyne
Alcohol	-ol	R–OH	pentanol
Aldehyde	-al	$$\underset{\text{R–C–H}}{\overset{\overset{\displaystyle O}{\|}}{}}$$	pentanal
Ketone	-one	$$\underset{\text{R–C–R}}{\overset{\overset{\displaystyle O}{\|}}{}}$$	pentanone
Carboxylic acid	-oic	$$\underset{\text{R–C–OH}}{\overset{\overset{\displaystyle O}{\|}}{}}$$	pentanoic acid

2. Locate the substituent(s) present, and number the longest chain including the substituent in such a way that the substituent receives *the lowest possible number*. Functional groups take on the parent name. If more than one functional group exists, the groups are *prioritized*; the one with greatest priority takes on the parent name, and the others are treated as substituents. Functional groups are listed in order of *decreasing priority* as follows:

   - Carboxylic acids and their derivatives [esters (-oate), amides, nitriles (-nitrile), -C(N), acid halides (-yl halide), anhydrides]
   - Aldehydes
   - Ketones
   - Alcohols
   - Amines
   - Alkynes
   - Alkenes
   - Halogens and alkyl groups

3. Use dashes to separate numbers from words, and commas to separate numbers from numbers. If a group appears more than once as a substituent, use the prefixes *di-*, *tri-*, and *tetra-* in addition to the numbers (example: 2,2-dimethyl-3-heptene).

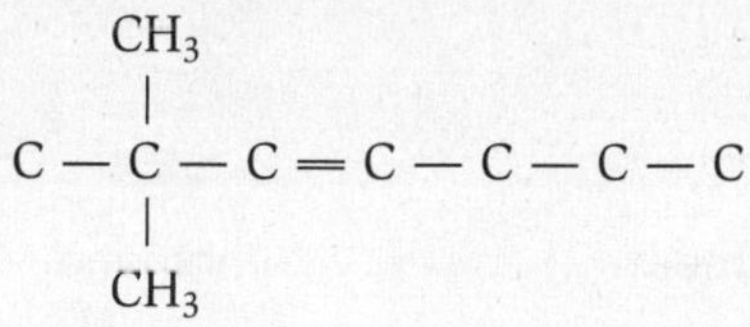

$$CH_3$$
$$|$$
$$C - C - C = C - C - C - C$$
$$|$$
$$CH_3$$

4. Name substitutents alphabetically when two or more exist (example: 2-ethyl-3-methylheptane). The prefixes *iso-*, *sec-*, *tert-*, and *neo-* are *included* in alphabetizing, but, *di-*, *tri-*, and *tetra-* are *excluded*.

5. For cylic compounds use the prefix *cyclo-*.

Examples of IUPAC nomenclature:

1. 3-Methylpentane

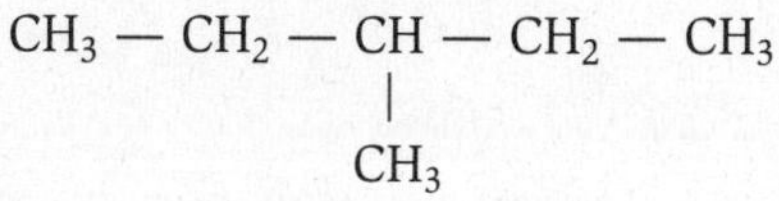

$$CH_3 - CH_2 - CH - CH_2 - CH_3$$
$$|$$
$$CH_3$$

2. 3-Bromo-2-chloropentane

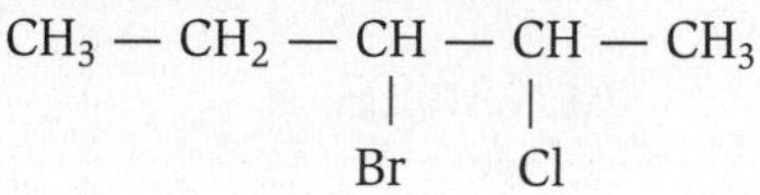

$$CH_3 - CH_2 - CH - CH - CH_3$$
$$|\qquad|$$
$$Br\quad Cl$$

3. 2-Heptene

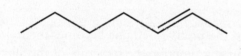

4. Cyclohexene

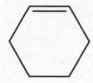

5. Butanal

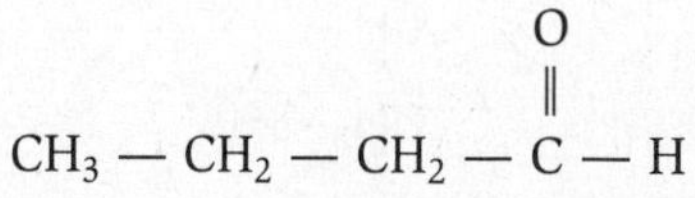

$$O$$
$$\|$$
$$CH_3 - CH_2 - CH_2 - C - H$$

6. Butanoic acid

$$O$$
$$\|$$
$$CH_3 - CH_2 - CH_2 - C - OH$$

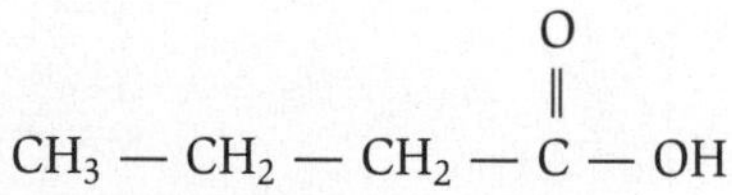

7. 3,3-Dimethyl-5-ethyl-6-propylnonane

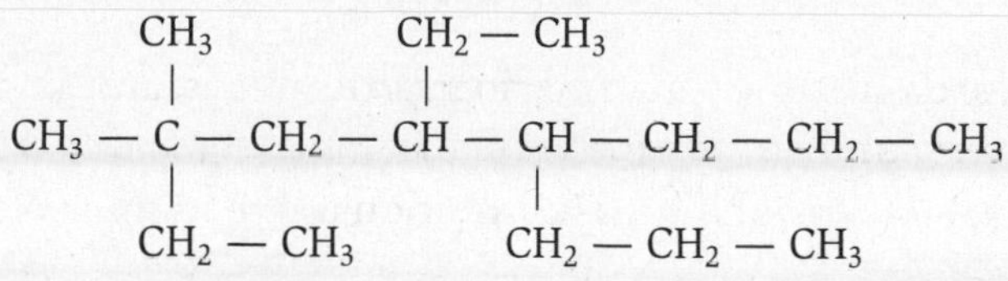

$$CH_3 \qquad\qquad CH_2 - CH_3$$
$$| \qquad\qquad\qquad |$$
$$CH_3 - C - CH_2 - CH - CH - CH_2 - CH_2 - CH_3$$
$$| \qquad\qquad\qquad |$$
$$CH_2 - CH_3 \qquad CH_2 - CH_2 - CH_3$$

Number of Carbon Atoms	Prefix	Name	Molecular Formula
1	meth-	methane	CH_4
2	eth-	ethane	C_2H_6
3	prop-	propane	C_3H_8
4	but-	butane	C_4H_{10}
5	pent-	pentane	C_5H_{12}
6	hex-	hexane	C_6H_{14}
7	hept-	heptane	C_7H_{16}
8	oct-	octane	C_8H_{18}
9	non-	nonane	C_9H_{20}
10	dec-	decane	$C_{10}H_{22}$

General Molecular Formulas

ALKANES

The general formula for alkanes is C_nH_{2n+2}. This means that, for any given number of carbon atoms, there are 2 more than twice that number of hydrogen atoms. The names of alkanes have the suffix *-ane*.

Alkyl Substituents

Alkyl substituents are named by adding *-yl* to the prefix (methane becomes methyl). *Iso-*, *sec-*, *tert-*, and *neo-* are prefixes used to further describe the structure of the alkyl substituent. Some common alkyl substituents are listed below.

Number of Carbon Atoms	Name	Structural Formula
1	methyl-	CH_3-
2	ethyl-	CH_3-CH_2-
3	propyl-	$CH_3-CH_2-CH_2-$
3	isopropyl-	$CH_3-CH-CH_3$ (with bond below center C)
4	butyl-	$CH_3-CH_2-CH_2CH_2-$
4	*sec*-butyl-	CH_3-CH_2-CH with CH_3 branch below
4	isobutyl-	CH_3 and CH_3 joined to $CH-CH_2-$

Number of Carbon Atoms	Name	Structural Formula
4	*tert*-butyl-	CH$_3$ | CH$_3$-C- | CH$_3$
5	pentyl-	CH$_3$-CH$_2$-CH$_2$-CH$_2$-CH$_2$-
5	*sec*-pentyl-	CH$_3$-CH$_2$-CH$_2$-CH- | C
5	isopentyl-	CH$_3$-CH-CH$_2$-CH$_2$- | CH$_3$
5	*tert*-pentyl-	CH$_3$ | CH$_3$-CH$_2$-C- | CH$_3$
5	neopentyl-	CH$_3$ | CH$_3$-C-CH$_2$- | CH$_3$

Rings

Carbon chains that form a ring have the same general molecular formula as alkenes, C_nH_{2n}. Two hydrogens are lost from the bond that forms the ring.

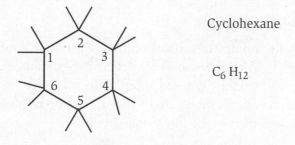

Cyclohexane

$C_6 H_{12}$

ALKENES

The general formula for alkenes is C_nH_{2n}. Alkenes have a *double bond* between two adjacent carbon atoms and therefore have *two fewer hydrogen atoms than alkanes*. The names of alkenes have the suffix *-ene*.

Cis and *Trans* Isomers

The terms *cis-* and *trans-* refer to the substituents of planar molecules that are not free to rotate because of pi bonds. These terms are used to identify the isomers. Cis alkenes have the larger substituents on the same side of the double bond, and trans alkenes have the larger substituents on opposite sides.

E and *Z* Isomers

IUPAC uses *E/Z* terminology to describe the placement of substituents on planar molecules. This nomenclature is another method of describing cis/trans isomers. *E* refers to opposite sides, or trans. *Z*, refers to the same side ("Zame side"), or cis.

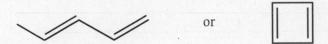

cis-3-Hexane   *trans*-3-Hexane

Dienes and Trienes

Alkenes that have two double bonds are dienes, and alkenes that have three bonds are trienes. If the double bonds are separated by a single bond, the structure is referred to as *conjugated*.

ALKYNES

The general formula for alkynes is C_nH_{2n-2}. Alkynes have a *triple bond* between two adjacent carbon atoms and therefore have *four fewer hydrogen atoms than alkanes*. The names of alkynes have the suffix *-yne*.

Naming Benzene Compounds

Without substituents, the fully conjugated six-carbon ring, with three double bonds, is called a *benzene* molecule (1,3,5-cyclohexatriene). Benzene is quite unique because of its overlapping *p* orbitals, and will be discussed at length in Section V on aromaticity. The prefixes *phenyl-* and *benzyl-* are often used when a benzene ring appears in a molecule as a substituent, rather than as the functional group.

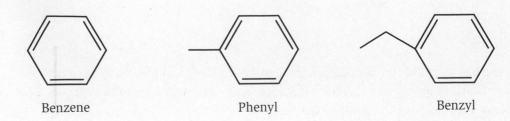

Benzene   Phenyl   Benzyl

MONOSUBSTITUTION

The following are common monosubstituted benzene rings:

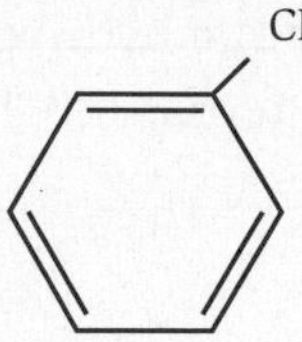

Toluene	Phenol	Aniline	Benzoic Acid	Benzaldehyde

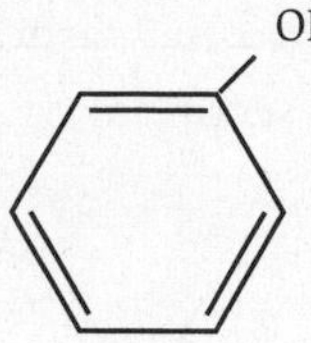

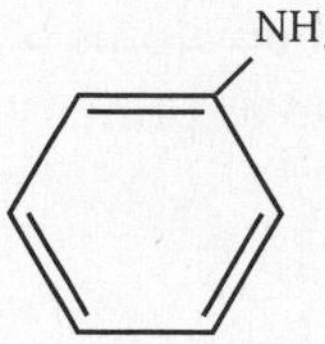

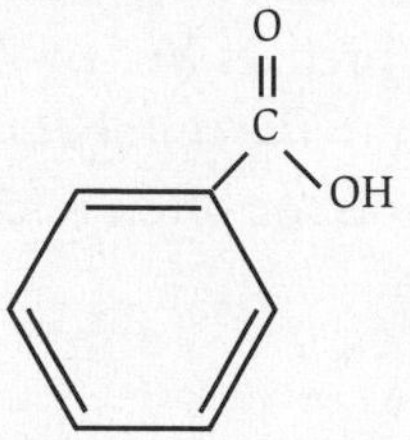

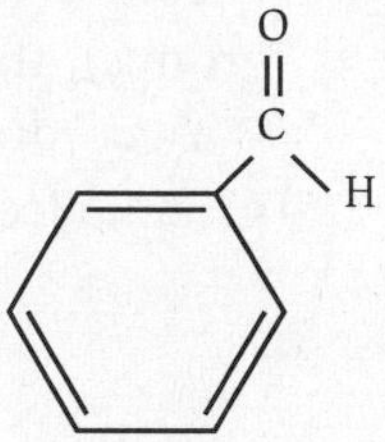

DISUBSTITUTION

Substituents are listed alphabetically in such a way that they receive the lowest number. The prefixes *ortho-*, *para-*, and *meta-* are used to describe disubstituted benzene rings.

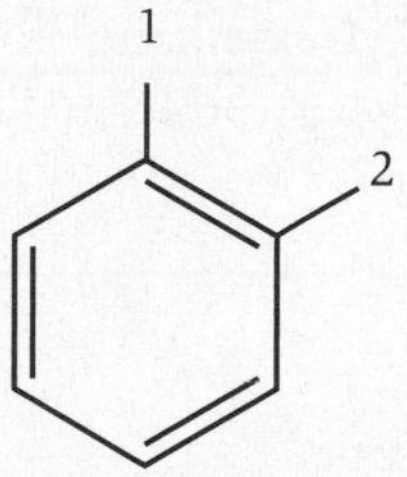

Ortho-
(1,2-disubstitution)

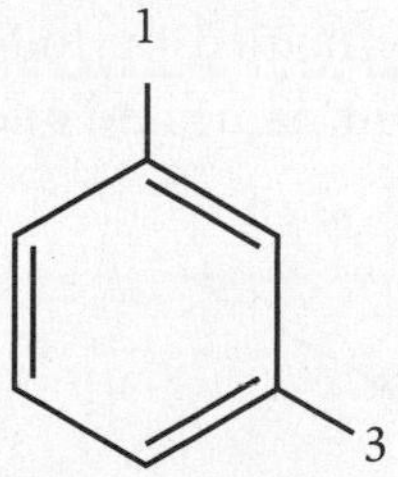

Meta-
(1,3-disubstitution)

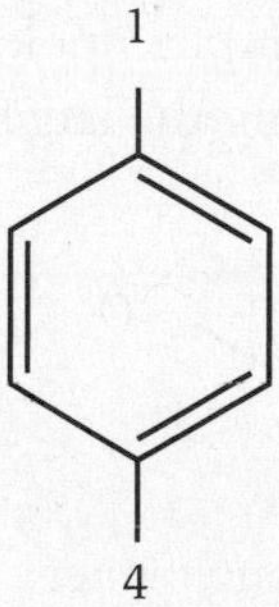

Para-
(1,4-disubstitution)

TRISUBSTITUTION AND OTHER SUBSTITUTIONS

Benzene rings that have more than two substituents cannot be described in terms of *ortho-*, *meta-*, *para-*. For these, the substituents are listed alphabetically in such a way that they receive the lowest possible number.

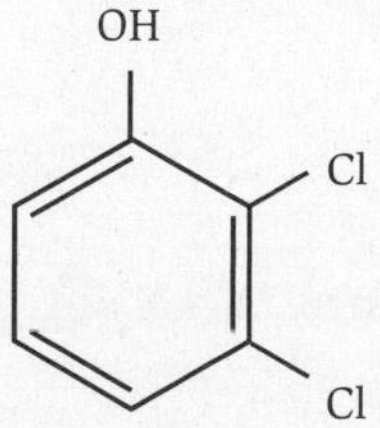

2,3-Dichlorophenol

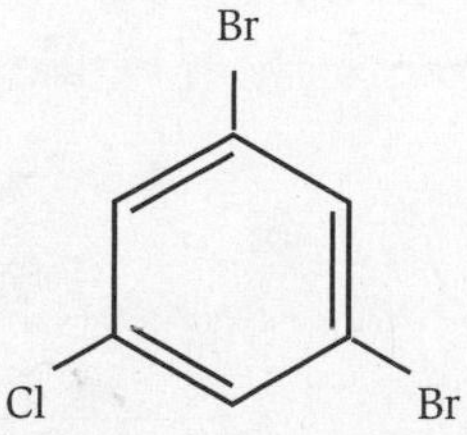

1,3-Dibromo-5-chlorobenzene

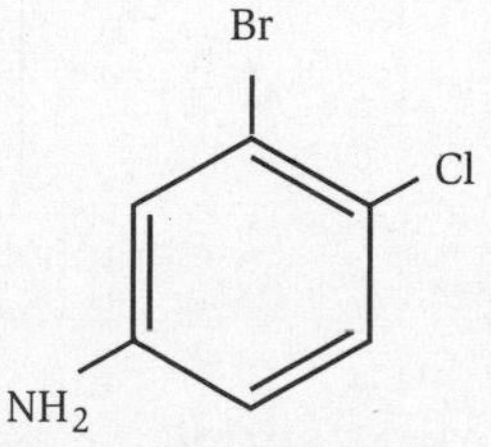

3-Bromo-4-chloro-analine

Alcohols: Primary (1°), Secondary (2°), Tertiary (3°)

Alcohols are named by adding the suffix *-ol.* For multiple *hydroxy groups* (–OH groups), the prefixes *di-*, *tri-*, etc., are added (diols and triols).

According to the number of carbon atoms bonded to the carbon with the hydroxy group, alcohols are often referred to as primary (1°), secondary (2°), or tertiary (3°).

Ethers

Ethers are named using two different methods. Simple molecules are usually named by listing the alkyl groups in order of increasing size and then adding the word *ether.* More complex molecules are usually named by following the "alkyl-*oxy*alkane" format, giving the larger group the parent name and adding the suffix-*oxy* to the smaller group.

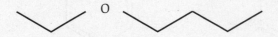

ethyl butyl ether   or   ethoxybutane

Carbonyl Compounds

In naming compounds with carbonyl groups (C=O), the Greek letters α, β, and γ are used to describe the relative positions of the carbon atoms attached to the carbonyl carbon.

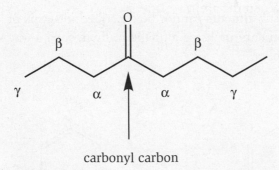

carbonyl carbon

ALDEHYDES

Identify the longest chain containing the aldehyde group, and number the chain starting at the carbonyl carbon. Add the suffix *-al.*

KETONES

Identify the longest carbon chain containing the carbonyl carbon. Number the chain so that the carbonyl carbon gets the lowest possible number. Add the suffix *-one*.

CARBOXYLIC ACIDS

Identify the longest chain containing the COOH group. Number the chain starting at the carbonyl carbon. Add the suffix *-oic* and "acid."

ESTERS

Ester nomenclature is similar to ether nomenclature in that the functional group divides the molecule into two parts that are individually named. The section of the molecule bonded to the oxygen is referred to as the alcohol portion and is the first part of the name. The part that is bonded to the carbonyl carbon is referred to as the carboxylic acid portion and is the second part of the name.

2, 3-Dimethylbutanal (an aldehyde)   2-Methylbutyl-3-methylbutanoate (an ester)

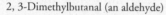

3-Pentanone (a ketone)   Propanic acid (an acid)

Amines and Amides

There are two ways of naming amines. When the amino group appears in a molecule as a branched side chain, it is given a number that identifies its position and the prefix *amino-*. Otherwise, the alkyl substituent is given the suffix *-amine*.

2-Aminobutane

Triethylamine

Special attention should be given to the naming of amides; this nomenclature is quite different. The base name is the longest carbon chain containing the amide, with the numbering starting at the carbonyl carbon. An N- is used to indicate each group bound to the nitrogen. (*Note:* Nitrogen forms a maximum of three bonds.)

3-Hydroxy-N-methylbutanamide

STEREOCHEMISTRY

General Information

The spatial relationships of atoms within a molecule can determine how the molecule as a whole reacts. Two molecules with the same number and type of atoms may have completely different properties, and therefore are truly different molecules. Some molecules, on the other hand, may be so similar in structure and properties that only certain tests can differentiate them.

IMPORTANCE: THE THALIDOMIDE EXAMPLE

The infamous example that illustrates the importance of stereochemistry is a drug called thalidomide that was prescribed in the 1960s to alleviate morning sickness. A mixture of *both* stereoisomers was administered to pregnant women. Later it became tragically evident that, while one stereoisomer in the mixture relieved morning nausea, the other caused severe birth defects.

STEREOISOMERS

For two molecules to be considered stereoisomers, they must have identical atoms and connectivity. Stereoisomers differ in the spatial configuration of their atoms. Stereoisomers are either *enantiomers* or *diastereomers*. Enantiomers are *nonsuperimposable mirror images of each other* (i.e., like a pair of gloves or a left and a right ear). Their difference lies in the orientation of atoms at one carbon. Diastereomers *are not mirror images of each other*. They differ in the orientation of atoms at two or more carbons.

CHIRALITY/CHIRAL CENTERS

An sp^3 carbon atom with four different substituents is asymmetric and has the property of *chirality*. This carbon is called the *chiral center* in an enantiomer. If a plane of symmetry can be drawn, the molecule is *achiral*.

OPTICAL ACTIVITY

Light waves normally exist in all planes, but if the light waves are filtered through a polarizer, only those oscillating in one plane pass through. This light is *plane-*

polarized light. Optically active compounds will rotate this light *counterclockwise/levoro-tary*, or *clockwise/dextorotary.* Enantiomers rotate light in equal amounts and in opposite directions. If equal amounts of two enantiomers are present (a *racemic mixture*), the *rotation will be zero. Meso compounds* have an internal plane of symmetry, are not optically active, and, in relation to optically active compounds, are diastereomers. No meso compounds are enantiomers.

A. Plane-polarized light

B. Rotation

C. Meso example

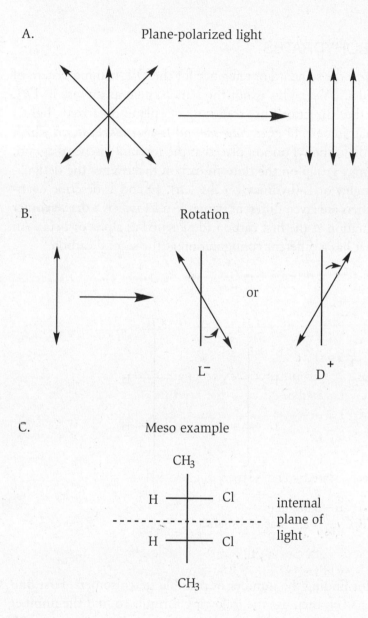

Fischer Diagrams

CONCEPTS

Often it is necessary to distinguish stereoisomers from each other. To illustrate the methods of doing so, we must first review *Fischer diagrams*. In a Fischer diagram, the vertical *y*-axis is representative of bonds going into the plane of the paper, and the horizontal *x*-axis is representative of bonds coming out of the plane of the paper.

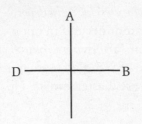
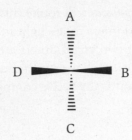

RELEVANCE TO CARBOHYDRATES

The molecule *glyceraldehyde* is the standard of reference for the D/L naming system of other carbohydrate molecules. (*Note*: This is not the same system as the use of D/L descriptors to identify the direction of rotation of plane-polarized light.) Glyceraldehyde has two enantiomers, D-*glyceraldehyde* and L-*glyceraldehyde*, on which this system is based. With the carbonyl carbon placed at the top of a Fischer diagram, the orientation of the hydroxy group on the bottom carbon determines the designation: D-(hydroxy on the right) or L-(hydroxy on the left). D and L describe enantiomers, whereas diastereomers are given different names. An *anomer* is a diastereomer that has a different configuration at the first carbon (designated as alpha or beta). An *epimer* is a diastereomer that has a different configuration at the second carbon.

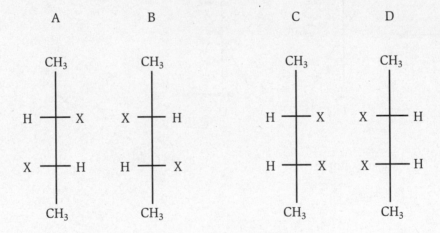

Therefore: A/B and C/D are enantiomers;
A/C, A/D, B/C, B/D are diastereomers

RULE OF 2^n

There is a quick method for finding the number of possible stereoisomers. First find the number of chiral centers (n); then use the following formula to find the number of possible diastereomers that exist for that molecule: number of diastereomers = 2^n.

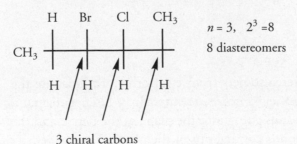

$n = 3$, $2^3 = 8$

8 diastereomers

3 chiral carbons

Absolute Configuration

To identify stereoisomers other than carbohydrates, it is necessary to assign an *absolute configuration* using the *R/S* system. The first step is to number the four different groups on the chiral carbon as 1, 2, 3, and 4 according to priority, 1 being the highest priority and 4 the lowest. The rules for assigning absolute configuration follow:

1. The atom directly bonded to the chiral carbon usually determines the priority of the group—*the higher the atomic number of this atom, the greater the priority of the group.*

2. If double or triple bonds exist, the atoms so bonded are considered to be doubled or tripled in atomic number.

The lowest priority group, usually hydrogen, is placed in the back, using a rotated Fischer projection—called the steering wheel approach. If the sequence is 1, 2, 3 *clockwise*, the molecule is designated as *R*; if c*ounterclockwise*, as *S*.

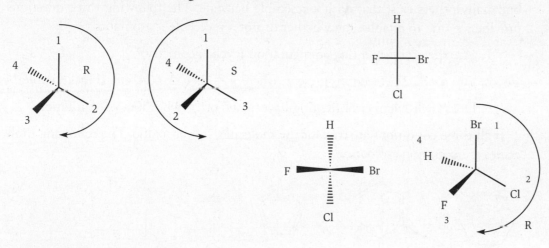

AROMATICITY

General Information

Before discussing the rules of aromaticity, it is necessary to state what these molecules have in common: *conjugation, resonance,* and *delocalization.*

CONJUGATION

A molecule that has double bonds separated by single bonds is *conjugated,* causing a linking of adjacent *p* orbitals. These *p* orbitals form two electron clouds: one above and one below the axis of the carbon-carbon bonding.

RESONANCE AND DELOCALIZATION

The linking of the *p* orbitals to form clouds of electrons is due to *resonance.* Besides being conjugated, the molecule must be in a planar configuration so that the *p* orbitals line up. The effect of resonance is a cloud of *delocalized* electrons, *yielding a very stable molecule.* Each *p* orbital has one electron. When six *p* orbitals are aligned with three conjugated pi bonds, the six electrons completely fill the lower energy bonding molecular orbital. This is a very favorable energetic situation. The molecule can be in a chain configuration or a ring configuration.

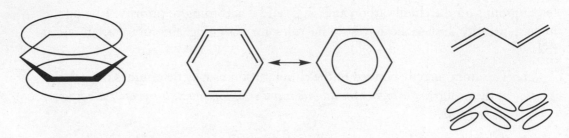

Rules for Determining Aromaticity

When the fully conjugated planar molecule, with overlapping *p* orbitals, is present in a ring, the term *aromatic* is applied. Benzene is the most commonly found aromatic, but many others exist that do not resemble benzene. The following three questions provide a guide to establishing whether or not a molecule is aromatic:

1. Are the atoms in a ring configuration (cyclic geometry)?

2. Are $4n + 2$ pi electrons present, where $n = 0, 1, 2, 3, 4$, etc. (Huckel's rule)?

3. Does each member of the ring have an sp^2 or sp hybridized configuration?

If all three conditions are true for the molecule, it is aromatic. The following molecules are common aromatics:

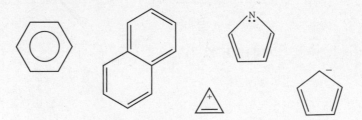

These molecules are *not* aromatic:

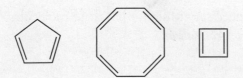

Electrophilic Aromatic Substitution (EAS)

GENERAL CONCEPTS AND MECHANISM

It should be obvious that aromatic molecules are perfect targets for electrophiles. The molecule is electron rich, and the electron cloud is quite accessible. The electrophile draws an electron from the ring forming, a resonance-stabilized *carbocation* (a positively charged carbon molecule). To reestablish aromaticity, the nonaromatic intermediate is deprotonated; that is, it loses the hydrogen bound to the carbon that accepted the electrophile. The loss of the proton causes the extra electron maintained in the system to eliminate the carbocation.

The electrophilic aromatic substitution (EAS) can be illustrated as follows:

TYPES, REAGENTS, AND PRODUCTS

Knowledge of the reagents used in the various types of EAS reaction can assist in quickly predicting the products.

Type of EAS	Reagent	Product
Friedel-Crafts acylation	CH_3COCl / $AlCl_3$	$CH_3C=O$
Halogenation	X_2 / FeX_3	$-X$ (Cl, Br)
Nitration	HNO_3 / H_2SO_4	$-NO_2$
Alkylation	RX / AlX_3	$-R$ (1°)
Sulfonation	SO_3 / H_2SO_4	$-SO_3H$

Effects of Substituents on Electrophilic Aromatic Substitution

GENERAL CONCEPTS

When EAS occurs with a substituted benzene ring, the characteristics of the ring in reactions are changed. These benzene substituents, classified as activators/electron-donating groups or deactivators/electron-withdrawing groups, will polarize the electron clouds and therefore alter the orientation (ortho/para or meta) and speed at which groups will add through EAS. *It is the substituent(s) on the benzene ring that determine the orientation and rate of reaction of the incoming group.* Because of their importance, these substituents are classified so that the products of the reaction can be predicted.

ACTIVATORS AND DEACTIVATORS

The activators and deactivators are listed in a prioritized method according to the strength with which they affect incoming groups. This is important when there is more than one substituent already on the benzene ring and one substituent directs ortho/para orientation and the other directs meta. Halogens are an exception to the rule that ortho/para directors are activators and meta directors are deactivators. This anomaly is due to the strong electronegativity of halogens.

Activators	Deactivators
1. are electron-*donating* groups,	1. are electron-*withdrawing* groups,
2. *increase* the rate of reaction,	2. *decrease* the rate of reaction,
3. are *ortho, para* directors.	3. are *meta* directors.

Classification	Examples	Priority
Ortho/para activators	$-NH_2$, $-OH$, $-NHR$, $-OCH_3$, $-C_6H_5$ ($-Ph$), $-CH_3$	High
Ortho/para deactivators	Halogens ($-F$, $-Cl$, $-Br$, $-I$)	Medium
Meta deactivators	NO_2, $-COOH$, $-CN$, $-NH_3+$, $-SO_3$, $-CHO$	Low

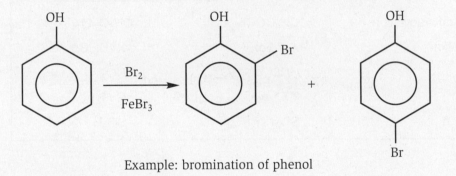

Example: bromination of phenol

CHEMICAL AND PHYSICAL PROPERTIES OF MOLECULES

General Concepts

POLARITY

The *polarity* of a molecule determines in part how the molecule will react with other molecules. Polarity is due to the geometric configuration of the molecule, often a result of hybridization. The physical properties common to a species are a result of intermolecular interactions determined mostly by the net polarity of the molecule.

No Net
Dipole

Net Dipole

SOLUBILITY

Solubility is a measure of how readily a compound will dissolve in another compound. The *solvent* (dissolving medium of a solution) is generally added to the *solute* (substance dissolved in the solution). The important concept to remember is that *polar compounds solvate polar compounds* and *nonpolar compounds solvate nonpolar compounds*.

Alkanes, Alkenes, and Alkynes

ALKANES

Alkanes are *nonpolar hydrocarbons* that are *insoluble in water*. Their melting and boiling points are relatively low. The *higher the molecular weight* (the greater the number of carbons), the *higher the boiling point*. The interaction of the electrons with each other, due to what are called *van der Waals* forces, causes this increase in boiling point. If two alkanes have the same formula weight (differing only in connectivity of atoms), the one that has more extensive branching has the lower boiling point because the branching prevents the molecules from being packed together as tightly as occurs in a straight chain. This results in weaker intermolecular forces and therefore a lower boiling point. Branching often has the reverse effect on the melting point. Usually the melting point increases because of an increase in symmetry, which aids in the formation of crystal lattices.

Alkanes with 1–4 carbons are gases; alkanes with 5–17 carbons are liquids; alkanes with 18 or more carbons are solids. *Combustion* of alkanes due to oxidation yields water and CO_2 and is an *exothermic* reaction.

ALKENES AND ALKYNES

The melting points and boiling points of alkenes and alkynes increase with an increase in molecular weight. In general, alkenes and alkynes have physical properties similar to those of alkanes. However, the presence of the double bond in alkenes creates cis/trans isomerization, as previously discussed. This can affect the net polarity of the molecule and therefore affect intermolecular interactions.

Alcohols, Ethers, and the Carbonyl Compounds

ALCOHOLS

Alcohols have higher boiling points than alkanes because of the hydrogen bonding of the hydroxy group. The lone pairs of electrons on the oxygen are free to bond to neighboring hydroxy hydrogens. As the carbon chain grows in length, the polarizing effect of the hydroxy group diminishes and the molecule acts as a nonpolar molecule. Alcohols that have five or fewer carbons exhibit a net dipole and are water soluble. Alcohols react with acids, which protonate the oxygen, creating a positive charge that reacts with a nucleophile.

ETHERS

Ethers cannot form intermolecular hydrogen bonds as alcohols do because, in place of the hydroxy hydrogen, ethers have an alkyl group. Therefore, in comparison to alcohols of similar weight, ethers have lower melting and boiling points. An increase in the carbon chain length increases the melting point and boiling point because of van der Waals forces. Solubility in water decreases with increasing carbon chain length. Ethers react with acids, which protonate the oxygen, creating a positive charge that reacts with a nucleophile.

ALDEHYDES

All carbonyl compounds have higher boiling points than comparable alkanes because the polarity of the carbonyl group creates strong intermolecular forces. Aldehydes have melting and boiling points higher than those of ketones, but lower than those of carboxylic acids.

KETONES

Ketones have low boiling and melting points because they lack the hydrogen that the other carbonyl compounds use to hydrogen-bond to adjacent molecules. The boiling and melting points of ketones are lower than those of comparable alcohols.

CARBOXYLIC ACIDS

Because of extensive hydrogen bonding, carboxylic acids have higher melting and boiling points than aldehydes and ketones. Also, as a result of their very strong polarity, these acids have higher melting and boiling points than alcohols. Resonance at the carbonyl group creates an electrophilic carbon and a nucleophilic oxygen.

Carbohydrates, Lipids, and Amines

Carbohydrates, lipids, and amines are referred to as the organic molecules of biological importance. These are the molecules that make up our living tissues and biological chemicals, and their reactions are vital to life-sustaining processes.

CARBOHYDRATES

The oxidation of carbohydrates, which are polyhydroxylated molecules comprised of aldehydes and ketones, is responsible for the metabolism of stored energy and the formation of ATP. *Mutarotation* (change from axial to equilibrial positions) is responsible for the equilibration of the alpha and beta forms of the cyclical molecule.

LIPIDS

Lipids include a variety of compounds some of which are phospholipids, waxes, and fatty acids. A lipid is a nonpolar molecule with a carboxyl head and a long hydrocarbon tail (the polarity created by the carboxyl is overshadowed by the large number of nonpolar hydrocarbons). If the chain contains double bonds, it is either unsaturated (contains one double bond) or polyunsaturated (contains more than one double bond). Fats are the primary energy-storage molecules. The large number of carbon-hydrogen bonds, which release energy when metabolized, explains why fats provide twice as much energy per gram as do carbohydrates and proteins.

Micelles are spherical bodies comprised of many fatty acid soap molecules. The carboxylate groups are hydrophilic and polar; these ends point outward. The hydrophobic and nonpolar hydrocarbon ends point inward. Micelles are soluble in water because the nonpolar ends are shielded. A micelle can trap a nonpolar molecule (i.e., grease, fats, dirt) by engulfing it into the nonpolar internal region while remaining solvated in the polar medium.

AMINES

Amines are nitrogen-containing compounds derived from ammonia. The lone pair of electrons on the nitrogen affects many properties of amines. As expected, the electrons are involved in hydrogen bonding, giving amines high melting and boiling points. The electrons enable the amine to react as a nucleophile.

Optically Active Stereoisomers

All optically active stereoisomers have the same physical properties with the exception of the rotation of plane polarized light. In other words, enantiomers show the same IR and NMR spectroscopic results and have the same boiling points, melting points, and solubility.

ACID-BASE CHEMISTRY

General Information

RELEVANCE TO UNDERSTANDING REACTIONS

A thorough review of acid-base chemistry could very well be the best approach in preparing for the organic chemistry section of the DAT. In most reactions, the acidity or basicity of the reactants determines the products. The ability to predict the way in which a compound will react with another compound is a necessary tool for success on test day. In addition, resonance and inductive effects, two favorites of the ADA Department of Testing Services, are covered in this section as related topics. You will find it very difficult to grasp the information presented in Sections VIII and IX on mechanisms, reactions, and synthesis if you have not mastered the fundamentals of acid-base chemistry. *Therefore, be sure to spend adequate time and effort in reviewing this section—there is a high probability that this investment will equate to a better score on the DAT.*

REVIEW OF DEFINITIONS

Brönsted-Lowry Acid and Base

A Brönsted-Lowry *acid* can *donate a proton*. A Brönsted-Lowry *base* can *accept a proton*. Under the Brönsted-Lowry definitions, acids and bases equilibrate into conjugate acids and conjugate bases. The conjugate base of an acid is usually a molecule that has given off a proton and has taken on a negative charge, therefore becoming a Brönsted-Lowry base. The conjugate acid of a base is usually a molecule that has taken on a proton, becoming positively charged and likewise a Brönsted-Lowry acid.

Brönsted-Lowry reactions involve two acids and two bases in equilibrium, as is easily seen with the addition of an acid to water. The *dissociation equilibrium* must shift to the right for an acid to be characterized as strong. The following equation illustrates that strong acids exist on the right side of the equilibrium. In calculating the K_a, this increases the value of the numerator, and therefore strong acids have large K_a values.

$$HA + H_2O \leftrightarrow H_3O^+ + A^-$$
$$acid + base \leftrightarrow conjugate\ acid + conjugate\ base$$

or

$$Conjugate\ acid + conjugate\ base \leftrightarrow acid + base$$
$$K_a = \frac{[H_3O^+]\ [A^-]}{[HA]}$$

Lewis Acid and Base

A Lewis *acid* is *an electron pair acceptor*. A Lewis *base* is *an electron pair donor*. Whenever a lone pair of electrons exists in a Lewis dot structure, the molecule is a base. Whenever a vacant *p* orbital exists, the molecule is an acid. When dealing with ions, remember that cations are acids and anions are bases.

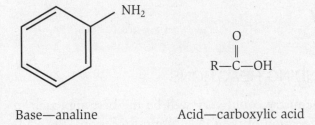

Base—analine   Acid—carboxylic acid

STRENGTH AND STABILITY OF ACIDS AND BASES

The stronger the conjugate base, the weaker the acid, and the stronger the conjugate acid, the weaker the base. To evaluate the strength of an acid or a base, it is necessary to evaluate the stability of its conjugate. Resonance, inductive effects, and electronegativity will affect the stability of the conjugate.

Resonance

TERMS AND CONCEPTS

To understand resonance and to be able to draw resonance forms, it is necessary to understand that *electrons are not static*. Electrons are constantly moving from one atom to the next. Learning what will cause the electrons to leave an atom is crucial. When electrons move around within the atomic framework of a molecule, this phenomenon is referred to as *resonance*. Pictorial representations of the positions that electrons may have are called *resonance forms*. A combination of these resonance forms is a representative structure called a *resonance hybrid*.

Resonance increases the stability of a molecule. The more stable an individual resonance form is, the greater its contribution to the resonance hybrid. Delocalization of electrons can occur with adjacent *p* orbitals connected by pi bonds. In the case of benzene, it was shown that through delocalization the electrons were spread over the cyclical structure, forming what were described as electron clouds above and below the ring. It was also mentioned that all aromatic compounds are extremely stable molecules.

RULES FOR DRAWING RESONANCE FORMS

It is important to be able to draw resonance structures quickly. The following rules should help in understanding which electrons move where and why:

- Atoms do not move; only electrons move.

- A molecule that has a charge does not lose the charge unless there is interaction with another molecule.

- The total number of electrons does not change.

- The Lewis structures of molecules must remain accurate when electrons move.

- Electrons will move toward a positive charge.

- Negative charges prefer to be on electronegative atoms.

- A resonance form with a greater number of covalent bonds is more stable than one with fewer covalent bonds.

- A resonance form that has fewer charges is more stable than one with a greater number of charges.

- A resonance form with complete octets is more stable than one that lacks complete octets.

> **TIP**
>
> **Remember:**
> Resonance increases stability, and strong acids have stable conjugate bases.

EFFECTS OF RESONANCE ON ACIDITY

One method of determining the strength of an acid is to evaluate the resonance of the conjugate base.

A.

B.

Inductive Effects and Electronegativity

When the electron density of a molecule shifts toward the more electronegative atom, a partially positive charge is created. This charge can help stabilize the conjugate base of an acid that is deprotonated. When the electronegative atom bonds to a hydrogen atom in the acid (HF or HBr), the effect increases the stabilization of the conjugate. When, however, there are atoms between the electronegative atom and the hydrogen (Cl–CH$_2$–COOH or Cl–CH$_2$–CH$_2$–OH), the *effect is termed inductive*. The shift of electron density is simply polarization due to a highly electronegative atom. The farther the hydrogen is from the electronegative element, the less the effect.

MECHANISMS AND REACTIONS OF THE MAJOR FUNCTIONAL GROUPS

General Information

BRIEF REVIEW

A very brief reminder of some concepts from Section XII on kinetics of the general chemistry chapter is included in this section. *You should review the relevant topics of general chemistry before reviewing this section.*

A reaction that gives off heat is *exothermic*, and one that absorbs heat is *endothermic* (a change in *enthalpy* occurs). Some reactions do not proceed directly from reactants to products; these reactions create *intermediates* in *transition states*. The difference between the energy levels of the reactants and the intermediates is the *activation energy*. *Catalysts* (enzymes) lower the activation energy. Gibbs free-energy diagrams graphically illustrate these concepts.

STRUCTURE AND STABILITY OF RADICALS

Very often the intermediates in reactions are radicals, and an assessment of their stability is necessary in order to predict the products. The determinants for stability hold true for determining the stability of radicals as well. In general, the more substituted the alkyl radical, the more stable it becomes. The following diagram indicates, in order of stability, the radicals most frequently encountered.

Alkane Reactions

FREE-RADICAL HALOGENATION OF ALKANES

This reaction involves three steps: initiation, propagation, and termination. *Initiation* is the formation of a halogen radical. These initial halogen radicals are formed by heat or light in an *endothermic* process, requiring much energy. *Propagation* is a chain reaction in which a product and another halogen radical are formed. In this homolytic cleavage, the halogen radical bonds with hydrogen, creating HX and an alkyl radical. The radical produced in the propagation step splits a nearby X_2 molecule, and the reaction continues until the reactant is fully exhausted or all the radicals bind in the termination step. The *termination* step, which involves two radicals coming together to form a bond, is exothermic and creates a lower, more stable, and therefore more desirable energy state. The general reaction sequence is as follows:

1. Initiation

$$X_2 \xrightarrow[\Delta]{h\upsilon} X - X \longrightarrow 2X\overset{\bullet}{}$$

2. Propagation

$$X\overset{\bullet}{} \quad H - H_2 C - R \longrightarrow R - \overset{\bullet}{C}H_2 + HX$$

$$R - \overset{\bullet}{C}H_2 \quad X - X \longrightarrow R - CXH_2 + X\overset{\bullet}{}$$

3. Termination

$$2 \; R - \overset{\bullet}{C}H_2 \longrightarrow RCH_2CH_2R$$

$$R - \overset{\bullet}{C}H_2 + X\overset{\bullet}{} \longrightarrow R - CXH_2$$

$$2X\overset{\bullet}{} \longrightarrow X_2$$

NUCLEOPHILIC SUBSTITUTION AND ELIMINATION

The Basics

Four types of reactions occur when electron-rich and electron-deficient compounds come into contact. The first two reactions result in substitution on alkanes, whereas the second two result in elimination and therefore the formation of alkenes. Substitution and elimination have characteristic trends that help in determining which type of reaction will occur. Rate-determining steps, first- and second-order rates, and steric considerations are evaluated for each reaction. A rate-determining step is the step in a reaction that requires the most activation energy. First-order rates of reaction are determined by the concentration of one reactant. Second-order reaction rates are determined by the concentrations of two of the reactants. (*Note*: Zero-order-rate reactions occur regardless of the concentrations of the reactants.)

S_N1

This is a *two-step, unimolecular, first-order reaction.* The first step involves the formation of a carbocation intermediate by the dissociation of a leaving group. The second step, as logic predicts, involves an attack by a nucleophile (any carbocation is an obvious target for a nucleophile). This nucleophile becomes the substituted part. S_N1 reactions are first order: they depend only on the concentration of the substrate. The stability of the carbocation determines its reactivity. If a more stable carbocation can be formed in this transition state, formation will occur through a process called *carbocation rearrangement*. It is important to note, when reviewing the mechanism of the S_N1 reaction, that the carbocation can be attacked by the nucleophile from either side, causing a *racemic mixture* (two stereoisomers are produced). This reaction prefers bulky electrophiles (3° < 2° < 1°) and favors *protic solvents*—protons readily available for hydrogen bonding.

S_N2

This is a *one-step, bimolecular, second-order reaction* in which the nucleophile attacks the bond of the electronegative leaving group and there is *no formation of a carbocation*. Just as the leaving group dissociates, the incoming nucleophile bonds. This one-step reaction has *no rate-determining step*.

One of the easiest ways to determine whether a reactant favors the S_N1 or S_N2 reaction is to evaluate the bulk of the reactant. *Inversion of configuration occurs with S_N2.* The *steric hindrance* of large groups physically prevents both the leaving group and the nucleophile from reacting in one step. Therefore, *only primary and secondary carbons will react via S_N2. Tertiary carbons will react only by S_N1.* The S_N2 reaction favors *aprotic solvents*—free of protons for hydrogen bonding.

$E1$

This is a *two-step, unimolecular, first-order reaction* similar to the S_N1 reaction. $E1$'s first step is the dissociation of the leaving group, forming the carbocation. Rather than adding a nucleophile in the next step, however, the compound loses a proton to the nucleophile (strong base). The most *substituted double bond forms, trans preferably*. The rate-determining step is the formation of the carbocation. The $E1$ rate is determined by the concentration of the substrate.

$E2$

This is a *one-step, bimolecular, second-order reaction* similar to the S_N2. The $E2$ is a more effective elimination reaction than the $E1$. The term antiperiplanar, used to describe the position of the proton in reference to the leaving group, refers to the proton's being on the partially positive end. Because of steric hindrances $E2$ reactions do not occur with bulky groups. No rearrangement occurs. The rate is determined by the concentrations of both the nucleophile/base and the substrate.

Here is a comparison of the characteristics of nucleophilic substitution and elimination reactions:

S_N1 vs. $E1$:	$E1$ favors higher temperatures.
S_N2 vs. S_N1:	S_N1's are typically more polar and protic, and have increased substitution, weak nucleophiles, and a low concentration of nucleophiles.
S_N2 vs. $E2$:	$E2$ favors bulky bases with increased branching and heat.
$E1$ vs. $E2$:	$E2$ favors a stronger base and a higher concentration of the base.

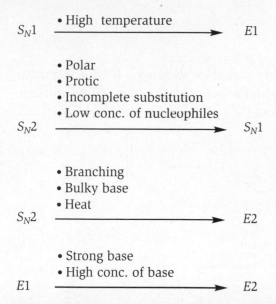

S_N1　• High temperature　⟶　$E1$

S_N2　• Polar
　• Protic
　• Incomplete substitution
　• Low conc. of nucleophiles　⟶　S_N1

S_N2　• Branching
　• Bulky base
　• Heat　⟶　$E2$

$E1$　• Strong base
　• High conc. of base　⟶　$E2$

Alkene and Alkyne Reactions

The electrons in the pi bonds of alkenes and alkynes are responsible for the reactions with other compounds. Generally, these two types of substances react as electron-rich compounds.

MARKOVNIKOV'S RULE—HX ADDITION

Markovnikov's rule states that the electrophilic addition of a hydrogen to a double bond will occur at the carbon that has the greatest number of hydrogens. Stability of the carbocation intermediate dictates the placement of substituents in this addition reaction.

$$CH_3 — CH_2 — CH = CH_2 \longrightarrow CH_3 — CH_2 — CH^+ — CH_3 \longrightarrow CH_3\ CH_2\ CHCH_3$$

$$\underset{\text{HCl addition}}{} \qquad\qquad\qquad \underset{\text{Major product}}{\overset{\displaystyle |}{Cl}}$$

ANTI-MARKOVNIKOV REACTIONS—RADICAL HALOGENATION

In an anti-Markovnikov reaction, a radical halogen first bonds to the lesser substituted carbon of the alkene. The resulting radical reacts with the hydrogen of a hydrogen halide forming an anti-Markovnikov product and another halogen radical. Thus, the hydrogen bonds to the carbon with fewer hydrogens in an anti-Markovnikov reaction.

Reactions of Oxygen-Containing Molecules

In the presence of acids, the hydroxy group is replaced in a substitution reaction or removed in an elimination reaction.

ALCOHOLS

Oxidation to Aldehydes

With a weak oxidizing agent, such as pyridinium chlorochromate (PCC), a primary alcohol can be oxidized to an aldehyde. With further oxidation the alcohol will continue to react until it forms a carboxylic acid.

PCC as Oxidizing Agent

Dehydration to Alkenes

Dehydration is one method of creating alkenes. The hydroxy group and a hydrogen leave in an elimination reaction, producing water and an alkene.

$$H_3C - CH_2OH \xrightarrow[H_2SO_4]{Heat} H_2C = CH_2 + H_2O$$

Formation of Esters from Alcohols and Carboxylic Acids

In the most common method of creating an ester, the alcohol hydroxyl group and the proton from the acid leave and the alkyl group from the alcohol bonds to the resonance-stabilized deprotonated carbonyl group on the acid. The hydroxyl group from the alcohol and the proton from the acid combine to form water, leaving behind an ester.

$$R - COOH + R' - OH \underset{\longleftarrow}{\overset{H^+}{\longrightarrow}} R - \overset{\overset{\displaystyle O}{\|}}{C} - OR' + H_2O$$

ALDEHYDES AND KETONES

Aldehydes and ketones are subject to nucleophilic attack.

Reactions with Grignard Reagents

When Grignard reagents and other nucleophiles come in contact with aldehydes and ketones, addition reactions occur. These reactions result in the formation of a number of alcohols. Grignards are alkylmagnesium halides with the general formula RMgX.

$$HCHO + RMgBr \longrightarrow R-CH_2-OMgBr \xrightarrow{H_2O} R-CH_2OH$$

Reactions with Alcohols

When the electrophilic carbon is attacked by an alcohol, the aldehyde or ketone undergoes a nucleophilic addition reaction and adds to the carbonyl group. When one alcohol reacts, the result is either the formation of a hemiacetal from an aldehyde or the formation of a hemiketal from a ketone. When a second molecule reacts, the hemiacetal and hemiketal form the acetal and ketal, respectively.

1.

$$R-CHO + R'-OH \xrightarrow{H^+} \begin{matrix} OH \\ | \\ R-C-OR' \\ | \\ H \end{matrix} \qquad \text{Hemiacetal}$$

2.

$$\begin{matrix} OH \\ | \\ R-C-OR' \\ | \\ H \end{matrix} \xrightarrow[H^+]{R'OH} \begin{matrix} OR' \\ | \\ R-C-OR' \\ | \\ H \end{matrix} \qquad \text{Acetal}$$

3.

$$\begin{matrix} O \\ \| \\ R-C-R' \end{matrix} + R''OH \xrightarrow{H^+} \begin{matrix} OH \\ | \\ R-C-R' \\ | \\ OR'' \end{matrix} \qquad \text{Hemiketal}$$

4.

$$\begin{matrix} OH \\ | \\ R-C-R' \\ | \\ OR'' \end{matrix} \xrightarrow{R''OH, H^+} \begin{matrix} OR' \\ | \\ R-C-R' \\ | \\ OR'' \end{matrix} \qquad \text{Ketal}$$

Oxidation

The oxidation of aldehydes involves two common reagents, Tollen's and Benedict's. Note that the oxidation of alcohols with Tollen's reagent is often referred to as the silver mirror test. Since, whenever there is oxidation there is reduction (and vice versa), Tollen's reagent forms silver metal from the reduction of a silver salt *only in the presence of an aldehyde.*

Tollen's reagent

$$RCHO + Ag(NH_3)_2 \xrightarrow{OH^-} \begin{matrix} O \\ \| \\ RCO^- \end{matrix} + Ag^+$$

Benedict's reagent

$$RCHO + Cu^{2+} \xrightarrow{OH^-} \begin{matrix} O \\ \| \\ RCO^- \end{matrix} + Cu_2OH$$

Aldol Condensation

When an aldehyde and a ketone come together in the presence of a dilute acid or base, the two molecules combine. The products are either hydroxyaldehydes or hydroxyketones.

O
R
R'
O⁻
Base
H
OH
Δ

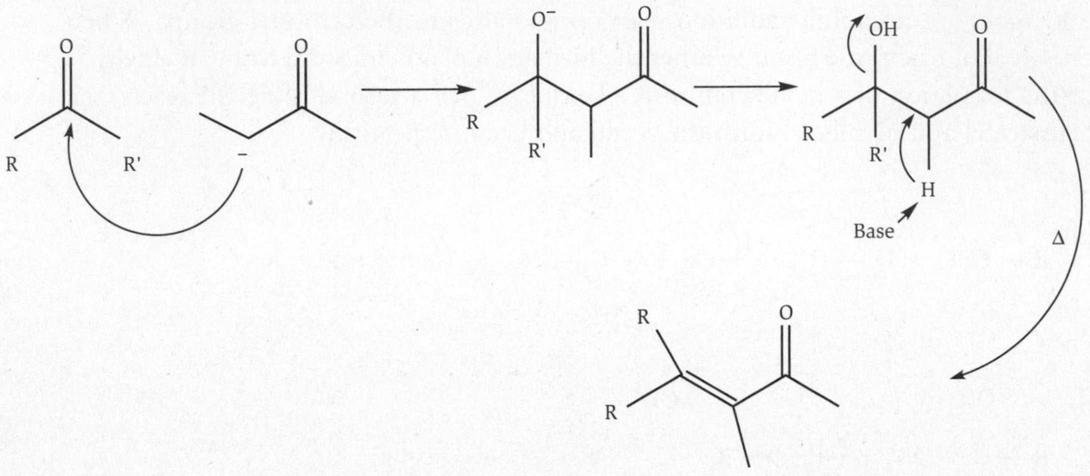

Keto-Enol Tautomerism

Any carbonyl compound with an alpha hydrogen is subject to interconversion between keto and enol forms. (*Note*: the term *enol* refers to a compound that contains a double bond and an alcohol.) The conversion is referred to as tautomerism. The keto form is more stable.

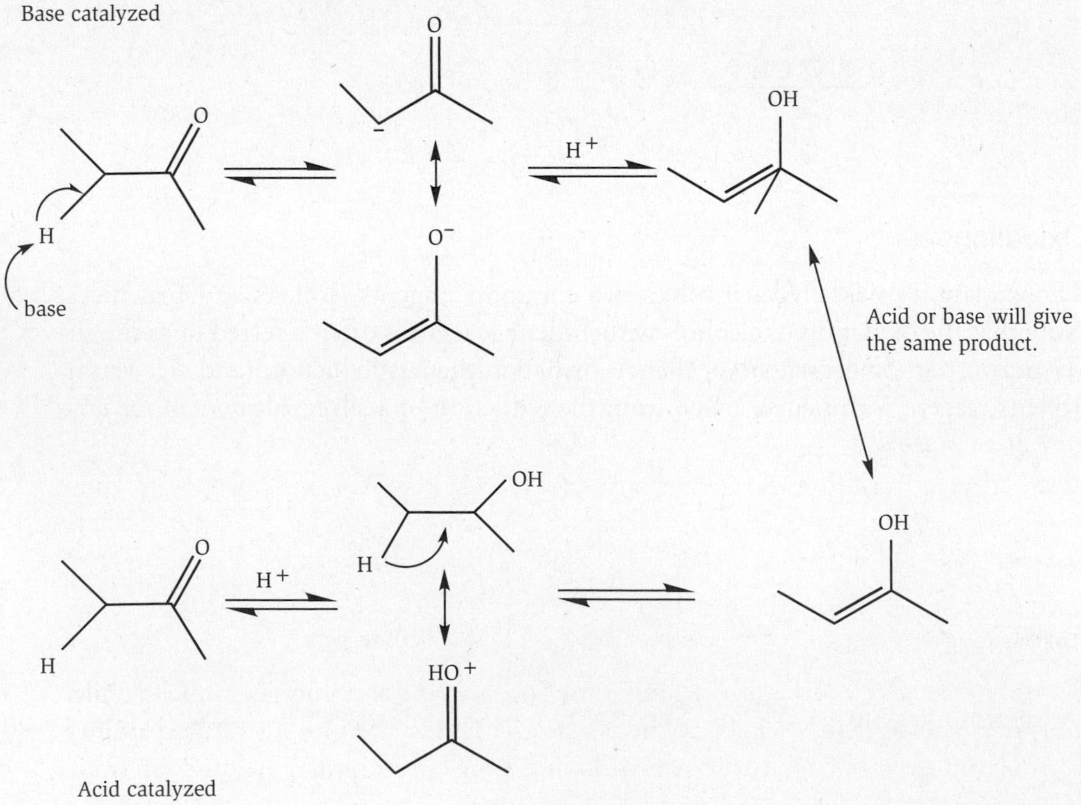

Base catalyzed
O
H
base
O⁻
H+
OH
Acid or base will give the same product.
H+
HO+
Acid catalyzed

CARBOXYLIC ACIDS

Carboxylic acids are acidic because of the stability of the carboxylate ion, the conjugate base.

Nucleophilic Substitution Reaction

Whereas aldehydes and ketones prefer nucleophilic addition reactions, carboxylic acids prefer nucleophilic substitution reactions. The general reaction is as follows:

$$X = Cl^-, Br^-, {}^-OR, {}^-NH_2$$

Esterification

The reaction of a carboxylic acid with an alcohol results in an ester and water.

$$RCOOH + R'OH \xrightleftharpoons{H^+} R - \overset{\overset{\displaystyle O}{\|}}{C} - OR + H_2O$$

Formation of Anhydrides

The reaction of two carboxylic acids creates a special type of molecule referred to as an *anhydride*.

$$2\ RCOOH \longrightarrow R - \overset{\overset{\displaystyle O}{\|}}{C} - O - \overset{\overset{\displaystyle O}{\|}}{C} - R + H_2O$$

Reactions of Carbohydrates and Amines

CARBOHYDRATES

There are three reactions to note for carbohydrates: glycoside formation, ether formation, and ester formation. Glycosides are nonreducing sugars (i.e., negative Tollen's silver mirror test). They are acetals that do not undergo mutorotation.

AMINES

The lone pair of electrons in an amine make this compound act as a nucleophile. Ammonia and primary amines are the best nucleophiles; in more substituted amines the electrons are not able to react with incoming electrophiles because of steric hindrances. Amines react with electrophiles and carbonyls to form *imines* and *amides*, respectively.

1.

2.

SYNTHESIS

General Information

Methods of synthesis are given for various types of organic compounds. Note that there are multiple methods of creating compounds. Some methods yield higher percentages of the desired product, while other methods may work only under special conditions. It is important to learn what reagent will convert one species to another. Familiarity with the basic types of synthesis reactions is far more important than memorization of all of the mechanisms of formation.

Alkanes—Wurtz Reaction

The Wurtz reaction, in which the two alkyl groups from the alkyl bromides are joined and sodium bromide is formed as a side product, is used to make longer chains of hydrocarbons.

$$2RBr + 2Na \rightarrow RR + 2NaBr$$

Alkenes and Alkynes

ALKENES

The substitution of the alkane starting material dictates which method is used to create the pi bond present in alkenes. All three methods involve elimination reactions.

Dehydrohalogenation

Dehydrohalogenation involves the removal of hydrogen and a halogen from an alkane with a halogen substituent. Here is an example:

$$CH_3CH_2Br + KOH \longrightarrow CH_2 = CH_2 + H_2O + KBR$$

Dehydration

In dehydration, a hydroxy and a hydrogen are removed, forming an alkene and water. The starting material is an alcohol.

Dehalogenation

Dehalogenation occurs when adjacent carbons of an alkane are substituted with halogens. Here is an example:

$$BrCH_2CH_2Br + Zn \longrightarrow CH_2 = CH_2 + ZnBr_2$$

ALKYNES

Dehydrohalogenation

The dehydrohalogenation process is basically similar to that for the formation of alkenes. The difference is that there is more KOH to remove the alkene hydrogens forming the second pi bond of the alkyne.

Dehalogenation

The dehalogenation process is basically similar to that for the formation of alkenes. The difference is that the alkane starting material has two halogens on each of the adjacent carbons, permitting the formation of two pi bonds.

Alcohols, Aldehydes, and Ketones

ALCOHOLS

Hydration of Alkenes

The hydration of alkenes follows Markovnikov's rule:

Grignard Reagents

The formation of alcohols using magnesium bromide in the presence of anhydride and ether follows:

1.

$$RMgBr + HCHO \xrightarrow[\text{Ether}]{\text{Anhydride}} RCH_2OMgBr \xrightarrow{H^+} RCH_2OH$$

2.

$$RMgBr + R'CHO \xrightarrow[\text{Ether}]{\text{Anhydride}} \underset{H}{\overset{R'}{RC-OMgBr}} \xrightarrow{H^+} \underset{H}{\overset{R'}{RC-OH}}$$

3.

$$RMgBr + R'-\overset{R''}{C}=O \xrightarrow[\text{Ether}]{\text{Anhydride}} R'-\underset{R}{\overset{R''}{C}}-OMgBr \xrightarrow{H^+} R'-\underset{R}{\overset{R''}{C}}-OH$$

Reduction of Aldehydes and Ketones

Formation of an alcohol is easily accomplished by the reduction of carbonyl compounds by $LiAlH_4$ or $NaBH_4$. Ketones reduce to secondary alcohols and aldehydes, and carboxylic acid derivatives reduce to primary alcohols. Some milder reducing agents can reduce carboxylic acid derivatives to aldehydes, but not to alcohols.

ALDEHYDES

Mild Oxidation of a 1° Alcohol

This oxidation reaction proceeds as follows:

$$RCH_2OH \xrightarrow{Cu, \Delta} R-CHO$$

Oxidation of a Diol

The formation of two aldehydes results from the splitting of a diol, a molecule with two hydroxy groups.

$$R-\overset{OH}{\underset{}{CH}}-\overset{OH}{\underset{}{CH}}-R' \xrightarrow{HIO_4} R'-CHO + R'-CHO$$

KETONES

Mild Oxidation of a 2° Alcohol

This oxidation reaction proceeds as follows:

$$\xrightarrow[\text{H}_2\text{SO}_4]{\text{CrO}_3}$$

Ozonolysis

The starting material for ozonolysis can be linear or cyclic. Depending on the substitution of the double bond, an aldehyde or ketone is formed.

Formation of ketone or aldehyde

Decarboxylation of Carboxylic Acids

The decarboxylation reaction proceeds as follows:

$$2RCOO \xrightarrow{\text{ThO}_2, \Delta} R - \overset{\overset{\displaystyle O}{\|}}{C} - R + CO_2$$

Carboxylic Acids, Esters, and Ethers

CARBOXYLIC ACIDS

Oxidation of Alkenes

This oxidation reaction proceeds as follows:

$$R{-}CH = CH{-}R' \ + \ KMnO_4 \longrightarrow R{-}\underset{\underset{\displaystyle OH}{|}}{\overset{\overset{\displaystyle H}{|}}{C}}{-}\underset{\underset{\displaystyle OH}{|}}{\overset{\overset{\displaystyle H}{|}}{C}}{-}R' \xrightarrow{\text{KMnO}_4} RCOOH \ + \ R'COOH$$

Grignard Reagent with Carbon Dioxide

The two-step formation of a carboxylic acid using carbon dioxide and Grignard reagents proceeds as follows:

$$RMgBr \ + \ CO_2 \longrightarrow R - \overset{\overset{\displaystyle O}{\|}}{C} - OMgBr \xrightarrow{H^+} R - \overset{\overset{\displaystyle O}{\|}}{C} - OH$$

Oxidation of 1° Alcohols

This oxidation reaction proceeds as follows:

Saponification of Esters

This saponification reaction proceeds as follows:

$$R - \overset{\overset{\displaystyle O}{\|}}{C} - O - R' \ + \ NAOH \ \rightleftharpoons \ R'OH + R - \overset{\overset{\displaystyle O}{\|}}{C} - ONa \ \xrightarrow{H^+} \ R - COOH$$

ESTERS—ACID AND ALCOHOL

See the reactions of alcohols.

ETHERS

Williamson Ether Synthesis

In Williamson ether synthesis, the reaction between an alcohol and a strong base results in an alkoxide that reacts via an S_N2 process to form an ether.

Dehydration

The result of the dehydration of two alcohols is the formation of an ether:

$$2CH_3 - CH_2OH \ \xrightarrow{H_2SO_4, \ \Delta} \ CH_3 - CH_2 - O - CH_2 - CH_3$$

ORGANIC ANALYSIS

General Concepts

All too often the desired product of a chemical reaction is accompanied by undesirable secondary products. The following section discusses tests to determine what organic substances are present and how to separate them to produce a pure yield of the desired product.

Some Simple Chemical Tests

TIP

Remember: Aqueous acids extract organic bases, and aqueous bases extract organic acids.

When compounds have different solubilities, *extraction* can be used to separate them. Often the compounds are chemically altered to create a species soluble in aqueous solution.

Distillation is used to separate compounds with different boiling points. When two compounds in a liquid mixture are heated, the one with the lower boiling point will vaporize first, leaving behind the higher boiling point compound, which will also vaporize once its boiling point is reached. The vapors can be condensed and collected, yielding two pure compounds.

Crystallization is a type of purification involving the heating of a solid in a solution until the solvent evaporates. The crystallization of a precipitate follows as the supersaturated solution cools.

Chromatography is the separation of the components of a mixture based on differences in solubility and polarity. Chromatography involves the distribution of solutes between a moving phase and a stationary phase. There are four types of chromatography.

1. *Thin-layer chromatography (TLC)* incorporates a thin layer of stationary phase (typically silica gel) on a flat surface, usually a glass or plastic plate. The distances traveled by the components of the mixture because of capillary action permit the identification of these components on the basis of characteristic polarity.

2. *Column chromatography* can be thought of as inverted TLC. Rather than traveling across a plate because of capillary action, in column chromatography the mixture runs down a column. The mobile phase can be altered, changing its affinity for the polarity of a solvent.

3. *Gas chromatography* requires the evaporation of a mixture. The vapors are passed through inert gas, the mobile phase, and through a column with the stationary phase.

4. *High-performance liquid chromatography* is done at high pressure with liquids as the mobile phase. Depending on the solid material in the column, applications include reverse phase chromatography, molecular sieving, ion exchange chromatography, and affinity chromatography.

Chromatography is a very useful method of identification and separation in the laboratory.

Infrared (IR) Spectroscopy

CONCEPT OF OSCILLATION FREQUENCIES

The bonds of a molecule can be stretched and bent. The frequency of bond vibrations can be used to identify unknown specimens. Atoms slow the vibrations according to their mass. Each functional group has a range of oscillation frequencies that is determined by the numbers and types of bonds and atoms. When infrared electromagnetic energy passes through a molecule, the molecule will vibrate or absorb the energy, if the natural frequency of the molecule equals the energy, according to this formula:

$$E = h(c/\lambda)$$

Then, since $c/\lambda = v$,

$$E = hv$$

COMMON IR SPECTRUMS

You should memorize the absorbencies of the major functional groups. The units are reciprocal centimeters (cm^{-1}).

Functional Group	IR Absorbance (cm⁻¹)
–CH	2850–2960
=CH	3020–3100
≡C–H	3300
–C=C–	1650–1670
–C≡C–	2100–2260
Aromatics	1500–1600
–C≡N	2210–2260
–O–H	3400–3640, broad
–N–H	3310–3500, broad
C=O	
Aldehyde	1690–1740
Ketone	1680–1750
Esters	1735–1750
Amides	1630–1690
C–O; Ethers and esters	1080–1300

Nuclear Magnetic Resonance (NMR) Spectroscopy

NMR AND THE CONCEPT OF CHEMICAL SHIFT VALUES

Electrons spin, and this spin creates a magnetic field. If a molecule is placed in a magnetic field, some of the protons spinning in the same direction will align with the applied field, whereas others will spin in a direction that creates a field that opposes the applied field. The direction can be changed if a proton spinning against the field absorbs the electromagnetic radiation. At this point, an NMR tracing signal, referred to as a chemical shift value, can be observed.

It is important to note that the *number* of signals describes the number of different protons. The *position* of the signals describes the environment of the proton. The *intensity* of the signals indicates how many of each kind of proton exist. The *splitting* of a signal describes the proton's environment in relation to other protons and is further discussed in the next section.

Here is an example of an NMR tracing.

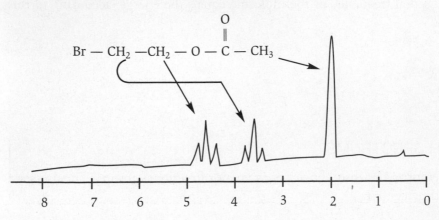

SPIN-SPIN SPLITTING

The effect of adjacent and neighboring hydrogens on adjacent carbons is explained in spin-spin splitting. The direction of spin of the nearby proton creates a magnetic field that will oppose or align with that of a given proton. The number of different ways in which the spins can occur determines the number of signal splits that will result. A lone proton signal will be split into four signals, a quartet (one signal is a singlet; two signals, a doublet; three signals, a triplet), if three protons are adjacent. This situation is explained by illustrating the possible spins.

	❶	❷	❸	❹
1.	↑	↑	↑	↑
2.	↑	↑	↑	↓
3.	↑	↑	↓	↓
4.	↑	↓	↓	↓

Also, note that like protons will not split each other. Like protons must be chemically and magnetically equivalent. Only one signal results from equivalent protons.

SHIELDING AND DESHIELDING

The electrons create a magnetic field. If this field reduces the strength of the applied field, the proton is shielded; if it enhances the applied field, the proton is deshielded. Shielding creates an upfield shift, to the right, and deshielding creates a downfield shift, to the left.

CHEMICAL SHIFT VALUES

You should memorize the following chemical shift values of the major functional groups.

Functional Group	NMR Chemical Shift (δ)
$R-CH_3$	0.8–1.0
$R-CH_2-R$	1.2–1.4
$Ph-CH_3$	2.2–2.5
$R-CH_2-Cl$	3.6–3.8
$R-CH_2-Br$	3.4–3.6
$R-CH_2-I$	3.1–3.3
$R-O-CH_3$	3.3–3.9
$R-CO-CH_3$	2.1–2.6
$RCHO$	9.5–9.6
$Ph-H$	6.0–9.5
$RC{\equiv}CH$	2.5–3.1
$R_2C{=}CHR$	5.2–5.7

Perceptual Ability Test Review

OUTLINE

OVERVIEW

What Is the Perceptual Ability Test?

The Perceptual Ability Test (PAT) is perhaps the most unusual component of the DAT. It is a measure of your ability to perceive and consider two- and three-dimensional forms and is probably unlike any other type of test you have taken. The test is composed of six parts that appear in the following order: aperture passing, orthographic projection, angle discrimination, paper folding, cubes, and form development.

Details of the Test

The PAT is administered second, directly following the Survey of Natural Sciences. There is a total of 90 items on the PAT, divided evenly among the six parts (15 questions each). Although there are 90 questions, only 75 of them are scored. The remaining 15 are experimental questions that are scattered randomly throughout the PAT sections. You will *not* be able to identify these experimental questions. You are given 60 minutes to complete the 90 questions.

The six parts of the PAT are arranged in sections of 15 questions. However, even though the sections are discrete, they are administered as a unit with no time breaks between them. This means that you have the freedom to skip ahead to a particular section first, if you wish, and later return to address the skipped sections. Within the 60-minute time frame, you may address the PAT as you wish.

Taking the Test

Considering the allotted time and the number of test items, you have an average of 40 seconds to complete each question and an average of 10 minutes to complete each section. As you will come to discover through practice, some questions are quite time consuming, while others have answers that seem readily apparent.

There is no right number of seconds or minutes to spend on each question and section. Perhaps the best rule to follow is that you should progress through the test to completion at a productive pace. If you find yourself spending too much time on a difficult item and thus failing to maintain your established pace, you should leave that question and later, time permitting, return to it. As you take the practice tests in this book, you should time yourself on at least one of the two tests. It might be useful to complete one test at a comfortable pace, but record precisely how long you spent on each perceptual ability section. This will give you an index of the relative time it took you to complete each group of questions.

Perceptual Ability? I Just Want to Become a Dentist

In examining the utility of the PAT, the American Dental Association ran a study to assess the correlation between performance on this test and preclinical performance in laboratory settings that require a high degree of manual dexterity. The result is not surprising—performance on the PAT and preclinical performance in laboratory settings are indeed significantly correlated. The study and the practice of dentistry demand the ability to conceive of objects spatially. A strong performance on the PAT reflects the sort of mental agility useful in the profession.

Additionally, it should be mentioned that, in light of the correlation between PAT scores and performance in dental school, Admissions Committees hold the PAT score in high regard. These committees examine with particular care two scores that reflect performance on the DAT: (1) total academic and (2) perceptual ability. Arguably, since several individual scores are figured into the total academic score, the perceptual ability score is the single most important score on the DAT.

How Can I Improve My Perceptual Ability?

You will quickly come to learn that perceptual ability (as it is measured by the PAT) is not something that you either *have* or *don't have*. It is a quality that can be nurtured, developed, and enhanced through training. The following review is a comprehensive preparation guide that addresses the details of what to expect on the test and provides explanatory figures and practice exercises.

The components that you need to perfect are: visual perception and visualization and mental imagery. Even if you have perfect vision, you will find that discipline and practice are needed in order to perceive minuscule details. (If you suspect that you don't have very good vision, now is a good time to invest in a pair of glasses.)

The ability to make use of visualization and mental imagery also improves with practice. As you are preparing for the PAT, continue to challenge yourself with mental imagery tasks even after you close this book. Imagine, for example, how the room you are sitting in would be oriented if the entire unit (the room and all its contents) were rotated and flipped. Try to identify the new positionings of various objects in the room. Exercises like this one will help keep your *mind's eye* active throughout the day.

There are also several creative activities, such as origami, that rely on the same skills you will be refining for the PAT. Origami, the Japanese art of paper folding, is a discipline that requires a lot of structure and precision. The intricate origami folds transform a flat piece of paper into a multidimensional form. Involvement in origami will expand your ability to recognize how flat paper can take on a multitude of forms. This activity is most applicable to the part of the PAT called "form development" but will also contribute to your preparation for the paper-folding questions.

Be creative in choosing supplementary activities for your additional practice. By stacking sugar cubes or children's building blocks, you can create cube formations like those illustrated in this book or can create your own. This offers further practice for the painted-surface-counting questions in the cube section of the PAT. Additionally, by using dice, you can practice imagining the location of the surface dots after repositioning each die. This will contribute to enhanced performance on aperture passing and form development questions.

Preparing for the PAT can actually be quite enjoyable. The following preparation review offers clear, easy to understand approaches to each part of the PAT. In each section of the review are highly useful descriptions of the nature of the test questions and appropriate practice exercises. While the additional activities suggested above will help you to generally improve your perceptual abilities, the exercises in each review section are designed to "target train" your perception, visualization and mental imagery, and logical reasoning skills as they apply specifically to the questions on the DAT.

APERTURE PASSING

Introduction

The first section of the Perceptual Ability Test is aperture passing. Here you will be presented with an image of a three-dimensional object and the outlines of five different apertures. Your task is to identify the aperture (or opening) that could accommodate the insertion of the solid object.

An aperture is much like a keyhole. It is an opening through which an object can pass. An aperture-passing item as it appears on the DAT is governed by a number of rules, which are outlined below.

- Although the object is presented in a particular position, it may be turned in any direction prior to insertion.

- Once the object has been started through the opening, it may not be rotated, turned, or twisted in any way.

- Both the aperture and the object are drawn to the same scale.

- There are no irregular or surprising shapes in any portion of the object that are not in clear view as is presented in the three-dimensional rendering.

- The correct aperture is always the exact shape of the object's silhouette.

- In each group of apertures, there is only one aperture that can be used to pass the solid object.

A thorough understanding of these parameters will further enhance your ability to make use of strategy. Perhaps more so than on any other section of the Perceptual Ability Test, the questions on aperture passing exploit your understanding of the rules.

Each rule stated above has a number of consequences that can help you locate the correct answer quickly. Also, when in doubt, application of the rules will help you to eliminate one or more incorrect answer choices, thus improving your chances of selecting the correct response.

The Rules, Their Consequences, and Your Strategy

Although the object is presented in a particular position, it may be turned in any direction prior to insertion. Usually the three-dimensional form will need to be turned or oriented in a position different from the initial presentation. The aperture-passing questions are largely a test of your ability to mentally maneuver obscure forms and to identify appropriate corresponding silhouettes. For this reason, you should assume that most times a degree of maneuvering is required. You may need to imagine either turning the object to align a particular side, or rotating the object horizontally or vertically in order to accommodate the orientation of the aperture.

Each object has six distinct sides: top, bottom, left, right, front, and rear. This first rule implies that the object may be inserted into the aperture top first, bottom first, or any of the sides first. You need not consider any angular insertions that deviate from a distinct side or top entry. Below is an example of an aperture-passing question. The object is pictured at the left.

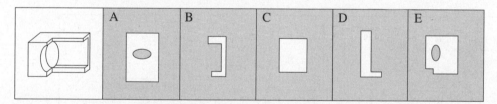

Before examining the possible apertures, choices A–E, it is important that you identify the significance of each line in the three-dimensional drawing. The subtleties of the lines are often overlooked. Also, the aperture shapes can bias your viewing, causing you to overlook the intricate detail of the object. You set yourself up for failure if you examine the apertures before thoroughly understanding the drawing.

The subtleties that you should look for in the drawing are reflected in the following questions:

- Are the outermost surfaces of the object (front, rear, top, bottom, and left and right sides) flat, or are there slopes or protrusions?

- From which direction are protrusions noticeable and unnoticeable?

- Are there any holes or recesses in the form? Where are they?

- Are there any stairlike edges? Are the stairs of equal height?

The second rule states that, *once the object has been started through the opening, it may not be rotated, turned, or twisted in any way.* Although there are six sides to choose from as the entry side, in actuality you need to consider only three sides. Remember that, not only must a side be able to enter the aperture, but also the entire form must be able to follow through. Thus, you need consider only three possibilities: a top/bottom entry and the two different side entries (see figures below).

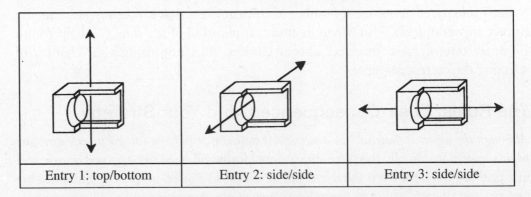

| Entry 1: top/bottom | Entry 2: side/side | Entry 3: side/side |

After you are familiar with the form of the object, you should begin to identify what each of the three silhouettes looks like. A silhouette is an outline of a form that contours the outermost edge. Keep in mind that a silhouette is a contour on a single plane that does not reveal any information about the object's depth. Although the depth of the object is not indicated on a silhouette, all of the points of the object (including the ones that recede into space) will take part in the formation of the silhouette if they extend beyond the image created from the surface being considered. In the following illustration, each of the three silhouettes corresponds to one of the images presented above:

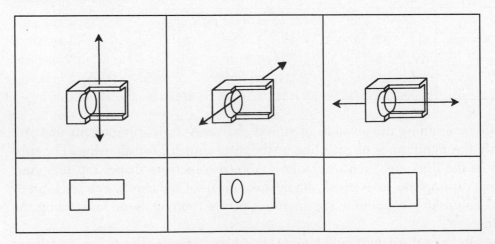

Since, as the third rule states, *both the aperture and the object are drawn to the same scale,* you need to rely heavily on precise comparison between the projected silhouette and the aperture opening. The aperture must accommodate the size of the silhouette. A perfect but smaller silhouette would not allow the three-dimensional shape to be inserted. Hence, it is possible for the aperture to be the same shape but too small for the object. According to the publishers of the DAT, the differences in size are "large enough to be judged by [the precise] eye." You are cautioned, however, to take great care in looking for small differences in size.

Although you are presented with a drawing in which three sides are exposed, there are portions of the object that are not visible in the view that is displayed. The fourth rule states that *there are no irregular or surprising shapes in any portion of the object that are not in clear view as is presented in the three-dimensional rendering.* If, however, the object has symmetric indentations, the hidden portion will be symmetric with the part shown. As a rule, enough information will be presented to allow you to make an informed decision concerning the appropriate opening.

According to the last two rules, *the correct aperture is always the exact shape of the object's silhouette* and *in each group of apertures, there is only one aperture that can be used to pass the solid object.* These rules are clearly to your advantage. Unlike questions that challenge you to select the *best* answer, your task here is to select the *only* answer. Regarding the last rule, if you find that two openings appear to accommodate the object, you are probably overlooking a detail of form or have failed to recognize that one opening is too small. Consider, if you are stumped by multiple answer choices, that you are committing one of the above errors.

With all six of these rules in mind, the appropriate answer to the aperture passing question on page 225 is easily located. Careful consideration of the silhouette helps to eliminate choices B, D, and E. Choice A closely approximates "Entry 3: side/side," but the darkened oval shape is slightly misplaced. Choice C shows the correct aperture through which the object under consideration could pass (see "Entry 3: side/side," on page 226).

Lines as "Builders of the Form"

You need to practice the discipline of attending to lines as "builders of the form." There is a human tendency to approach an oddly shaped, irregular drawing with a mental stereotype of a familiar (household or geometric) form. A desire to deal with the familiar often overshadows the reality of what is presented. If you approach this section of the PAT by attending to lines as "followers of the form," you will unfortunately overlook quite a bit. Most likely you will never before have experienced the oddly shaped form in question. The bias to project ideas about familiar forms will undoubtedly cause you to overlook the actual lines in the drawing.

Keep in mind that all of the forms presented in the aperture-passing section are irregular. They are irregular in the sense that they are not easily describable and correspond only indirectly to familiar geometric shapes. For this reason, you need to take inventory of each line. Overlooking one subtle but important line is often the cause of error in this section. Practice attending to the details offered by each line in the following figure:

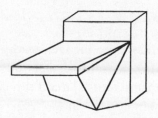

This is a highly complex figure. What makes it so difficult to deal with is the heavy reliance on the lines that is required in order to determine the many spatial planes. Below is the same figure reproduced with visual cues and spatial guidelines.

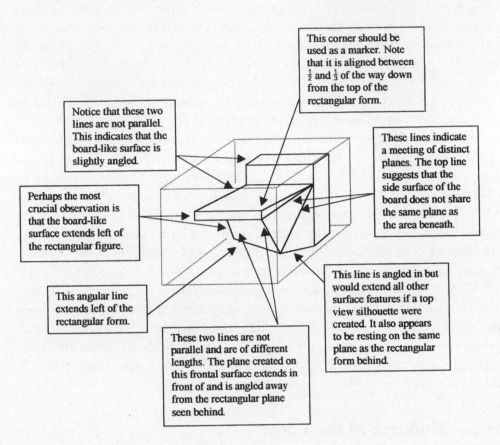

This corner should be used as a marker. Note that it is aligned between $\frac{1}{2}$ and $\frac{1}{3}$ of the way down from the top of the rectangular form.

Notice that these two lines are not parallel. This indicates that the board-like surface is slightly angled.

These lines indicate a meeting of distinct planes. The top line suggests that the side surface of the board does not share the same plane as the area beneath.

Perhaps the most crucial observation is that the board-like surface extends left of the rectangular figure.

This angular line extends left of the rectangular form.

This line is angled in but would extend all other surface features if a top view silhouette were created. It also appears to be resting on the same plane as the rectangular form behind.

These two lines are not parallel and are of different lengths. The plane created on this frontal surface extends in front of and is angled away from the rectangular plane seen behind.

Now consider the various silhouettes that would be produced from both side/side angles and from the top/bottom angle.

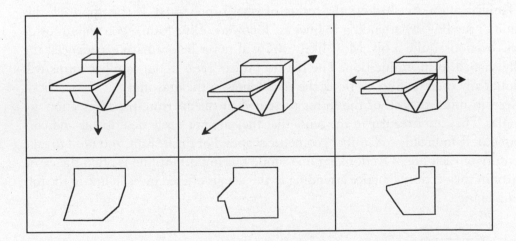

As you work through this section of the PAT, try to maintain a productive, steady pace. Do not let any one question drain you of too much time. If you find that you are stumped on a question, it is to your advantage to move on and return later if time permits. Often, a second consideration of a complex three-dimensional form will bring a fresh perspective if you allow yourself to concentrate on other forms in the meantime.

Review

- Although the object is presented in a particular position, it may be turned in any direction prior to insertion. The three-dimensional form will most often need to be turned or oriented in a position different from the initial presentation.

- You may need to imagine either turning the object to align a particular side, or rotating the object horizontally or vertically in order to accommodate the orientation of the aperture.

- The object may be inserted into the aperture top first, bottom first, or any side first. You need not consider any angular insertions that deviate from a distinct side or top entry.

- Always examine the intricate lines of the object prior to reviewing the aperture choices. The aperture shapes can bias your viewing, causing you to overlook subtle details of the object.

- After you are familiar with the form, you should identify what each of the three silhouettes looks like—side/side, side/side, and top/bottom. Recall that the aperture and the object are drawn to the same scale. Hence, the aperture must be no smaller than the silhouette.

- Only one of the possible five apertures will allow the object to be inserted. If you find that two openings appear to accommodate the object, you are probably overlooking a feature detail or have failed to recognize that an opening is too small.

- Carefully attend to each line. Remember that the forms in aperture passing are highly irregular. Consider the lines to be "builders of the form" rather than "followers of the form."

- Parts of the object that are out of view will not contain any surprising shapes. However, if the object has symmetric indentations, the hidden portion will be symmetric with the part shown.

- Keep to a productive, steady pace. If you find that you are stumped on a question, move on and return later if time permits.

EXERCISE 1

Examine the form presented in each framed box. After carefully studying the lines of the form, create a silhouette for every direction of viewing in the boxes below. Practice visualizing and representing each silhouette scaled to the size of the small image with arrows.

1.

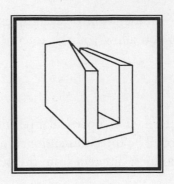

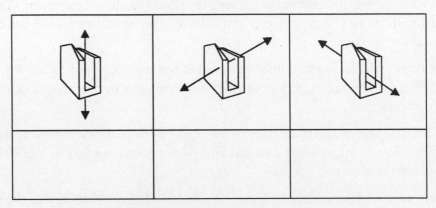

2.

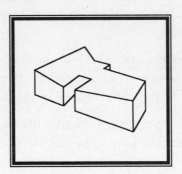

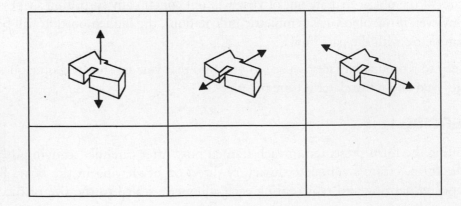

3.

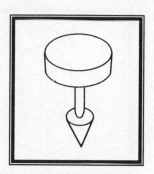

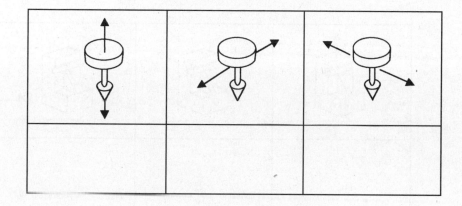

4.

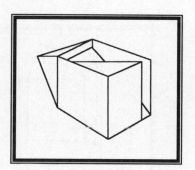

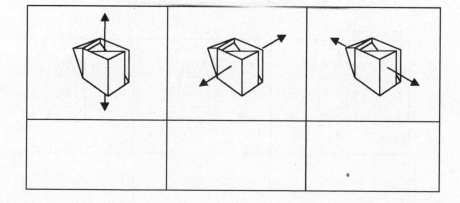

5.

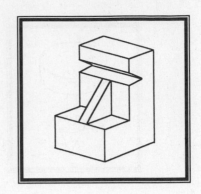

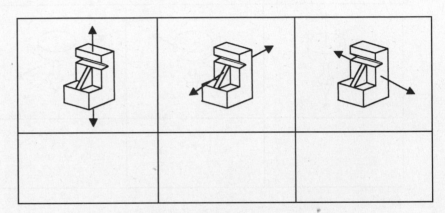

6.

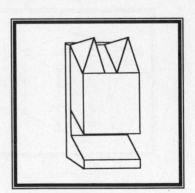

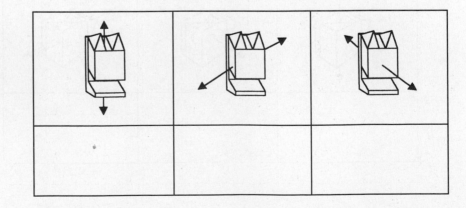

7.

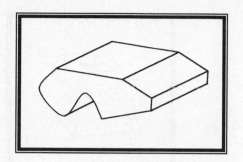

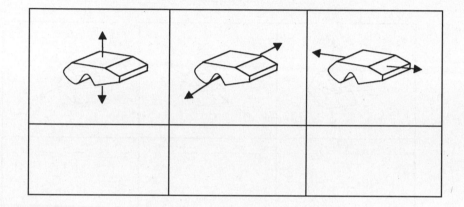

8.

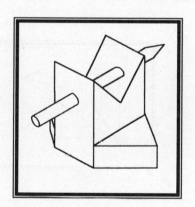

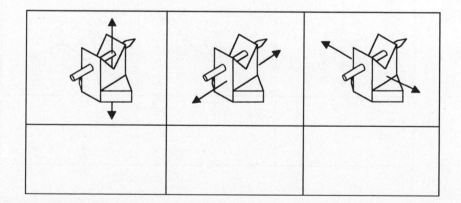

9.

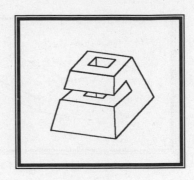

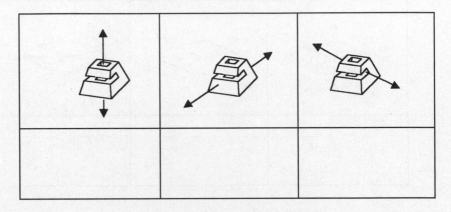

10.

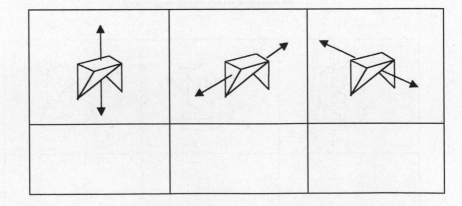

EXERCISE 2

This exercise follows the same format and directions that apply to the aperture-passing questions on the Perceptual Ability Test. Examine the figure shown to the far left. Then choose the aperture that would allow the object to completely pass through the opening if the proper side was inserted first.

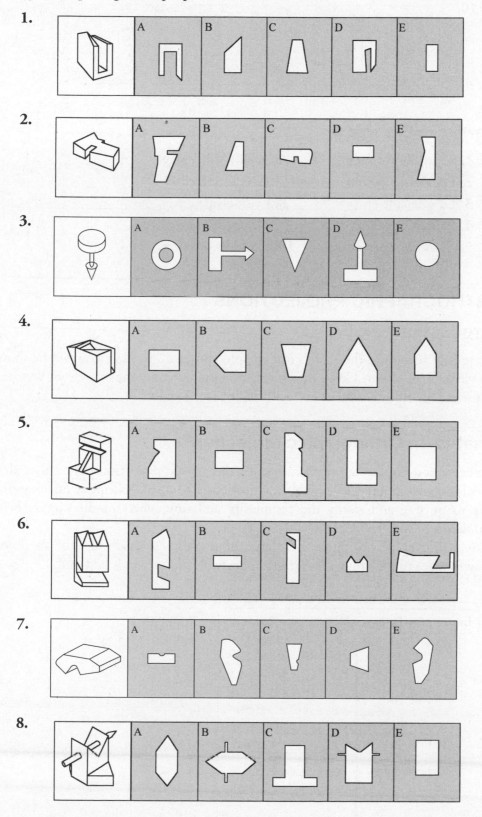

9.

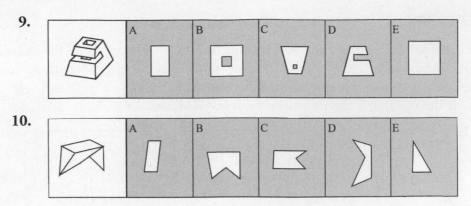

10.

Answers to Exercise 2

1. C, top/bottom entry	**6.** A, side/side entry
2. E, side/side entry	**7.** E, side/side entry
3. D, side/side entry	**8.** C, side/side entry
4. E, side/side entry	**9.** E, top/bottom entry
5. E, top/bottom entry	**10.** C, side/side entry

ORTHOGRAPHIC PROJECTIONS

Introduction

The second section of the PAT is orthographic projections. Here you will be shown two views of an object. Given the information presented by the two views, your task is to select the third view that correctly describes the object.

What Is an Orthographic Projection?

Engineers and architects heavily rely on orthographic projections when they draft plans for construction. Orthographic projections are sets of descriptive drawings that serve to portray and clarify the complexity and uniqueness of the objects being considered.

An orthographic projection is a series of two-dimensional views of an object. Below is an example of how an orthographic projection series is laid out.

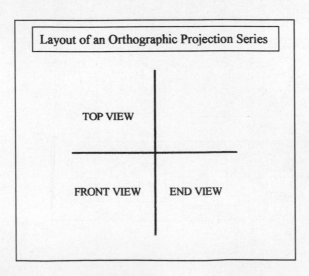

The orthographic projections on the DAT are composed of three views: the top view, front view, and end view. Each of the views is rendered *without perspective*. In other words, each view is drawn as it would appear head on with its planes parallel to the viewer.

In the example of a brick below, examine both the labeled brick shown at the left and its corresponding orthographic projection at the right.

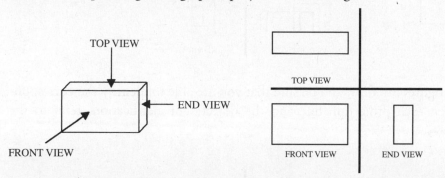

Notice the orientation of each projected image. It is as though the viewer examined each side in turn, walking around the object so that a perfect head-on view could be seen of each face (top, front, and end). Consider each display box (created by the crossed lines) to be a frame for the projection as seen from that particular viewing direction.

On the DAT, the projection layout is identical to that in the example above. The projection looking down at the object is displayed in the upper left hand corner of the projection layout and is labeled "TOP VIEW." The projection looking at the object from the front is displayed in the lower left corner and is labeled "FRONT VIEW." Lastly, the projection looking at the object from the end (or side) is displayed in the lower right corner and is labeled "END VIEW."

The use of both hidden and visible lines is a convention standard to the practice of creating and interpreting an orthographic projection. Visible lines are represented by the solid lines; hidden lines, by dashed lines. Most of the questions in this section of the PAT challenge your understanding and logical reasoning skills concerning the use of solid and dashed lines. Crucial to your success in this section is a strong understanding of when each of the two lines is used.

The Visible Line

As mentioned, a visible line is represented by a solid line. Visible lines are lines that are exposed to you when you view a particular side face on—simply put, visible lines are *visible* to you. Changes in form that are visible *only* from the view being considered and the outline of the object as seen from that view are represented by solid lines.

Examine the use of solid lines to represent visible lines in the following two examples:

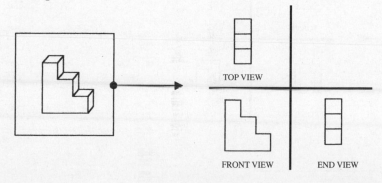

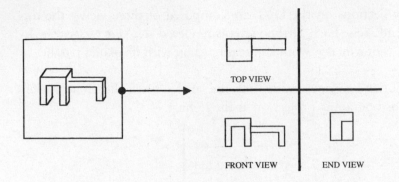

Study the figures carefully, and be sure that you are able to identify the correspondence between each projection line and the object. For clarification, refer to the following:

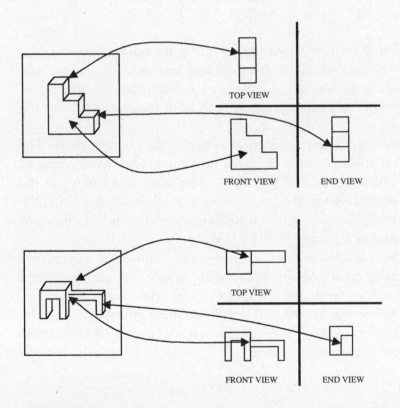

Now notice the slight modification of the second object that has occurred. Instead of a benchlike extension, this object now has a slide that extends from the central unit.

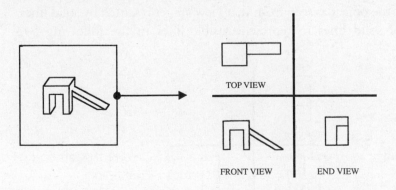

Comparison between the projection series before and after modification reveals that only the front view changes. It is most important to understand why the end view does not change. Examine the line that is highlighted by the arrow in the figure below.

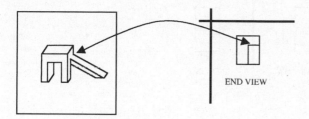

It may not be initially obvious why the end view does not change. To fully understand the use of the solid line (or the *visible line*), you must first understand how it is used in the end view of the modified object. In the figure, the slide extends from the flat surface that is just above it and is parallel to the plane on which the projection is rendered. Any deviation from this parallel plane results in a visible line at the point where the transition from parallel to angular takes place. Creases in the form that are visible from the projection view will always result in a solid line.

Lastly, the point should be made that, to fully describe some highly complex forms, additional projections may be necessary. For example, none of the views examined thus far addresses the wide hidden leg of the second example. In preparing for the PAT, you need be concerned only with mastering the three views discussed (top, front, and end). The end view will refer to the right side of the object in each projection series.

The Hidden Line

A hidden line is represented by a dashed line. Hidden lines refer to edges that cannot be seen because they are either inside or behind the object. These lines provide meaningful cues about an object's depth. In the following examples dashed lines indicate the presence of hidden lines.

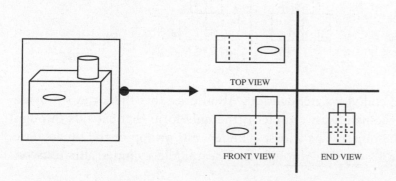

In the first example, the drawing at left shows only a brick with an object on top and an oval on the side. The orthographic projection views reveal that these oval shapes are tubular and travel through the height and width of the brick.

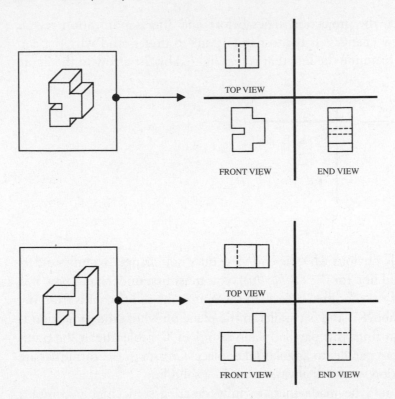

In the second and third examples, notice that the width of the object can be identified by the vertical lines; solid and dashed, in the top view. The lengths of these lines match the width in the end view.

Now examine the following series:

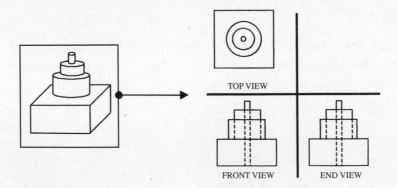

Here, the front and end views are identical. Also notice that these views provide the information that the narrowest cylinder is the only form that extends through the entire height of the object. The widest cylinder rests on top of the square base with the middle cylinder passing through it. The middle cylinder also rests on the base.

Note: When a hidden line is exactly behind a visible line, the part of the dashed line that coincides with the solid (visible) line remains solid. When two hidden lines overlap, the resulting line remains dashed.

Completing the Orthographic Projection Series

On the Perceptual Ability Test, you will be provided with two of the three views discussed above. You will *not* be presented with a perspective drawing; but given the information contained in the views, you will be able to choose the appropriate view that completes the series.

On the PAT the orthographic projection series is laid out with two views and a question mark in place of the third, missing view. This section is much like trying to complete a puzzle. In the absence of a guiding image, you will need to examine each possibility in order to see what logically fits the given arrangement. It is highly unlikely that, by seeing the two views, you will be able to imagine the appropriate third view before examining the answer choices. There will be many third-view possibilities that could satisfy the conditions of the first two. Your job in this section is to examine the answer choices and identify the only correct view by eliminating the three incorrect choices.

Expect to see several types of each missing view question. The following is an example of an orthographic projection question as it would appear on the PAT:

Choose the correct END VIEW.

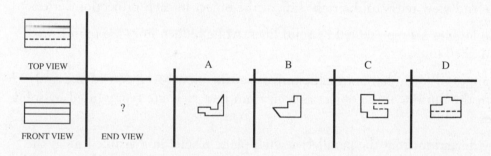

Your first strategy should be to identify the number of visible lines and hidden lines in one of the two views given. In this example, the top view has five horizontal lines. The top and bottom line are always exterior outlines, so the interest lies in the three interior lines. From top to bottom, the order of these lines is visible, visible, and hidden. With this information in mind, you should immediately begin eliminating incorrect answer choices. When examining the choices, take great care to count the sequence of visible and hidden lines in the proper order. As a rule, if you identify horizontal lines in the top view from top to bottom, their order of appearance in the end view will be from right to left. The first round of elimination leaves answers A and B as the only possible choices.

The next step is to use the information given by the other view in the same way. The front view has a total of four horizontal lines, two of which are interior visible lines. Choice A can now be eliminated because the front view that would correspond to its end view would have the following lines from bottom to top: visible, hidden, visible, and visible (not including the outlines). Choice B is the correct answer.

If after counting the number and pattern of visible and horizontal lines you have a match between two or more answer choices, verify for each choice that the lines are in the proper locations relative to each other and to the perimeter of the side being considered. For each group of projections, there will be only one answer that satisfies the conditions set forth by the two given views.

This strategy of identifying the number, order, and placement of appropriate lines can be highly effective and time saving. It will be necessary, however, to fully understand the logic of projected lines so that you can easily make transitions among different views.

If you find that you have difficulty with transitions among different types of absent views, it is suggested that you identify the projection series that you can most easily solve. Then, to remain clearly focused throughout this section, first solve the sets that you are most comfortable with; for example, solve all the problems that have a top and front view. Then return to all of one of the remaining types, for example, the front and end view problems. Lastly, address the questions of the third type (absent front view). This approach will help you to keep track of each perspective and will serve to "warm you up" for questions of greater challenge.

Review

- The orthographic projections on the PAT are composed of three views: the top view, front view, and end view. Each of the views is rendered without perspective.

- The end view refers to the right side of the object in each projection series.

- Visible lines are represented by solid lines, while hidden lines are represented by dashed lines.

- Changes in form that are visible only from the view being considered and from the outline of the object as seen from that view are represented by solid lines.

- Any deviation from the parallel viewing plane results in a visible line at the point where the transition from parallel to angular takes place. Creases in the form that are visible from the projection view always result in solid lines.

- Hidden lines, shown as dashed lines, refer to edges that cannot be seen because they are either inside or behind the object.

- When a hidden line is exactly behind a visible line, the part of the dashed line that coincides with the solid (visible) line remains solid. When two hidden lines overlap, the resulting line remains dashed.

- Your job in this section is to examine the answer choices and identify the only possible view by eliminating the three incorrect choices.

- When examining answer choices, take great care to count the sequence of visible and hidden lines in the proper order.

- The strategy of identifying the number, order, and placement of appropriate lines is highly effective and time saving.

EXERCISE 1

In each case, examine the three-dimensional image presented in the box. Then, to the right of each image, draw in the appropriate views. Use of a straightedge is suggested for this exercise.

1.

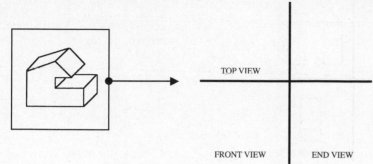

2.

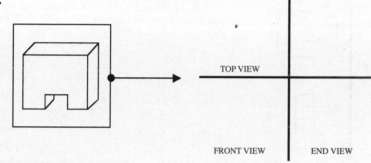

3.

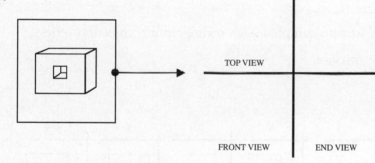

Answers to Exercise 1

1.

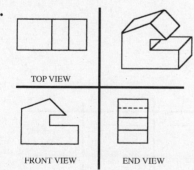

2.

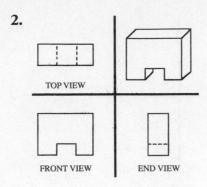

3.

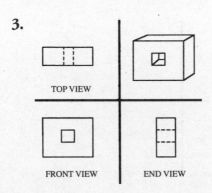

EXERCISE 2

Choose the correct view to complete each orthographic projection series.

1. Choose the correct END VIEW.

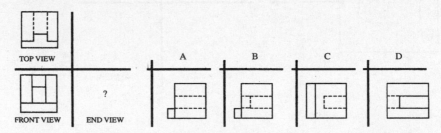

2. Choose the correct TOP VIEW.

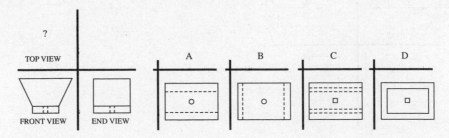

3.

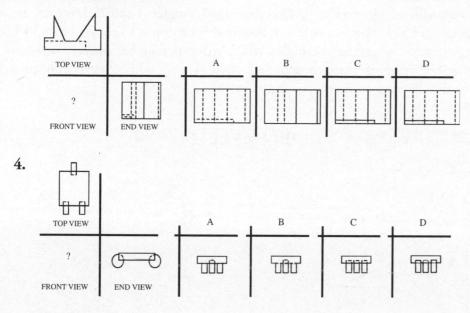

4.

Answers to Exercise 2

1. B   **2.** B   **3.** D   **4.** D

ANGLE DISCRIMINATION

Introduction

The third part of the Perceptual Ability Test is angle discrimination. This is the only portion of the PAT that involves flat renderings representing two-dimensional space that you need not mentally rotate.

Angle discrimination questions ask you to rank angles by size, from smallest to largest. With practice, you will be able to sharpen your angle-estimation skills and thus to avoid pitfalls that are meant to complicate the task of discriminating between similar angles.

Angle Ranking

As a warmup to this section, spend some time reviewing the illustrations below. Begin by ranking the four angles in each of the following examples from smallest to largest.

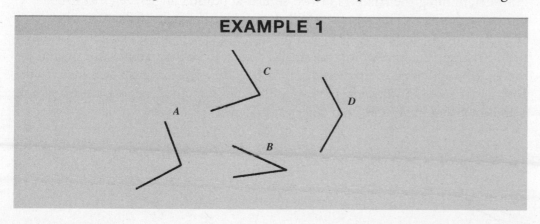

EXAMPLE 1

The correct ranking is *B, C, A, D*. Most likely, you were able quickly to choose angle *B* as the smallest angle and angle *D* as the largest. Angles *A* and *C*, however, are relatively close in size. The first rule to follow in this section is to always begin by identifying the smallest and largest angles, which will generally be apparent upon initial inspection. Even if just the largest angle is obvious, your odds of answering correctly have been increased (more on this later).

EXAMPLE 2

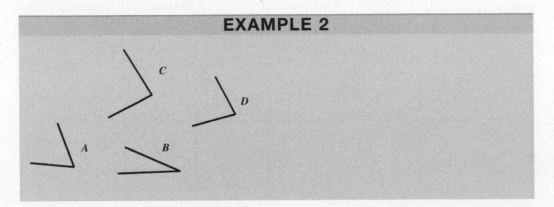

The correct ranking is *B, A, D, C*.

The angles in the following example are closer in size.

EXAMPLE 3

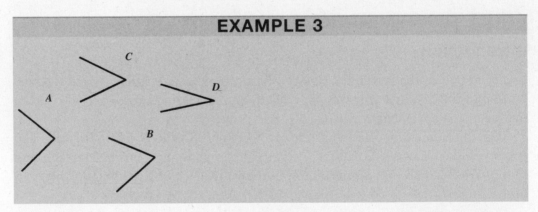

The correct ranking is *D, C, B, A*. In this example, the two angles closest in measurement are *B* and *A*. Angle *D* clearly appears smallest, but it is somewhat unclear which angle is largest.

In determining the rankings of two similar-appearing angles, refer to Exercise 1. One strategy that is often useful is called "parking the angle." When you have two angles of varying degrees, one angle (the larger angle) will always be able to "house" the other angle. In other words, the smaller angle can be inserted into the opening of the larger angle. Hence, the notion of *parking the angle* can help you identify the rankings of angles. To illustrate the application of this method, angle *C* from Example 1 above may be "parked" within angle *A* as follows:

Employment of the parking method depends largely on mental imagery. Asking the question, "Could angle *X* fit within angle *Y* or vice-versa?" often helps illuminate an intuitive hunch that one angle is smaller than the other. The concept of parking the angle applies also to angles with varying leg lengths. Basically stated, *a larger angle will always accommodate a smaller angle regardless of the length of the angles' legs.* From Example 3, angle *B* is parked within angle *A* as shown below.

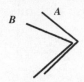

EXERCISE 1

In each of the following 10 sets of angles, determine which angle is larger.

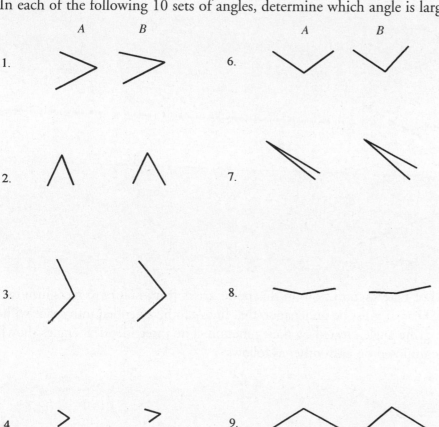

Answers to Exercise 1

1. A   **2.** B   **3.** A   **4.** A   **5.** B   **6.** A   **7.** B   **8.** B   **9.** A   **10.** B

If you have identified several of the larger angles incorrectly, return to the angle sets repeatedly until you are able to perceive the subtle differences. It is often helpful to review these angle sets several times before moving on to further examples and explanations.

An angle is created by the joining of two distinct legs. Crucial to your success on the angle discrimination section is an understanding of the following rule: *The length of an angle's legs is independent of its angular measurement.* To fully grasp this rule, examine the angles below, which share the same angular measurement.

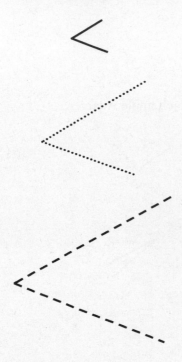

For most test-takers, confusion on this point arises from failure to recognize two main points. First, it must be understood that lines can be extended into space without disturbing the angle created by their junction. The three identical angles shown above can be imposed on each other as follows:

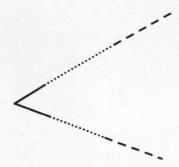

<table>
<tr><td>

TIP

The length of an angle's legs is independent of its angular measurement.

</td><td>

The three sets of legs (or rays) are extensions of the same angle.

</td></tr>
</table>

The second crucial point is concerned with how an angle is measured. On the DAT you will not be permitted to make use of any measuring device (including your fingers and test-taking materials). You must rely on visual acuity to "eyeball" relative sizes. One method of eyeing an angle is to examine the mouth at a set distance from the joining point of the legs. This technique can be helpful as long as you use great caution. To implement the procedure correctly, *you must compare all the angles at the same distance from the joining point.* The following figure illustrates this point.

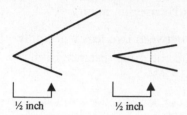

½ inch   ½ inch

It can be inferred that the angle on the left is the larger angle. *When comparing angles, a greater measured distance between two legs will imply a larger angle if and only if the measurement is taken at the same distance from each angle's vertex.*

To practice your understanding of this rule, examine the two angles below.

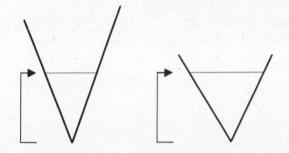

When the horizontal dotted lines at the same distance from each angle's vertex are compared, it is readily apparent that the angle on the right is larger. Keep in mind that you will not be permitted to use any measurement devices on the DAT. The horizontal lines shown in the figures above are there to illustrate the viewing path that you may take when comparing angles.

Where to Look

Another useful method of angle comparison relies heavily on viewing only a discrete area of the angle, namely, the niche. The niche of the angle is the tightest part of the corner created by the two joining legs. This method also takes practice. Since your eye wants to traverse the extended lines away from the vertex, you must practice the restraint necessary to make angle comparisons at the niche. In the following examples, which highlight the viewing of an angle's niche, the angles are ordered from small to large:

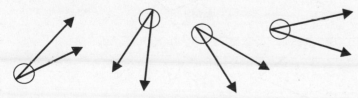

Paramount to your success on the angle discrimination questions is a solid understanding of the basic laws and methods of angle comparison:

- Always begin by establishing a largest or smallest angle, or both if possible.

- Regardless of leg size, a smaller angle can always be inserted within the opening of a larger angle. Hence, the method of "parking an angle" can be useful in conceptualizing the task at hand.

- The length of an angle's legs is independent of its angular measurement.

- When comparing angles, a greater measured distance between two legs will imply a larger angle if and only if the measurement is taken at the same distance from each angle's vertex.

Complex Arrangements

The task of comparing angles is made slightly more complex by oblique positioning. Certainly it will not be possible to rotate the computer screen in order to view the angles at similar positions. For this reason, as you practice the comparison of angles, refrain from angling the book to accommodate your view of particular angles.

The following arrangement is made with identical angles. Notice how the oblique positioning of angles coupled with varying leg lengths affects your visual sensibility.

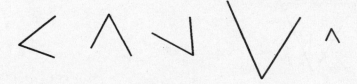

With repeated practice, you will overcome any tendency to allow distortions of angle orientation and leg length to interfere with your reasoning.

EXERCISE 2

The following exercise will help you overcome distortion interference. In each set of three angles, two angles are identical and one angle is different. Select the angle that is different from the other two angles; then determine whether it is smaller or larger.

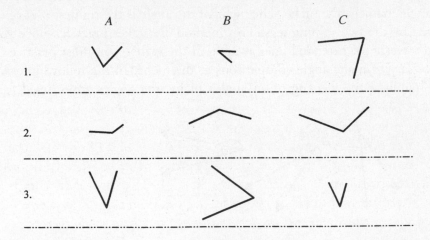

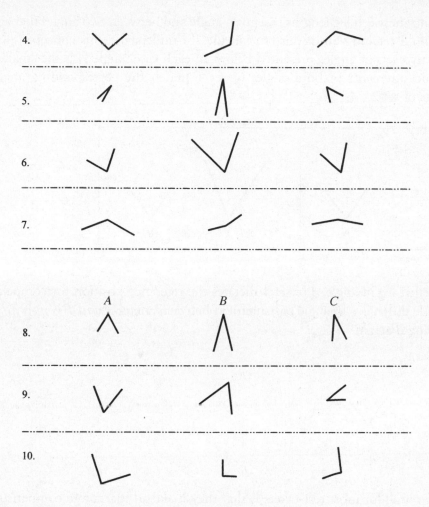

Answers to Exercise 2

1. B (smaller) **2.** C (smaller) **3.** B (larger) **4.** A (smaller) **5.** C (larger)
6. A (larger) **7.** A (smaller) **8.** A (larger) **9.** C (smaller) **10.** C (larger)

You are not expected to score perfectly on this exercise. With continued exposure to these and other angle discrimination problems, however, you will develop the agility necessary to move from angle to angle with a keen eye.

Varied Leg Lengths in an Angle

You have now been exposed to a variety of angles positioned uniquely and having different leg lengths. Another form of perceptual interference is due to a mixed set of leg lengths in a given angle. If, however, you are careful to employ the techniques discussed thus far, you will find that angles with mixed leg lengths are actually helpful. Since your eye tends naturally to rush to the end of the line to make the angular comparison, the presence of a shorter leg helps you to avoid making an inaccurate comparison at the end of the line. Recall that, when comparing angles, a greater measured distance between two legs implies a larger angle *if and only if the measurement is taken at the same distance from each angle's vertex.*

A discrepancy between leg lengths in a given angle and between two angles that are compared should remind you of this crucial rule. To understand this concept fully, compare the two sets of angles presented below. In each case, angle *A* is the smaller angle. The measurements of both angles of set 1 match the corresponding angle measurements of set 2.

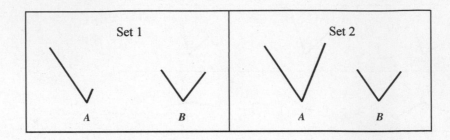

The shortened leg in angle *A* of set 1 dictates the reference position for comparison. The subtle difference in angle measurement between angles *A* and *B* is indicated in the following diagram.

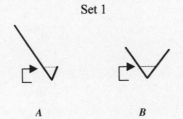

Again, the pitfall for most test-takers is that they make an inaccurate comparison at the end of the leg lengths, leading to an incorrect response. Below is an example of this *faulty* reasoning taken from set 2.

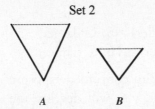

General Strategy

Without becoming unduly suspicious, be aware that both the angles and answer choices on the PAT may tempt faulty reasoning. Rely heavily on the methods discussed, and rehearse the implementation of visual reasoning skills on angles you encounter.

Questions on the PAT show sets of four angles. You are asked to select, from four choices, the correct ranking of the angles from small to large. With a bit of test-taking logic and your heightened awareness of discriminating between like angles, you will be able to greatly improve your odds of scoring highly on these questions.

As already mentioned, you first should identify the smallest or largest angle, or both if possible. Then, before proceeding, examine the answer choices. Many times you will be able to eliminate one or two choices before examining the remaining angles. If the angle you selected as smallest is represented in two choices as the smallest angle, you can begin eliminating the other choices. Next examine whether the angle you think is largest is also listed as largest in one of the two choices you are considering. At this point, you may be able to select the correct answer.

Maintaining a fast pace throughout this section will allow you to concentrate longer on other items of the Perceptual Ability Test that require additional time. In order to stay organized while working quickly, it is recommended that you keep track of your angle discrimination decisions on the erasable board provided. For example, upon your initial inspection for the largest and smallest angles, write down any decisions you can make before looking at the answer choices.

To keep track of choices that you have eliminated and answers you are still considering, you should jot down the answer choices on your erasable board, and cross numbers off as you delete the corresponding choices. Simply writing "1," "2," "3," and "4" will enable you to stay organized, and it should take you only a few seconds to make these notes. Under test-taking circumstances, you can easily become confused in your decision making without these and similar brief notations. Most students who are skilled test-takers make use of minimal notes such as the ones suggested here.

Because of the computer format of the DAT, you will not be able to mark decision-making notations directly on the test. Hence, part of your preparation for the DAT should include practice in using scratch paper effectively. Below is an example of a typical PAT angle discrimination question and the use of the erasable board.

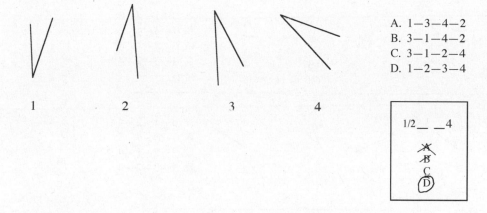

A. 1—3—4—2
B. 3—1—4—2
C. 3—1—2—4
D. 1—2—3—4

Review

- The length of an angle's legs is independent of its angular measurement.

- You must compare all the angles at the same distance from the joining point of the legs. When comparing angles, a greater measured distance between two legs will imply a larger angle if and only if the measurement is taken at the same distance from each angle's vertex.

- A useful method of angle comparison relies heavily on viewing only a discrete area of the angle, namely, the niche. The niche of the angle is the tightest part of the corner created by the two joining legs.

- When ranking angles, you first should identify the smallest or largest angle, or both if possible. Then begin eliminating answer choices.

EXERCISE 3

The following sets of angles are provided for your additional practice. They are structured in the same manner as angle discrimination problems from previous versions of the DAT. In each case, select the ranking that appropriately orders the angles from small to large.

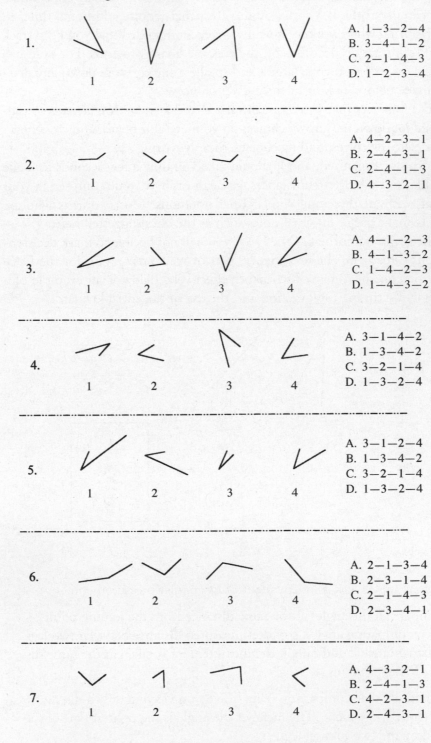

1.
    A. 1—3—2—4
    B. 3—4—1—2
    C. 2—1—4—3
    D. 1—2—3—4

2.
    A. 4—2—3—1
    B. 2—4—3—1
    C. 2—4—1—3
    D. 4—3—2—1

3.
    A. 4—1—2—3
    B. 4—1—3—2
    C. 1—4—2—3
    D. 1—4—3—2

4.
    A. 3—1—4—2
    B. 1—3—4—2
    C. 3—2—1—4
    D. 1—3—2—4

5.
    A. 3—1—2—4
    B. 1—3—4—2
    C. 3—2—1—4
    D. 1—3—2—4

6.
    A. 2—1—3—4
    B. 2—3—1—4
    C. 2—1—4—3
    D. 2—3—4—1

7.
    A. 4—3—2—1
    B. 2—4—1—3
    C. 4—2—3—1
    D. 2—4—3—1

8.

| 1 | 2 | 3 | 4 |

A. 2—4—1—3
B. 1—2—3—4
C. 4—3—2—1
D. 3—2—1—4

9.

| 1 | 2 | 3 | 4 |

A. 2—1—3—4
B. 2—4—3—1
C. 1—2—3—4
D. 2—1—3—4

10.

| 1 | 2 | 3 | 4 |

A. 4—1—2—3
B. 1—4—2—3
C. 1—4—3—2
D. 4—1—3—2

Answers to Exercise 3

1. C, 2 – 1 – 4 – 3   **6.** D, 2 – 3 – 4 – 1
2. B, 2 – 4 – 3 – 1   **7.** D, 2 – 4 – 3 – 1
3. D, 1 – 4 – 3 – 2   **8.** B, 1 – 2 – 3 – 4
4. D, 1 – 3 – 2 – 4   **9.** B, 2 – 4 – 3 – 1
5. A, 3 – 1 – 2 – 4   **10.** C, 1 – 4 – 3 – 2

PAPER FOLDING

Introduction

The fourth section of the perceptual ability test is paper folding. Beginning with a square, you are presented with a series of progressive folds that the initial square undergoes. After the folds have been completed, a hole is punched somewhere in the final form. The task of this section is to mentally unfold the paper and determine the precise positioning of the one or more holes resulting from the punch.

Rules

The parameters of paper folding are straightforward:

- The initial paper will always be square.

- The paper will never be twisted.

- The orientation of the paper will remain the same.

- All folds will result in forms that are contained within the imaginary perimeter of the initial square.

- Dashed lines indicate the absence of paper due to a fold.

- Solid lines indicate either a crease or the paper's edge.

- Only after all folds have been completed will a hole be punched.

- One or more holes may be punched.

- The hole may penetrate one layer or multiple layers of the paper.

Success on the paper-folding section relies heavily on the understanding of a few basic principles. With practice, you should be able to answer the paper-folding questions in a short time and with little error.

Format of the Folding Sequence

The paper-folding sequence is presented as a series of two to four images arranged side by side. The series is laid out progressively, beginning with the first fold, then the second, and so on. Although not shown, the starting form is always assumed to be a square. The final image of the sequence is identical to the next to last image but shows the placement of the hole punch.

Below is an example of a typical paper fold sequence.

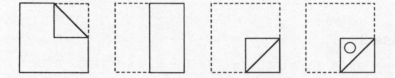

The dashed lines indicate absence of the paper (due to folding) from the original square. A solid line marks either a crease in the paper (seen only from frontal viewing) or the paper's edge. In the last image, the circle marks the location of the hole punch.

The following illustration includes guide arrows for clarification.

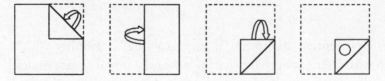

In this sequence, there are three folds. Prior DATs indicate that you can expect to see mostly two- and three-fold sequences.

The Punch Grid

Presented with the folding sequence are five possible answers as to where the punched holes are located on the paper. These choices are presented in the form of punch grids. The blackened circles on the grid indicate the locations of punched holes. Below are five possible answer choices for the sequence presented above.

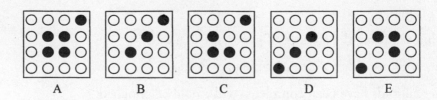

A   B   C   D   E

The punch grid is a standard configuration that is used in all types of folding sequences. Examination of the general punch grid offers important information concerning the nature of the types of folds that can be used in folding series.

The punch grid is composed of 16 possible holes, evenly arranged in rows and columns. A folding pattern will never result in hole punches that stray from the possibilities offered in the punch grid. With this fact in mind, it is evident that the folds must maintain the integrity of the four ordered rows and columns.

EXERCISE 1

The following exercise will help you better understand the relationship between folding patterns and punched hole outcomes. Remove the exercise punch grids found in pages 265–270. Using these punch grids and a hand-held hole puncher, complete each of the following folding patterns and punch a hole in the place as indicated. Blacken the appropriate holes of the answer punch grid for each sequence *after* unfolding the hole-punched exercise punch grid.

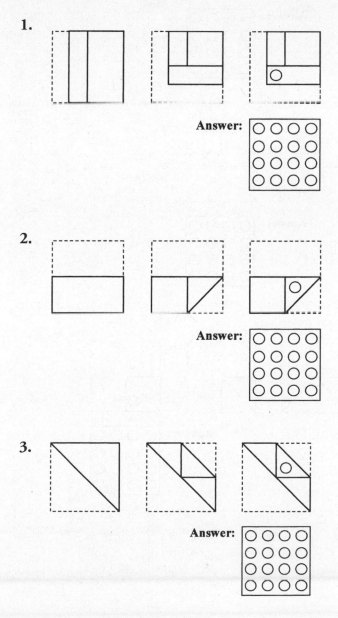

4.

5.

6.

7.

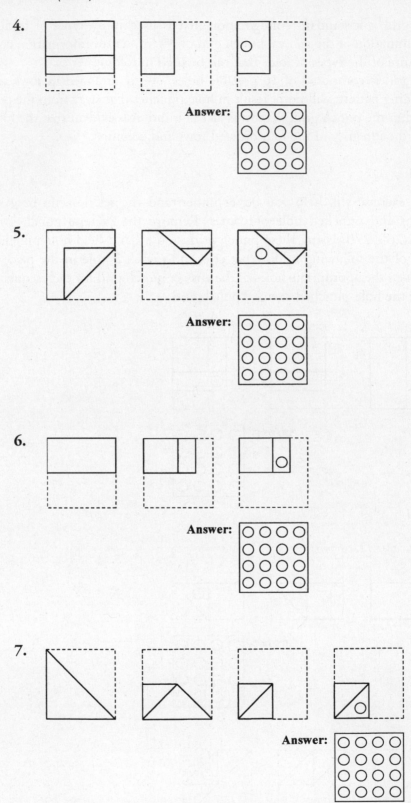

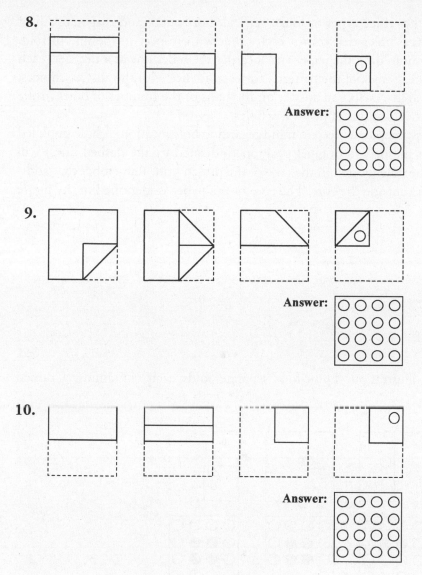

8.

Answer:

9.

Answer:

10.

Answer:

The Logic of Folds and Holes

With an understanding of the basic logic that underlies this section, you will be able to quickly identify the correct answer from the array of choices presented. Having completed Exercise 1, you have probably made the basic observation that *the number of resulting holes is equivalent to the number of paper layers through which the hole is punched.* You will often find that several answer choices can be disregarded as having too few or too many holes. In some cases, you may be left with only one choice, thus allowing you to select the correct answer without even considering the location of the holes. For this reason, your initial step should be to determine the number of paper layers *at the location of the punched hole.* Then quickly scan the answer choices to identify the punch grids that have the same number of blackened holes as the number of paper layers you identified.

The next step in arriving at the correct answer efficiently is to pinpoint the locations of holes. If you have narrowed the answer choices to just a few candidates, it may not be necessary to identify the locations of all the points.

You will encounter three types of folds: vertical, horizontal, and diagonal. All of these folds will reveal holes that mirror each other with respect to the line of fold. Begin by mentally unfolding the paper and locating the holes one at a time. As each hole is identified, keep track of the pattern's correspondence with the answer choices. Often you will be able to select an answer on the basis of the number of holes in the final pattern and the locations of just a few holes.

There are a few principles to keep in mind regarding hole location. A hole punched within the core of the paper's original position (indicated by the dashed lines) will result in at least one hole located in the core of the punch grid. Remember that additional holes may lie outside the core. The core of the paper is identified in the figure below.

The following illustration shows four separate folds each containing a punch within the core.

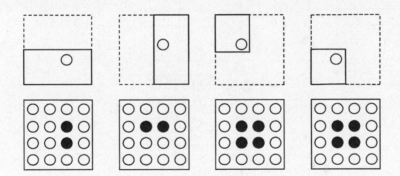

As previously mentioned, although a hole may be punched within the core, holes may also occur around the perimeter of the paper. For example, examine the following sequence:

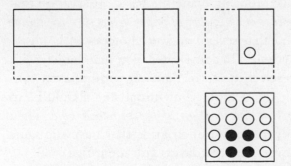

As a general rule, if the final form has a hole punched within the core of the form created by the original square (indicated by the dashed lines), the resulting punch grid will have at least one core hole. This general rule may be used to eliminate improbable answer choices.

Holes punched around the perimeter of the original square will result in forms that have at least one perimeter hole. Perimeter hole punches may be located in any of the positions indicated below.

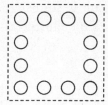

The restraint that the paper must stay within the confines of the original square makes it difficult to obtain an interior core hole from a perimeter punch. With this restriction, the only way to obtain interior core holes from a perimeter punch is to have a folding segment that quarters the length or width of the paper to the edge of the original square. Examples of the resulting forms are seen in the figure below.

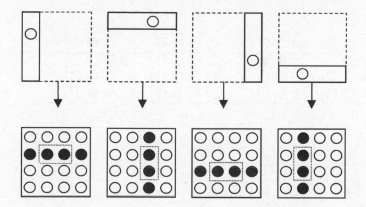

Most of the folds necessary to create an interior core hole from a punch around the perimeter would resemble those in the following sequence:

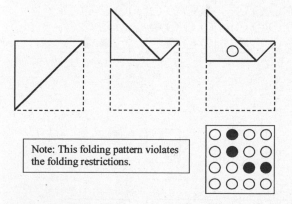

Note: This folding pattern violates the folding restrictions.

Review

• First establish how many paper layers were penetrated by the hole punch.
  Eliminate answer choices that have too few or too many holes.

- Identify the locations of the punched holes. Remember that each fold will produce mirrored holes with respect to the line of fold.

- If the final form has a hole punched within the core of the form created by the original square (indicated by the dashed lines), the resulting punch card will have at least one core hole.

- Holes punched around the perimeter of the original square will result in forms that have at least one perimeter hole and generally no core hole (see the illustration above for exceptional folds).

EXERCISE 2

The following folding sequence questions are provided for your additional practice.

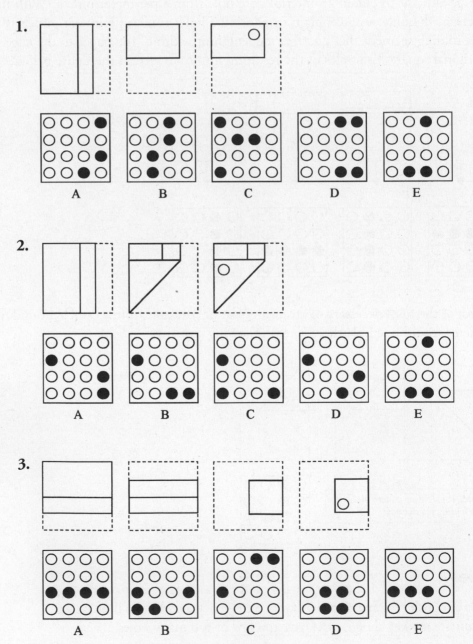

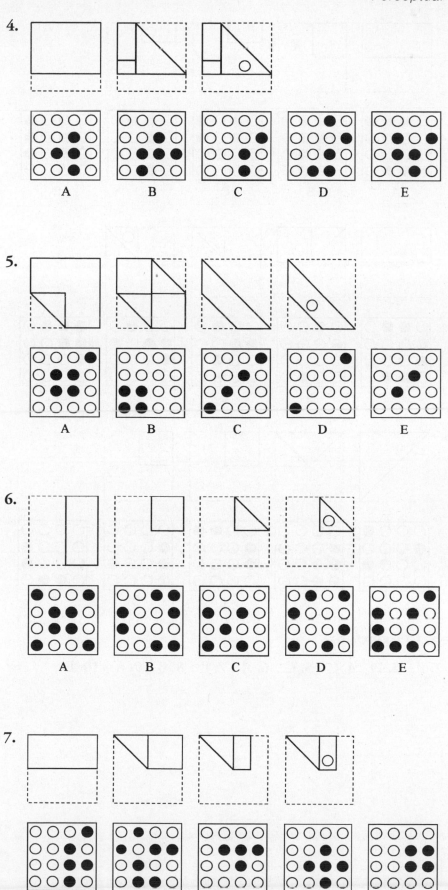

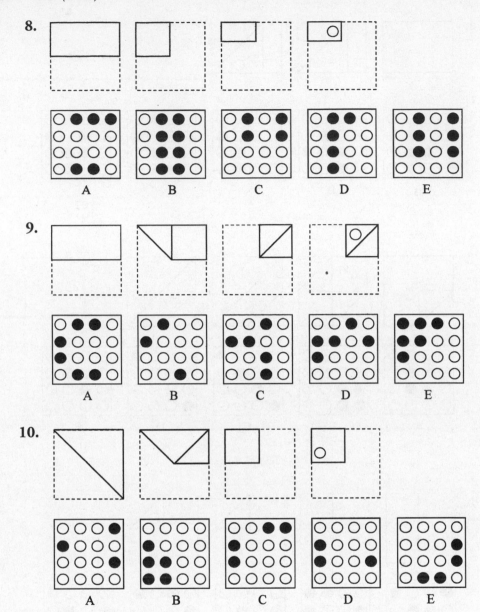

8.

9.

10.

Answers to Exercise 2

1. D **2.** B **3.** D **4.** C **5.** C **6.** A **7.** E **8.** B **9.** A **10.** E

The following punch grids are provided for use in the folding exercises. Using scissors, cut along the perimeter of each grid.

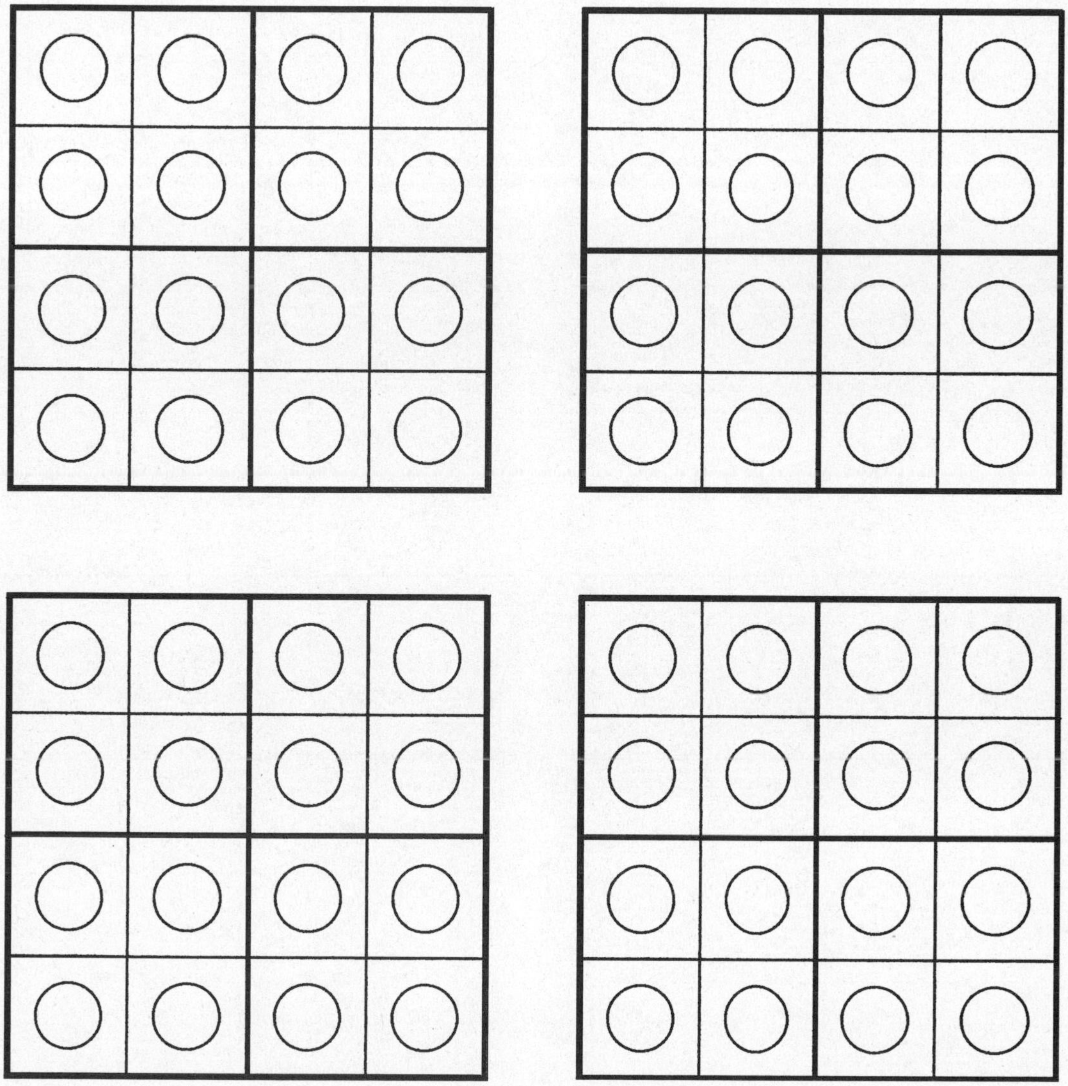

CUBES

Introduction

The fifth section of the Perceptual Ability Test involves counting the painted surfaces of cubes. In this section, you will be presented with formations of stacked cubes. Groups of questions will correspond to the cube formations. The questions will ask you to determine how many cubes have a particular number of painted surfaces.

What distinguishes this section is the ease with which an answer can be quickly generated. For most test-takers, this section presents the fewest difficulties. In fact, with careful preparation and strategy, you can expect to answer these questions both efficiently and accurately. Because of the relative ease of this section in comparison to the other perceptual ability sections, you are cautioned to *not overlook* the use of strategy and preparative measures necessary for exceptional scoring. A high score on this group of questions will play an important role in achieving an overall high score on the PAT. Remember as you review for the cube questions that you are aiming for a nearly perfect score on these questions, which count no less than other, seemingly more difficult questions in the perceptual ability section of the DAT.

Cube Counting

Below is an example of a basic cube formation. This example is used to illustrate the basic assumptions that should underlie your reasoning throughout the cube section. The cube formations on the actual test will not be labeled and will be more complex than the simple example that follows. Further testlike examples will be offered after the introductory explanations.

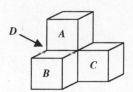

Notice that there appear to be three cubes in the above formation. In this section, you must pay careful attention to any hidden or obscured cubes. Realizing that cube *A* is above cubes *B* and *C*, you should infer that there exists cube *D*, which is out of view. Hence, there are four cubes in this simple formation. The assumption of *necessary support,* that is, that any cube above the first level must be supported by underlying cubes, is the first crucial assumption that you should make throughout this section.

To review your understanding of this basic assumption, practice counting the number of cubes in the following formation.

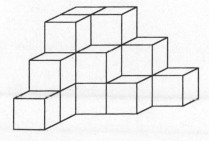

If you counted 18 cubes, you have answered correctly. If you failed to identify all 18 cubes, chances are that you either lacked organization as you counted or you did not attend to the assumption of necessary support. An organized count might begin at the top and work downward. (Additionally, for more complex arrangements, the direction of count would move from left to right for each level.) In this fashion, you would first identify the top 3 cubes. Then, following the assumption of necessary support, you would identify the 3 hidden cubes plus the additional 3 visible cubes on the second level. Thus, the second level has a total of 6 cubes. The bottom level has 6 hidden and 3 visible cubes, totaling 9 cubes. The grand total is $3 + 6 + 9 = 18$.

Again, practice arriving at a total cube count by using the following formation.

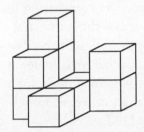

The correct answer is 10 cubes ($1 + 3 + 6 = 10$).

The second assumption that you should make in dealing with the cube section is that an *empty "ceiling" implies that there are no hidden cubes beneath.* For example, in the following formation examine the columns beneath the arrows. Of course, in real life a cube *could* exist on the first level that is out of view. On the PAT, however, an empty ceiling (top level) implies an empty column if the column is entirely out of view.

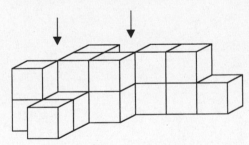

In the figure shown above, there are 6 cubes on the top level and 9 cubes on the bottom level. Here, the arrows draw your attention to empty columns. On the PAT, however, there will not be arrows to indicate empty columns. You will need to rely on your knowledge of the two assumptions discussed above in order to make appropriate judgments concerning the absence or presence of cubes out of view.

Now, try a more complex arrangement.

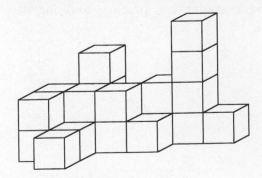

The correct answer is 21 cubes.

The initial counting of cubes is an important step that should precede any reasoning concerning the painted surface questions. Although no questions will ask you to simply identify the total number of cubes, an initial cube count takes little time and helps you avoid the trap of failing to identify hidden cubes. Additionally, the cube count will serve as a self-check in figuring your answers.

EXERCISE 1

The following cube formations are provided to help you achieve greater speed and accuracy in counting cubes.

How many cubes are there in each formation?

1.

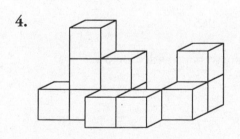

2.

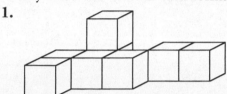

3.

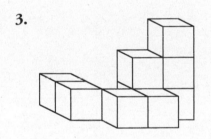

4.

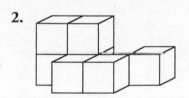

5.

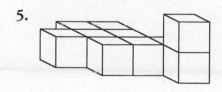

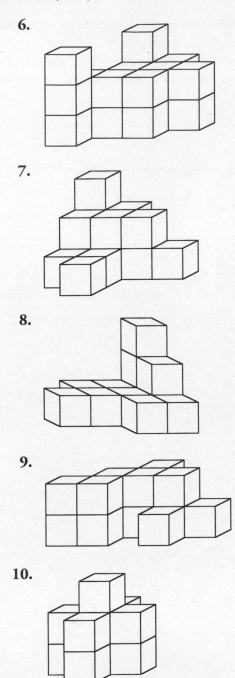

6.

7.

8.

9.

10.

Compare your cube count totals with the answers provided below:

Answers to Exercise 1

1. 8   **2.** 7   **3.** 9   **4.** 11   **5.** 10   **6.** 20   **7.** 15   **8.** 12   **9.** 14   **10.** 11

Counting Painted Surfaces

The task in the cube section of the PAT is to count painted surfaces. Imagine that the formation below has been painted with white paint on all exposed sides. The exposed sides are the sides that would reflect light if light were projected from the front, the back, and the left and right sides of the formation.

What is the total number of painted surfaces (or cube sides) in the formation shown below?

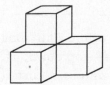

The total number of painted surfaces (or cube sides) of this formation is 15. In counting, it is a common mistake to overlook the exposed sides of blocks that are not visible to the respondent.

Below is a block separation of the basic figure considered above. Notice that the blackened areas are the surfaces that either sit on the imaginary floor or are shared between two blocks. These blackened areas are never to be counted as painted surfaces.

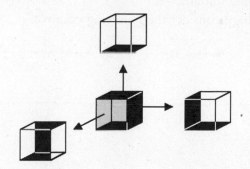

Actual painted surface questions that have appeared on previous DAT exams had this form:

In figure X, how many cubes have

    A. one of their exposed sides painted?
    B. two of their exposed sides painted?
    C. four of their exposed sides painted?

On the test approximately three painted surface questions refer to each formation. For this reason, it is crucial to follow a consistent methodology when counting painted surfaces. Failure to accurately identify all the cubes in a particular formation could result in incorrect responses to several questions.

Note that no cube should ever have six painted surfaces. Although there are six surfaces to a cube, the cube will always be resting against the imaginary floor or another cube. Also note that there will be instances in which a given cube will have no painted surface. This will occur when there are neighboring cubes on all sides and another cube rests above the cube in question. In general, your success in counting painted surfaces will depend on your ability to mentally meander around the far corners of the arrangement that are out of view. As is true for all sections of the DAT, with practice you will notice improvement.

Since the DAT will be administered on the computer, you will need to make good use of available scratch board. The painted cube questions, perhaps more than any other type, will reflect your ability to remain organized under test-taking circumstances.

Strategy

As stated previously, you should count the total number of cubes before addressing the issue of painted surfaces. (Remember to use an organized count—top down, left to right, and back in space.) This preliminary count will serve two purposes. First, it will help you identify all the obscured or hidden cubes. Second, the total cube count will serve as a self-check when you tally the numbers of painted surfaces. After establishing a total count, begin identifying (by cube) the number of painted surfaces on each cube. Follow the same pathway that you used to count the number of cubes (top down, left to right, and back in space). On your scratch paper create a vertical list that assigns a number of painted surfaces to each cube.

After counting the cube surfaces in the top level, draw a horizontal line to indicate the counting of cubes in a new level. Insert a horizontal line after each level. Finally, before answering the questions, check that the number of cubes you have tallied matches the total cube count that you identified initially.

To review the suggested counting methodology, consider the following example:

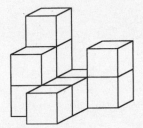

Although it is tempting to "break up" the cube formation into different sections for counting purposes (for example, to group the far left, middle, and right sections), this is *not* recommended. It takes only a few seconds to carry out the top down, left to right, and back in space procedure, and a consistent direction of count helps you to remain accurate from formation to formation despite the differences between formations. The use of an organized procedure such as the one recommended above and illustrated below helps ensure that you will properly identify all hidden cubes.

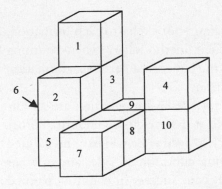

On your erasable board, note the total cube count before proceeding. Next, begin your vertical list of numbers that correspond to painted surfaces. For the above example, the list would be written as follows:

```
    5      (top level)
  ____
  ____

    4
    3      (middle level)
    5
  ____

    2
    2
    4      (bottom level)
    2
    2
    3

         total cubes= 10
```

As mentioned previously, the cube count serves as a means of self-checking. Before responding to questions, verify that the number of cube surfaces you have identified matches the total number of cubes. If you find that you have made a mistake at some point, recheck your scratch work level by level (as separated by the horizontal lines in your list) to find where the skipped item was omitted.

At this point, you are ready to efficiently answer questions regarding the numbers of painted surfaces. Consider the following questions:

In the figure above, how many cubes have two of their exposed sides painted?
How many cubes have three of their exposed sides painted?
How many cubes have four of their exposed sides painted?
How many cubes have five of their exposed sides painted?

A helpful method for combing your list is to employ a circle, the letter X, and a squiggle to identify like numbers. A basic method of this sort helps avoid the fatal flaw of overlooking a crucial number. Failure to identify how many cubes share a certain number of painted sides can lead to incorrect responses on the test. Using an active rather than a passive method at each stage of developing your final answer will enable you to avoid mistakes.

Below is an example of the circle, X, and squiggle method for establishing the final answers to the questions given above. You can develop additional forms of notation that catch your eye at a glance.

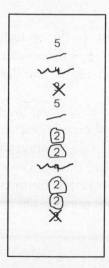

How many have two sides painted? 4
How many have three sides painted? 2
How many have four sides painted? 2
How many have five sides painted? 2

Review

- According to the assumption of necessary support, any cube above the first level must be supported by underlying cubes.

- An empty ceiling (top level) implies an empty column if the column is entirely out of view.

- The initial counting of cubes is an important step that should precede any reasoning concerning painted surface questions.

EXERCISE 2

Practice is necessary to develop speed and accuracy in the employment of the various methods discussed above. Turn to pages 273–274, and answer the following questions for each of the 10 formations:

a. How many cubes have one exposed side painted?
b. How many cubes have two exposed sides painted?
c. How many cubes have three exposed sides painted?
d. How many cubes have four exposed sides painted?
e. How many cubes have five exposed sides painted?

Answers to Exercise 2

1. 0, 1, 2, 4, 1
2. 0, 1, 2, 3, 1
3. 0, 1, 3, 4, 1
4. 0, 2, 3, 4, 2
5. 1, 2, 5, 1, 1
6. 3, 7, 6, 1, 2   (Note: One cube has no painted surface.)
7. 1, 6, 3, 3, 1
8. 2, 3, 4, 2, 1
9. 2, 3, 4, 5, 0
10. 0, 0, 4, 4, 1   (Note: Two cubes have no painted surface.)

FORM DEVELOPMENT

Introduction

The last section of the Perceptual Ability Test is form development. In this section, you are presented with a flat pattern that is to be folded into a three-dimensional form. Your task is to select the appropriate three-dimensional rendering of the flattened image from four possible choices.

This section has the power to consume a tremendous amount of valuable test time. One of your many goals for this section is to be able to recognize when it is prudent to skip questions too difficult to be solved at first try. Although form development is a challenge for most test-takers, it offers the opportunity to integrate the skills mastered for other sections of the PAT. This section need not be construed as formidable; careful use of strategy will enhance your ability to recognize the appropriate answer without delay.

The Flattened Image

The flattened image is a rendering of what you would have if a three-dimensional object was opened at its edges with each surface "unwrapped" and the whole form flattened on one plane. The following is an example of a flattened image.

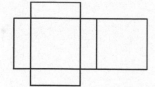

Notice that the flattened image is one complete unit. Although sides have been cut at the edges, each panel has at least one edge joined with another surface. On some flattened images, shaded regions or designs mark the surfaces. Keep in mind that each line that is part of the flattened image indicates one of the following: (1) a bend, (2) an edge, or (3) the outline of a shaded region.

Construction of the Three-Dimensional Image

Your task in the form development section is to select the correct or appropriate three-dimensional image constructed from the flattened figure. The three-dimensional figures will be rendered as isometric drawings. An isometric drawing is a representational drawing in which all faces of the image are shown with equal inclination and all the lines are drawn to their true lengths. Below is an example of a three-dimensional construction of the flattened image shown above.

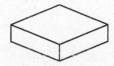

The orientation of the three-dimensional image will vary from question to question. After the form is constructed, it may be turned on its side or upside down. The following two examples illustrate how the same flattened image may be represented three dimensionally in two different ways.

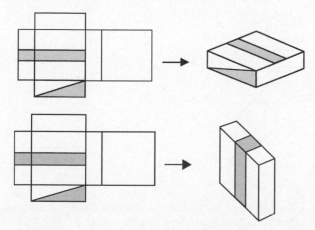

Likewise, there is no standard orientation of the flattened image that relates to the direction of fold used to construct the three-dimensional image. In the following example, the flattened pattern is oriented in four different positions. What is later perceived as the figure's top may seem to be a likely bottom when viewing the flat-tened image.

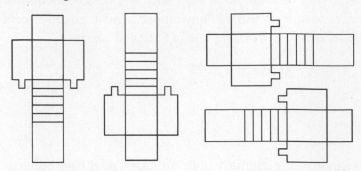

Any of the flattened images above could be used to describe *all* of the following three-dimensional forms:

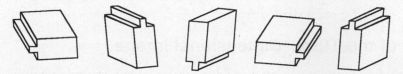

Often, the orientation of the flattened image biases your thinking in regard to where the folding begins and how you conceive of the folding direction. Such a bias may interfere with the ability to regard certain answer choices as possible accurate renderings. For this reason, it is important to develop a strategy that leads you to the correct answer regardless of the orientation or positioning of the flattened form or of the three-dimensional answer choices.

Attention to Detail

Perhaps the quickest way to identify an appropriate three-dimensional rendering of the flattened form is to utilize details of each drawing (flattened figures and three-dimensional answer choices). Consider the following flattened form and correspon-ding answer choices:

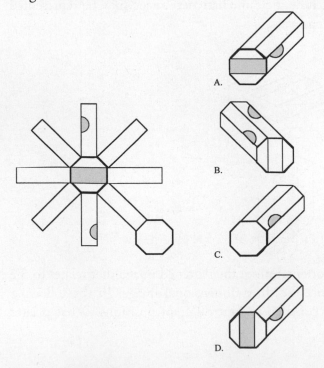

In this example, the details that stand out are the shaded half-circles and the shaded rectangle. *Whenever shading is used, first examine the answer choices to eliminate any that have an inappropriate positioning of the shaded region or design.* Take note of the precise positioning of a shaded region. It is not necessary to initially check each design for the positioning of each shaded region. Often you can eliminate several choices by checking the positioning of just one shaded region. As you narrow the choices, you can expand the degree of detail on which you will base your final judgment. In the example above, the first detail check might be to scan for the distance between the half-circle and the rectangular figure. Noticing that both half-circles are positioned closer to the blank hexagon than to the hexagon with the rectangle, you can eliminate choices A, B, and D. With little effort, you realize that the correct answer is C. This answer was arrived at without considering the angle of view or the spacing between marked sides. By keeping to a simplistic plan such as detail scanning, you save a tremendous amount of time and energy.

Although detail scanning is extremely helpful in questions that contain shaded regions or designs, in other questions you will be confronted with complex flattened images that contain no distinct feature markings.

Complex Forms

Some flattened forms will be difficult to visualize in three dimensions. The shape may be unusual, or the number of folds necessary to arrive at the final form may be unusually high. The form below would be considered complex in both regards.

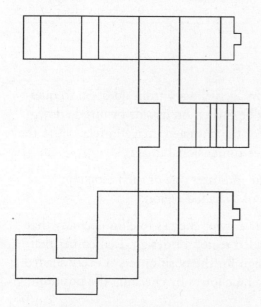

In such cases, rather than spending time trying to visualize the totality of the final three-dimensional form, concentrate on the elimination of unlikely answer choices. To begin the process of elimination, it is necessary to identify a reference shape in the flattened form. This reference shape should be easy to locate and unique in some regard.

One of many reference shapes that may be used is shown below:

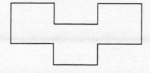

This particular form happens to be the largest unfolded portion of the flattened figure. It is also appears twice in the flattened image. Often, a pair of identical large regions serves the three-dimensional image as the sides or the top and bottom.

Once you have identified the reference shape you wish to use, examine the answer choices. Check each choice to see whether the shape is reproduced correctly, the neighboring sides make logical sense given the joining shapes in the flattened form, and the shape is repeated the correct number of times.

Now, considering the form given above, try these strategies on the answer choices below.

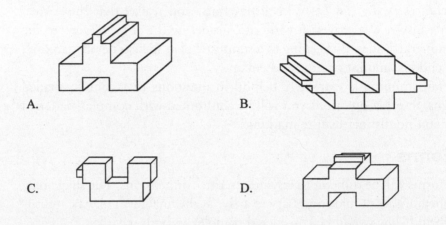

A.

B.

C.

D.

The correct answer is D.

Review

- The orientation of the three-dimensional image will vary from question to question. After the form is constructed, it may be turned on its side or upside down. Likewise, there is no standard orientation of the flattened image in relation to the direction of fold used to construct the three-dimensional image.

- Each line that is part of the flattened image indicates one of the following: (1) a bend, (2) an edge, or (3) the outline of a shaded region.

- Whenever shading is used, first search your answer choices to eliminate any that have an inappropriate positioning of a shaded region or design. Remember that it is not necessary to initially check each design for the positioning of every shaded region. You are often able to eliminate several choices by checking the positioning of just one shaded region.

- When confronted with a complex form, concentrate on the elimination of unlikely answer choices. To begin the process of elimination, identify a reference shape in the flattened form. Check each answer choice to see whether the shape is reproduced correctly, the neighboring sides make logical sense given the joining shapes in the flattened form, and the shape is repeated the correct number of times.

- Use your time carefully. Do not allow yourself to dwell on any one question. Skip a question if you cannot effectively eliminate answer choices at the first try.

EXERCISE 1

The following exercise makes use of both folding and design location skills. Paying particular attention to the locations of design markings, examine each flattened image. Below each flattened image, you will see an incomplete three-dimensional rendering. Add the appropriate marking to each cube so that it accurately represents the flattened image.

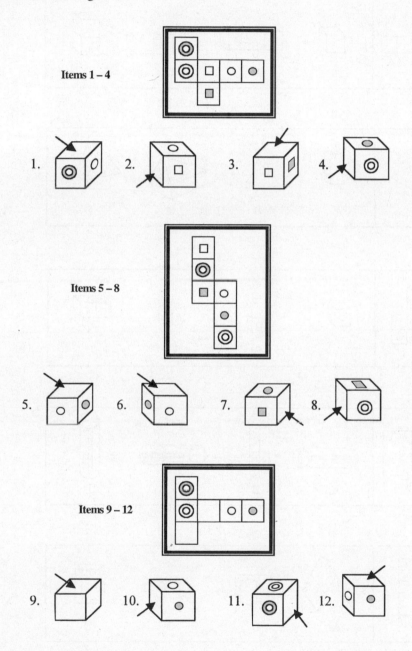

Answers to Exercise 1

1. Shaded circle	**2.** Shaded ring	**3.** White circle
4. Shaded square	**5.** White square	**6.** Shaded square
7. White ring	**8.** Shaded ring	**9.** White circle or white ring
10. (Blank)	**11.** Shaded circle	**12.** Shaded ring

EXERCISE 2

This exercise is formatted identically to the way in which form development questions appear on the DAT. In each case, choose the correct three-dimensional representation of the flattened image shown at left.

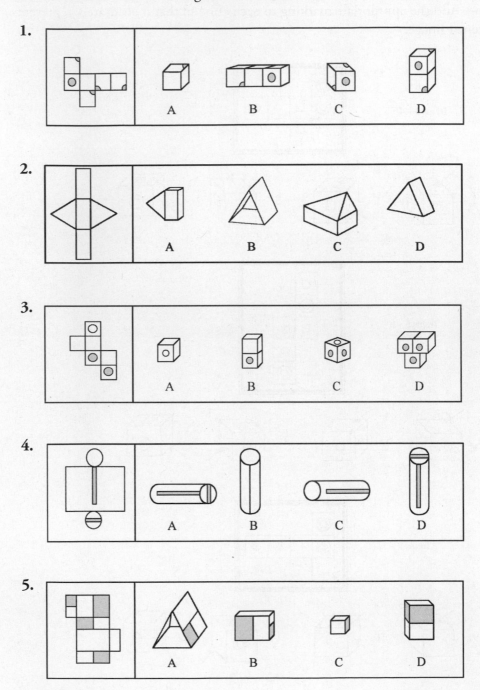

Answers to Exercise 2

(It is suggested that you complete Exercise 3 before checking your answers to Exercise 2.)

1. C **2.** D **3.** A **4.** B **5.** D

EXERCISE 3

On the following pages you will find reproductions of all the flattened forms discussed in the form development section. Carefully cut out each form and create three-dimensional forms by folding the cutouts. Then use the three-dimensional figures to review the strategic discussions and Exercises 1 and 2.

Carefully remove each flattened figure by cutting around its perimeter. Then construct a three-dimensional form by folding. Clear tape may be used to fasten the sides.

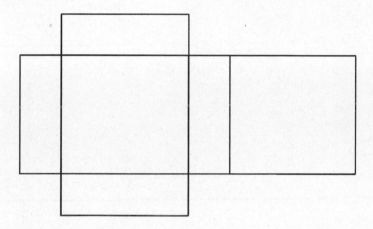

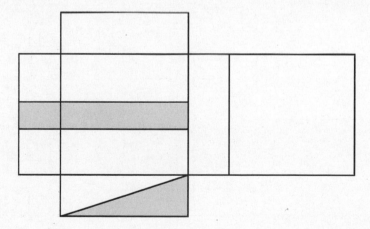

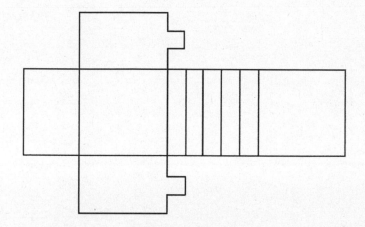

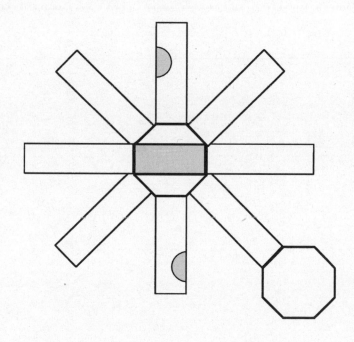

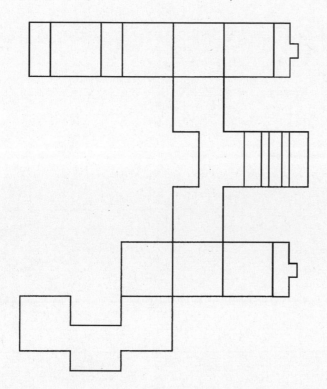

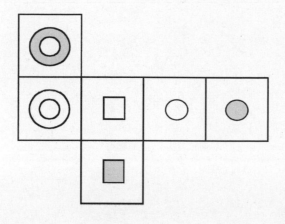

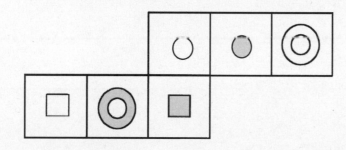

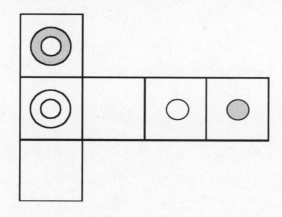

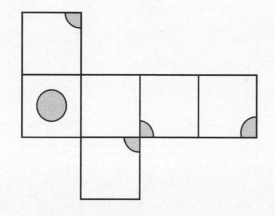

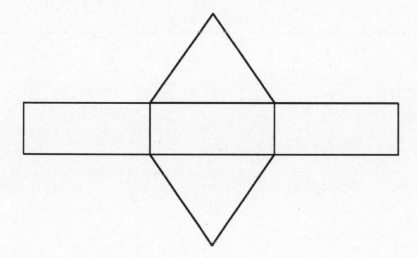

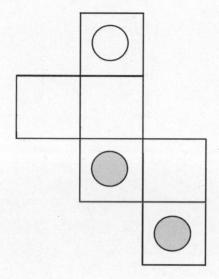

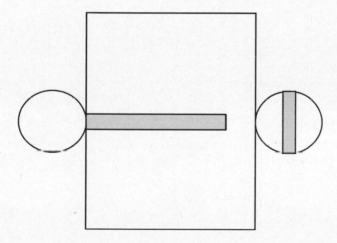

Reading Comprehension Test Review

OUTLINE

INTRODUCTION

This review will provide information on how to prepare for and take the Reading Comprehension Test (RCT) of the DAT. *Unlike reading comprehension sections on any other standardized exams, all of the reading comprehension passages on the DAT will be heavily technical and scientific.*

The RCT consists of three passages of about 1,300–1,500 words each. Dental school professors are hired by the ADA to write the passages on the actual DAT. These passages are representative of the type of material you will encounter in your first year of dental school. Following each passage are 16 or 17 multiple-choice questions for a total of 50 questions. You will have 60 minutes to complete this section.

THE IMPORTANCE OF READING COMPREHENSION

The Reading Comprehension Test is often regarded as the least important section of the DAT. There is some truth behind this view since most Admissions Committees tend to look for high marks on the sciences and the Perceptual Ability Test. However, reading comprehension also may be considered the most important section because your ability to read quickly and to comprehend what you have read will be a determining factor in how well you do in dental school.

During the first year of dental school you will be assigned more reading than you can possibly finish. You must be able to determine what readings are important, to read them at a good pace, and to retain a fair amount of what you have read. This is not to say that dental school is impossibly difficult, but rather that your ability to read well will be tested on a daily basis.

AN EASY TEST AND A HARD TEST

In one respect, you can think of the Reading Comprehension Test as the easiest part of the DAT. Just think: you do not need any outside knowledge, and all of the answers are provided in the passages. All that is required of you is to read the question, find the answer in the passage, and then mark the correct choice on the answer sheet. What could be easier?

As easy as the RCT is, it is also the test on which many people run into problems. The main problem is lack of time. It is not uncommon for test takers to find themselves with one minute left and five questions unanswered. This situation occurs, not because the questions are too difficult, but because the students did not have an efficient method for finding information in the passage.

WHY SOME STUDENTS DO POORLY

Many students believe that they do poorly on this test because they are slow readers, but this is not always the case. What is more important is how carefully you read and then how skillfully you go about finding the answers to the questions. Speed reading is not necessary for this section and may actually be counterproductive since many small facts may be missed.

There are only three passages on the exam, and each one is not excessively long. Therefore, even if you do not consider yourself a fast reader, you should still have no problem finishing the test. Where the majority of test takers lose the most time is in locating the answers in the text. It is imperative that you develop a method that allows you to read the passage, locate in the passage the answers to the questions, and then have 5–6 minutes left at the end to return to any questions you have skipped.

YOU CAN IMPROVE

It is completely reasonable to believe that with a little practice anyone can improve on the Reading Comprehension Test. You just have to be willing to put in some time. It is understandable that, with all the subjects you have to study, reading comprehension is probably not at the top of your list. You must learn, however, to budget your time and to set aside a certain amount of time each week to practice for this test.

You must remember that, just as with the other tests, practice will improve your RCT score. Just reading a lot will not guarantee a good score—although it will help. You must learn to quickly recall where you saw items in a passage so as to not waste time hunting for them.

METHODS FOR READING COMPREHENSION

Many methods have been proposed to help students achieve higher scores on the Reading Comprehension Test. All of these methods have positive and negative aspects, just as the one proposed in the next section surely does. It will be helpful now to mention several alternative methods and to explain why each is good and not so good.

One method suggests that you read the questions before reading the passage. This approach will help you in that it will provide you with some idea of what questions are being asked. Then, while reading the passage, you can be on the lookout for the answers to those questions. Thus, you may even be able to answer some of the questions while you are reading. There are, however, two drawbacks to this method. First, it is time consuming. If you have to read the questions twice, once before you read the passage and once after, you are wasting time. A second problem with this method is that there are 16 or 17 questions per passage. It is unlikely that you will be able to remember more than five or six of the questions while reading the passage.

A second method asks that you skim the passage once before reading. Skimming generally means that you read the first and last lines of each paragraph to try to get the main idea of the passage. This approach can be very useful, especially because there are usually a couple of questions that ask about the main idea. However, just as with the first method, this is time consuming. If you are having trouble making it through the RCT just reading each passage once, skimming is not likely to help you. A word of warning: If you decide to use this method, you must read the passage in its entirety after you have skimmed it. Do not just skim! Most questions pertain to specific facts that will be missed without careful reading.

A third method involves the order in which you answer the questions. All of the questions carry the same point value. If there were a quick way to find the easiest questions, so that these could be answered first, then this method would be worthwhile. Your best bet is to answer the questions in the order they are given, reading the question first and then the answer choices. This approach is less confusing, and you will be less likely to make a mistake when keying in your responses.

A final method suggests a system for marking the passage. The test taker is advised to mark the passage as he or she reads. Since this method is impossible on the computer, it is not discussed here.

THE "KEY" METHOD

This section will provide you with a detailed explanation of one possible method for taking the Reading Comprehension Test. As mentioned previously, this approach may not work for everyone. There are, however, two reasons why this method is preferable to the ones just discussed. The first reason is that it is easy to learn. With just a little practice you should be able to decrease the time required to complete the RCT while increasing the number of correct answers that you get. The second reason is that the method is easy and fast to use. It is not time consuming, and there is nothing extra that you will have to remember for test day.

This method is based on key elements, words, or numbers, which will be referred to as keys. Keys are any words that are important. The challenge is to determine which ones are important. Some obvious examples are scientific words or other words with which you are unfamiliar, such as *odontoblast* or *chondrocyte*. You don't have to worry about what these words mean. If a word is important, it will be defined in the passage. Other keys to look for are numbers or statistics because they often sum up the results of a study or give important data. Aside from these, it is up to you to determine what is important and therefore is a key. Don't worry—there are examples later on that will help to clarify what you should be looking for.

When you begin the RCT, the first thing you should do is read the first passage. Do not skim it, make sure you read every word. Use the following guides to create your *List of Keys*:

• As you read, look for keys and jot them down.

• Jot keys down in sequential order.

• Draw a short horizontal line in the left-hand margin to indicate paragraph breaks.

• For keys that are excessively long (10 letters or more) create your own form of shorthand to save time.

When writing keys, you must be careful to include only what is important; writing too many keys wastes time and can lead to confusion later on. When creating your list of keys choose for each key the one or two words that are most important.

Consider this sentence: "The olfactory nerve is the shortest of the twelve cranial nerves, spanning as several small bundles the short distance through the cribiform plate between the olfactory epithelium and the expanded olfactory bulb." It is easy to see that this sentence is important because it presents a term, *olfactory nerve,* and then a description of the nerve. If this were a text to be used for study purposes, you would highlight the entire sentence. On the DAT, however, you would just jot down the key, in this case *olfactory nerve* (or a shorthand version, *olfact n.*). This will allow you to find the description of the nerve quickly if it appears in a question later on. For this sentence you could also jot down *olfactory bulb* and *olfactory epithelium* (in shorthand, *olfact bulb/epith*); however, no information is given for these terms, so it may be better to skip them and go on. Continue this process until you have completed the passage; then move on to the questions.

EXERCISE 1

Read the following passage carefully and create a practice list of keys. Then compare your keys to those in the answer.

Achieving effective and predictable anesthesia of the mandibular arch has long been a formidable challenge for the dental professional. It is reported that the success rate for the inferior alveolar nerve block is 80% to 85%. Variations in the height of the mandibular foramen location coupled with the depth requirement of the needle penetration serve to reduce the success rate of the inferior alveolar nerve block. The density of the mandibular bone makes it imperative that the anesthetic solution be deposited to within 1 mm of the target nerve.

Alternatives to the traditional inferior alveolar block have been proposed. The Gow-Gates and Vazirani-Akinosi blocks provide regional anesthesia to the pulps of the mandibular teeth in a quadrant. The mandibular anterior teeth can be easily anesthetized with the incisive nerve block. It is a valuable alternative to the inferior alveolar nerve block when treatment is limited to these teeth; however, anesthesia of the mandibular molars is usually approached with a block injection.

Supplemental mandibular anesthesia techniques include the PDL injection. Although this supplemental injection can be used in either arch, it is most often used to anesthetize mandibular teeth.

Answer to Exercise 1

List of Keys

anesthesia of mand.

success rate	inf. <u>alveolar</u> n. block	80% to 85%.
height	mandibular foramen	
depth requirement	needle penetration	reduce the success rate
density mand. bone	anesth. sol. be deposited	

Gow-Gates and Vazirani-Akinosi
mandibular anterior teeth
<u>incisive nerve block</u>

Supplemental mandibular anesthesia
PDL injection

Start with the first question. Read the question and, as you did with the passage, look for a key. If you find one, try to match it with one of the keys you have listed from the passage. If you find a match, look for the corresponding answer choice. If you don't find a match, or an appropriate answer to the question, read the answer choices given and look for more keys. Then, once again, match those keys with ones you listed for the passage.

There is one more thing that you must do when reading each question: You must determine exactly what the question is asking. First try to figure out whether the question is asking for a specific fact or for a general understanding of the passage. If the question is asking for specific information, use your keys to find the answer. An example of this type of question could be: Which is the shortest cranial nerve? If, on the other hand, the question is asking for more general knowledge of the passage, keys may not be as helpful. *For these types of questions you will have to rely on your ability to comprehend what you have read.* Questions that require general understanding can pose more of a challenge for some test takers, and therefore it may be wise to skip them the first time around and return to them later. Be aware, though, that if you leave the general questions until the end of the test, you may not remember what the passage was about when you try to answer them. Your best bet is to answer as many of the questions as you can the first time through. If, however, you can not pick the correct answer, select the mark key on the screen and return to it later. If you have a best guess, mark it.

EXERCISE 2

Answer the following questions, using the passage from Exercise 1 to find the answers.

1. Which of the following could be used in place of a traditional inferior alveolar nerve block to anesthetize mandibular molars?

   A. PDL injection
   B. incisive nerve block
   C. mental nerve block
   D. Vazirani-Akinosi block
   E. greater palatine nerve block

2. For an inferior alveolar nerve block the anesthetic solution should be placed

   A. in the PDL
   B. directly on the target nerve
   C. in the mandibular bone
   D. no more than 1 mm from the target nerve
   E. no less than 1 mm from the target nerve

3. A PDL injection is most often used for

   A. anesthetizing mandibular bone
   B. anesthetizing mandibular teeth
   C. a Gow-Gates block
   D. primary mandibular anesthesia
   E. anesthetizing maxillary teeth

4. The success rate of the incisive nerve block is

   A. 80% to 85%
   B. dependent on the anesthetic used
   C. higher than that of an alveolar nerve block
   D. not given in the passage
   E. 60% to 70%

Answers to Exercise 2

1. **D**. For this question the key is "in place of." Refer to the passage for this phrase or one that is close to it. The closest match is "Alternatives." Now read the sentence in the passage that contains the key. Since no answer is given there, read the next sentence. Now check the answer choices. You could also read over the answer choices before reading the sentence in the passage. Either way is fine, so choose whichever works better for you.

2. **D**. Use the same method as above. Make sure to read the answer choices carefully. Answers D and E differ by only one word and can easily be confused.

3. **B**. The key is "PDL injection."

4. **D**. For this question there are two keys, "success rate" and "incisive nerve block." It is important that you locate all keys in the question; otherwise, you will end up with an incorrect answer. If you took only "success rate" as the key, you might choose A as the correct answer. That would be correct if you had

been asked about the success rate of inferior alveolar nerve blocks. Since no success rate was given for incisive blocks, answer D is the correct choice.

MAKING AN ANSWER GRID

Before you begin taking the DAT, there will be a lengthy tutorial (about 15 minutes) that provides you with instruction on taking the computer-based DAT. Because you will be intimately familiar with the exam, you can use this valuable time to prepare for the reading comprehension section of the DAT.

Using an erasable board provided by the testing center, make an answer grid similar to the one below. Across the top of the grid, you will have five columns headed by the letters A, B, C, D, and E. Each column represents one of five answer choices that you will select as the correct answer. You should also have 50 rows that run down the page—one row for each of the 50 questions that comprise the reading comprehension section of the DAT.

The answer grid is useful because it is impossible to physically eliminate answer choices because the DAT is a computer-based examination. You can use this grid to help you keep track of answer choices that you have eliminated for particular questions and can come back to when you reach the end of the section. This will save you time in the long run because you will not have to re-eliminate answer choices. Be aware, though. It takes practice to get accustomed to using an answer grid. Use it each time you take a mock DAT reading comprehension test. With practice, this system will help you to stay organized and manage time on test day.

	A	B	C	D	E
1					
2					
3					
4					
5					
6					
7					
8					
9					
10					
11					
12					
13					
14					
15					
16					

(*Continued*)

	A	B	C	D	E
17					
18					
19					
20					
21					
22					
23					
24					
25					
26					
27					
28					
29					
30					
31					
32					
33					
34					
35					
36					
37					
38					
39					
40					
41					
42					
43					
44					
45					
46					
47					
48					
49					
50					

Sample answer grid for reading comprehension section of the DAT.

MISCELLANEOUS TIPS

- Ensure that you have 5–6 minutes at the end of the reading comprehension section of the DAT to answer any skipped questions. Allow about 18 minutes to read each passage and answer the corresponding questions. This will leave about 6 minutes to answer skipped questions and review answers.

- Use the answer grid that you made on an erasable board during the DAT tutorial to make note of answer choices you have eliminated. As you are not penalized for incorrect answers, do not leave any question unanswered. If you still have any unanswered questions with one minute remaining on the test, use the answer grid to make "educated guesses." For instance, if your answer grid indicates that you eliminated answer choices A, C, and D for a particular question, you can make an educated guess by selecting answer choice B or E instead of guessing randomly.

- Practice reading longer scientific articles online (newspapers, journals). Reading a passage on a computer screen is markedly different than reading a printed reading passage. Also, on the computer-based DAT, you will not be able to see the entire reading passage on one screen and will have to use a scroll bar to scroll through the passage. Practice using the scroll bar when reading online scientific articles.

- All answers to DAT reading comprehension questions are found in the passage. If you have difficulty finding an answer, mark the question, and proceed to the next question. Regardless of difficulty level, all questions are worth the same. Do not get bogged down by any single question. Time management is very important in ensuring successful completion of the DAT reading comprehension section.

PRACTICE PASSAGE

Now try this practice passage. As you read the passage, create a list of keys on the erasable board provided (see page 301). Then use the keys to help you answer the questions that follow.

(Time limit 20 minutes)

Changes in Tissues Overlying Teeth

The initial change seen in the tissues overlying the teeth before eruption of the crown is the alteration of the connective tissue of the dental follicle to form a pathway for the erupting tooth. Usually, this is more prominent in erupting permanent teeth. Histologically, the coronal part of the dental follicle becomes heavily populated by numerous monocytes in parallel with osteoclasts to participate in bone resorption and formation of the eruption pathway. The future eruption pathway appears as a zone in which connective tissue fibers have disappeared, cells have degenerated and decreased in number, blood vessels have become fewer, and terminal nerves have broken up and degenerated. These changes are probably the partial result of the loss of blood supply to this area, as well as the release of enzymes that aid in degradation of these tissues. Clinically, tooth eruption may be accompanied by discomfort or pain, irritability, and/or a slight temperature increase. An altered tissue space or compartment overlying the tooth becomes visible as an innervated, funnel-shaped area. In the periphery of this zone, the follicle fibers direct themselves toward the mucosa and are defined as the gubernaculum dentis or gubernacular cord. Some authors believe that this structure guides the tooth in its eruptive movements.

For successful tooth eruption, there must be some resorption of the overlying bony crypt, which is in a constant state of remodeling as the tooth germ enlarges and the face grows anteriorly and laterally. The eruptive process can be considered part of this remodeling growth. Osteoclasts differentiate and resorb a portion of the bony crypt overlying the erupting tooth. The eruption pathway, which at first is small, increases in dimension, allowing movement of the tooth to the oral mucosa. Although the eruption of most permanent teeth is similar to that of primary teeth, the overlying primary teeth are an additional complication. The eruptive pathway of permanent incisors and cuspids is lingual to the corresponding primary teeth. This area shows a pronounced enlargement to accommodate the advancing crown.

Small foramina in the mandible and maxilla are evidence of eruption pathways of the anterior permanent teeth. These openings, the gubernacular foramina, are found lingual to the anterior primary teeth and are the sites of the gubernacular cords. The premolars are between the roots of the primary molars. Root resorption in primary teeth proceeds in much the same manner as bone resorptions. When the roots are fully resorbed, the attachment of the primary crown is lessened and the crown is shed. This produces an eruption pathway for the premolars. Most roots resorb completely; the primary pulps degenerate as well. During the period of mixed dentition (around 6 to 12 years of age), when both primary and permanent teeth are in the mouth, the phenomena of root resorption and tooth formation proceed side by side. These changes occur while the teeth still maintain chewing efficiency.

When the tooth nears the oral mucosa, the reduced enamel epithelium comes into contact with the overlying mucosa. Simultaneously, the oral epithelial cells and reduced enamel epithelial cells proliferate and fuse into one membrane. Further movement of the tooth stretches and thins the membrane over the crown tip. At this stage the mucosa become blanched because of a lack of blood supply to the area. Very soon, the tips of the teeth penetrate the area and appear in the oral cavity. Eruption is a gradual, as well as an intermittent, process. The tooth will erupt slightly, remain stationary for some time, and then erupt again. In this manner, the supporting tissues are able to make adjustments to the eruptive movements. Each eruptive movement results in more of the crown appearing in the oral cavity and further separation of the attachment epithelium from the enamel surface. Recent observations of human premolar eruption revealed that eruptive activity occurred mostly at night with a marked slowing or cessation during the day.

Changes in Tissues Around Teeth

The tissues around the teeth also undergo change during tooth eruption. Initially, the dental follicle is composed of delicate connective tissue. Gradually, as eruptive movements commence, collagen fibers become prominent, extending between the forming root and the alveolar bone surface. The first noticeable periodontal fiber bundles appear at the cervical area of the root and extend at an angle coronal to the alveolar process. At the same time, the alveolar bone of the crypt is remodeled to accommodate the forming root. As the large crown moves occlusally, the bone fills in to conform to the smaller root diameter. As eruption proceeds, other collagen fiber bundles become visible along the forming root. The area becomes more densely populated with fibroblasts. A special type of fibroblast, the myofibroblast, is said to have contractile capabilities. It has been reported to be present in the periodontal ligament. If present, the myofibroblast could aid in the force needed in tooth eruption. All ligament cells and fibers are currently believed to be important in the eruptive process. During eruptive movements, collagen formation and fiber turnover are very rapid (possibly 24 hours). Very early in the eruptive process, perforating givers attach to the cementum on the root surface and to the alveolar bone. Some fibers release as the tooth moves, then reattach to stabilize the tooth. In this manner, the tooth-stabilizing process is performed by the same group of fibers throughout tooth eruption. The fibroblasts are the cells active in formation and degeneration of collagen fibers. Alveolar bone remodeling is continuous during eruption. As the tooth moves occlusally, the alveolar bone increases in height and changes shape to accommodate passage of the crown. Because tooth crown has migrated occlusally, new bone is deposited around the root to reduce the size of the crypt. Above and around the crown, osteoclastic and osteoblastic actions occur. These actions are coordinated during the entire eruption process, as well as throughout life.

Changes in Tissues Underlying Teeth

Changes also occur in the follicular tissue underlying the developing tooth. These changes take place in the soft tissue and the fundic bone (bone surrounding the apex of the root). As the tooth erupts, space is provided for the root to lengthen, primarily because of the crown moving occlusally and the increase in height of the alveolar bone. Changes in the fundic region are thus believed to be largely compensatory to the lengthening of the root. During the preeruptive and early eruptive phases, the follicular fibroblasts and fibers lie in a plane parallel to the base of the root. The root moves more rapidly in the socket during prefunctional eruption than at any other period. Fine bony trabeculae appear in the fundic area. They compensate for tooth eruption and provide some support to the apical tissues. Some authors describe this as a bony ladder. The ladder becomes more dense as alternate layers of bone plates and connective tissue are laid down. At the end of the prefunctional eruptive phase, when the tooth comes into occlusion, about one third of the enamel remains covered by the gingiva, and the root is incomplete. At this time, the bony ladder is gradually resorbed, one plate at a time, to make space for the developing root tip. Root completion continues for a considerable time after the teeth have been in function; this process takes from 1 to 1.5 years in primary teeth and from 2 to 3 years in permanent teeth.

LIST OF KEYS

Questions

1. At what time is the crown of a primary tooth lost?

    A. when the underlying permanent tooth is fully formed
    B. when the crown is fully resorbed
    C. when the root is fully resorbed
    D. when the periodontal ligament is fully resorbed
    E. when the underlying permanent tooth erupts

2. What becomes prominent in the dental follicle during eruption?

    A. osteoclasts
    B. delicate connective tissue
    C. fundic bone
    D. erythrocytes
    E. collagen fibers

3. What is responsible for resorption of the bony crypt overlying the erupting tooth?

    A. reduced enamel epithelial cells
    B. osteoblasts
    C. dental follicle cells
    D. eruptive forces
    E. osteoclasts

4. As a tooth erupts, what happens to the alveolar bone?

    A. It remains constant.
    B. It increases in height.
    C. It decreases in height.
    D. It becomes more dense.
    E. It becomes less dense.

5. What makes up the bony ladder?

    A. bony trabeculae
    B. fundic bone
    C. compact bone
    D. osteoclasts
    E. cementum

6. What forms the gubernacular cord?

    A. osteoblasts
    B. follicle fibers
    C. the periodontal ligament
    D. oral epithelial cells
    E. monocytes

7. When do premolars show the most marked eruption?

   A. during periods of increased stress
   B. at no particular time; eruption is constant
   C. at night
   D. during mastication
   E. during the day

8. What is the bone surrounding the apex of the root called?

   A. alveolar bone
   B. periodontal bone
   C. fundic bone
   D. bony crypt
   E. follicular bone

9. What makes the myofibroblast unique?

   A. It can resorb bone.
   B. It aids in bone formation.
   C. It has immunological capabilities.
   D. It has contractile capabilities.
   E. It aids in pulp formation.

10. Once a permanent tooth has come into occlusion, what portion of the enamel is exposed?

    A. 1/2
    B. 1/3
    C. 2/5
    D. 2/3
    E. 1/5

11. What is necessary for successful tooth eruption?

    A. root formation
    B. enamel
    C. formation of the gubernacular dentis
    D. formation of the fundic bone
    E. resorption of overlying bone

12. What happens to oral epithelial cells and reduced enamel epithelial cells as the erupting tooth nears the oral mucosa?

    A. They fuse.
    B. They resorb.
    C. They remain the same.
    D. They form the enamel.
    E. They form the periodontal ligament.

13. Where is the eruption pathway of permanent incisors and cuspids in relation to corresponding primary teeth?

    A. facial
    B. distal
    C. lingual
    D. mesial
    E. The pathways are the same.

14. Where are the first periodontal fiber bundles seen?

    A. at the cervical area of the root
    B. at the apex of the root
    C. on the crown
    D. in the dentin
    E. within the bony crypt

15. What are changes in the fundic region attributed to?

    A. lengthening of the crown
    B. dentin formation
    C. tooth eruption
    D. loss of primary teeth
    E. lengthening of the root

16. During what ages does mixed dentition occur?

    A. 10–15 years
    B. 6–12 years
    C. 4–8 years
    D. 6–12 months
    E. There is no set age range.

Example of List of Keys

Changes over teeth	connective tissue, dental follicle
	monocytes
	gubernacular cord/dentis
Bony crypt	osteoclasts—resorb
	eruption pathway
	incisor/cuspids—lingual
Gubernacular foramina	root resorption
	mixed dentition 6–12 years
Near eruption	reduced enamel epi. + mucosa
	gradual, intermittent process
	night
Change around teeth	dental follicle
	collagen fibers
	periodontal fiber bundles
	fibroblasts/myofibroblasts
	collagen turnover 24 hours
Under tooth	fundic bone
	root — prefunctional stage
	bony ladder
	enamel covered by gingiva 1/3
	primary teeth 1–1.5 years
	permanent teeth 2–3 years

Practice Passage Answer Key

1. **C** Paragraph 3, sentence 5.
2. **E** Paragraph 5, sentence 3.
3. **E** Paragraph 2, sentence 3.
4. **B** Paragraph 5, sentence 19.
5. **A** Paragraph 6, sentences 7–9.
6. **B** Paragraph 1, sentences 7–8.
7. **C** Paragraph 4, sentence 10.
8. **C** Paragraph 6, sentence 2.
9. **D** Paragraph 5, sentence 9.
10. **D** Paragraph 6, sentence 11. Read each question carefully. You can avoid selecting incorrect answer choice B by focusing on the word "exposed." This requires you to subtract 1/3, the proportion of enamel covered by gingiva, from 1 (answer is 2/3).
11. **E** Paragraph 2, sentence 1.
12. **A** Paragraph 4, sentences 1–2.
13. **C** Paragraph 2, sentence 6.
14. **A** Paragraph 5, sentence 4.
15. **E** Paragraph 6, sentences 3–4.
16. **B** Paragraph 3, sentence 8.

Quantitative Reasoning Test Review

OUTLINE

XI. Trigonometry
   A. The Cartesian Coordinate System
   B. Trigonometry of the Right Triangle
   C. The Trigonometric Functions
   D. The Trigonometric Identities

XII. Applied Mathematical Problems
   A. Percent Word Problems
   B. Ratio and Proportion Word Problems
   C. Word Problems Involving Distance, Rate, and Time
   D. Word Problems Involving the Work Rates of Two Individuals
   E. Word Problems Using Odd and Even Integers
   F. Word Problems Involving Ages

INTRODUCTION TO QUANTITATIVE REASONING

The Quantitative Reasoning Test (QRT) contains 40 items. You will have 45 minutes to complete this last section of the DAT. To prepare successfully for the QRT, you need to develop your ability to reason with numbers, to manipulate numerical relationships, and to deal intelligently with quantitative materials.

Each test item is a question or an incomplete statement followed by suggested answers or completions. Read the test item and decide which choice is the best. In preparing for the test, the use of calculators, rulers, measuring devices, mathematical tables, and other study aids is not recommended because these aids are not permitted in the testing center.

SCOPE OF EXAMINATION

It is important to keep in mind that the goal of your review of quantitative reasoning is to score well on this section of the DAT. Mastering the fundamental concepts outlined in the scope of examination is the best method of preparation for the QRT. The following is the scope of examination, as defined by the ADA Department of Admission Testing:

- Algebra (equations and expressions, inequalities, exponential notation, absolute value, ratios and proportions, and graphical analysis)

- Numerical Calculations (fractions and decimals, percentages, approximations, and scientific notation)

- Conversions (temperature, time, weight, and distance)

- Probability and Statistics

- Geometry

- Trigonometry

- Applied Mathematics (word) Problems

Check off each topic on the outline as you review the material. Doing so will ensure that you have covered all the topics outlined in the ADA's scope of examination at the end of your review.

FRACTION SIMPLIFICATION AND OPERATIONAL MATH WITH FRACTIONS

A fractional number is a ratio of two numbers expressed as $\frac{x}{y}$, in which x can be any positive or negative number and y can be any positive or negative number except zero. A fraction is made up of two parts, the numerator and the denominator. In $\frac{4}{9}$ the numerator is 4, which indicates how many of the 9 equal parts are considered. In $\frac{3}{8}$, 8 is the denominator which indicates the number of equal parts.

When the numerator is less than the denominator, the fraction is called a proper function, otherwise the fraction is an improper fraction.

Proper fractions: $\frac{1}{4}, \frac{3}{5}, \frac{5}{8}, \frac{6}{9}$

Improper fractions: $\frac{4}{3}, \frac{6}{4}, \frac{8}{5}, \frac{9}{7}$

EQUIVALENT FRACTIONS

The value of a number is unchanged if you multiply or divide the number by 1. In a fraction, multiplying the numerator and denominator by the same nonzero number is the same as multiplying the fraction by 1; therefore, the fraction is unchanged. Similarly, dividing the numerator and denominator by the same nonzero number leaves the fraction unchanged.

EXAMPLE

Multiply $\frac{1}{3}$ by $\frac{2}{2}$.

$$\frac{1 \times 2}{3 \times 2} = \frac{2}{6}$$

REDUCING FRACTIONS

Generally speaking, when you work with fractions on the DAT, you'll need to put them in *lowest terms*. That means that the numerator and the denominator are not divisible by any common integer greater than 1. For example, the fraction $\frac{1}{2}$ is in lowest terms; but the fraction $\frac{2}{8}$ is not, since 2 and 8 are both divisible by 2. The method used to put such a fraction in lowest terms is called reducing.

EXAMPLE

Reduce $\frac{18}{27}$.

$$\frac{18}{27} = \frac{2 \times 9 \div 9}{3 \times 2 \div 9} = \frac{2}{3}$$

ADDITION AND SUBTRACTION OF FRACTIONS

Two fractions can't be added or subtracted directly unless they have the same denominator. Therefore, before adding or subtracting, you must find a common denominator. A common denominator is a common multiple of the denominators of the fractions. The *least common denominator* (LCD) is the least common multiple—in other words, the smallest positive number that is a multiple of all the terms.

EXAMPLE

Find the LCD of $\frac{1}{4}$ and $\frac{1}{5}$.

$\frac{1}{4}$ = 4, 8, 12, 20, 24

$\frac{1}{5}$ = 5, 10, 15, 20, 25

LCD = 20

EXAMPLE

Solve: $\frac{5}{6} + \frac{3}{4} - \frac{7}{8}$.

$$\frac{5}{6} + \frac{3}{4} - \frac{7}{8} = \frac{20}{24} + \frac{18}{24} - \frac{21}{24} = \frac{20 + 18 - 21}{24} = \frac{17}{24}.$$

MULTIPLICATION OF FRACTIONS

To multiply two or more fractions, multiply their numerators to obtain the numerator of the product, then multiply the denominators to obtain the denominators of the product.

EXAMPLE

Multiply: $\frac{9}{10} \times \frac{5}{4} \times \frac{2}{3}$.

Calculations are greatly simplified if the fractions are put in simplest terms by cancellation of common factors. Express all the numerators and denominators in the factored form, cancel the common factors, and carry out the multiplication of the remaining factors. Cancellation lets you work with smaller rather than larger numbers in the numerator and denominator, thus decreasing the chances of error.

$$\frac{9}{10} \times \frac{5}{4} \times \frac{2}{3} = \frac{3 \times 3}{2 \times \cancel{5}} \times \frac{\cancel{5}}{2 \times \cancel{2}} \times \frac{\cancel{2}}{\cancel{3}} = \frac{3}{2} \times \frac{1}{2} \times \frac{1}{1} = \frac{3}{4}$$

DIVISION OF FRACTIONS

Dividing is the same as multiplying by the *reciprocal* of the divisor. To get the reciprocal of a fraction, just invert the fraction by interchanging the numerator and the denominator. The reciprocal of fraction $\frac{x}{y}$ is $\frac{y}{x}$. It is important to emphasize that division by zero is impossible; therefore a fraction cannot have zero as a denominator.

EXAMPLE

Divide: $\frac{3}{5} \div \frac{2}{5}$.

$$\frac{3}{5} \div \frac{2}{5} = \frac{3}{5} \times \frac{5}{2} = \frac{3}{2}$$

COMPLEX FRACTIONS

A complex fraction is a fraction that contains one or more other fractions in its numerator or denominator. Treat the numerator and denominator separately. Combine the terms in each to get a single fraction on the top and a single fraction on the bottom. You are left with the division of the two fractions, which you perform by multiplying the top fraction by the reciprocal of the bottom one.

EXAMPLE

Divide: $\dfrac{\frac{7}{9} - \frac{1}{6}}{\frac{1}{3} + \frac{1}{2}}$

$$\frac{\frac{7}{9} - \frac{1}{6}}{\frac{1}{3} + \frac{1}{2}} = \frac{\frac{14}{18} - \frac{3}{18}}{\frac{2}{6} + \frac{3}{6}} = \frac{\frac{11}{18}}{\frac{5}{6}} = \frac{11}{18} \times \frac{6}{5} = \frac{11}{15}$$

MIXED NUMBERS

A mixed number is a number consisting of an integer and a fraction. For example, $5\frac{1}{4}, 3\frac{2}{3}, 8\frac{5}{6}$ are all mixed numbers. Fractions whose numerators are greater than their denominators may be converted into mixed numbers, and vice versa.

EXAMPLE

Convert $\frac{19}{3}$ to a mixed number.

$$\frac{19}{3} = \frac{18}{3} + \frac{1}{3} = 6\frac{1}{3}$$

EXAMPLE

Convert $5\frac{3}{4}$ to a fraction.

$$5\frac{3}{4} = 5 + \frac{3}{4} = \frac{20}{4} + \frac{3}{4} = \frac{23}{4}$$

COMPARING POSITIVE FRACTIONS

If the numerators of two fractions are the same, the fraction with the smaller denominator will have the larger value because the numerator is divided into a smaller number of parts. If the denominators are the same, the fraction with the larger numerator will have the larger value. If neither the numerators nor the denominators are the same, express all of the fractions in terms of some common denominator. The fraction with the largest numerator will be the largest.

PERCENT, DECIMAL, AND FRACTION CONVERSIONS

Percents are among the math relationships appearing most often on the DAT. Percent means "part of 100," one one-hundredth. Therefore, 21 percent (21%) means 21 hundredths, or 0.21, or $\frac{21}{100}$.

Percent is a special type of fraction with 100 as the denominator. A percent may always be reduced to a fraction, and then this fraction may in turn be expressed in decimal form. Thus, 25% represents the same fractional measure as $\frac{25}{100}$ or $\frac{1}{4}$, or the same decimal measure as 0.25.

DECIMAL TO PERCENT CONVERSION

To convert a decimal fraction to an equivalent percent, multiply the decimal fraction by 100. To do this, move the decimal point two places to the right.

EXAMPLE

Express 0.45 as a percent.

$0.45 \times 100 = 45\%$

FRACTION TO DECIMAL CONVERSION

To convert a percent to a decimal fraction, divide the numerator by the denominator.

$\frac{1}{4} = 0.25$	$\frac{1}{8} = 0.125$	$\frac{1}{5} = 0.20$	$\frac{4}{5} = 0.80$
$\frac{1}{2} = 0.50$	$\frac{3}{8} = 0.375$	$\frac{2}{5} = 0.40$	$\frac{3}{16} = 0.1875$
$\frac{3}{4} = 0.75$	$\frac{5}{8} = 0.625$	$\frac{3}{5} = 0.60$	$\frac{7}{8} = 0.875$

FRACTION TO PERCENT CONVERSION

To convert a fraction to a percent, convert the fraction so that its denominator is 100. The numerator of the new fraction is the percent.

EXAMPLE

Express $\frac{8}{25}$ as a percent.

Multiply by $\frac{4}{4}$: $\frac{8}{25} \times \frac{4}{4} = \frac{32}{100} = 32\%$

$\frac{1}{5} = 20\%$

$\frac{2}{5} = 40\%$ $\qquad$ $\frac{1}{6} = 16\frac{2}{3}\%$ $\qquad$ $\frac{1}{8} = 12\frac{1}{2}\%$

$\frac{1}{2} = 50\%$ $\qquad$ $\frac{1}{3} = 33\frac{1}{3}\%$ $\qquad$ $\frac{3}{8} = 37\frac{1}{2}\%$

$\frac{3}{5} = 60\%$ $\qquad$ $\frac{2}{3} = 66\frac{2}{3}\%$ $\qquad$ $\frac{5}{8} = 62\frac{1}{2}\%$

$\frac{4}{5} = 80\%$ $\qquad$ $\frac{5}{6} = 83\frac{1}{3}\%$ $\qquad$ $\frac{7}{8} = 87\frac{1}{2}\%$

WORD PROBLEMS USING PERCENT

Most percent problems can be solved by using one formula:

Percent $\times$ *Whole* = *Part*

This formula has three variables: percent, whole, and part. In percent problems, the *whole* usually follows the word *of* or a preposition; the *part* usually follows the word *is* or another verb. The percent can be represented as the ratio of the part to the whole, or the *is* to the *of*.

A percent problem usually gives you two of the variables and asks for the third. On the DAT, it is usually easiest to change the percent to a common fraction and solve from there.

EXAMPLE

What is 25% of 56?

Here you are given the percent and the whole. To find the part, change the percent to a fraction, then multiply. Use the formula above.

Since $25\% = \frac{1}{4}$ you are really asking what one-fourth of 56 is.

$\frac{1}{4} \times 56 = 14$

EXAMPLE

21 is $33\frac{1}{3}\%$ of what number?

Here you are given the percent and the part and are asked for the whole. If *Percent* $\times$ *Whole* = *Part*, then

$Whole = \dfrac{Part}{Percent}$

Since $33\frac{1}{3}\% = \frac{1}{3}$.

$$= \frac{21}{\frac{1}{3}} = 21 \times \frac{3}{1} = 63$$

EXAMPLE

24 is what percent of 8?

Here you are given the whole and the part and asked for the percent.

$$Percent = \frac{Whole}{Part}$$

Since the part and the whole are both integers, and you are looking for a percent, you will have to make the answer into a percent by multiplying by 100.

$$Percent = \frac{24}{8} \times 100 = 3 \times 100 = 300\%$$

WORD PROBLEMS USING PERCENT CHANGE

Percent change, percent increase, and percent decrease are special types of percent problems in which the difficulty lies in making sure to use the right numbers to calculate the percent.

$$Percent\ increase = \frac{Amount\ of\ increase}{original\ amount} \times 100\%$$

$$Percent\ decrease = \frac{Amount\ of\ decrease}{original\ amount} \times 100\%$$

EXAMPLE

An item is priced 20 percent more than its wholesale cost. If the wholesale cost was $800, what is the price of the item?

The original amount is $800, and the percent increase is 20%. Change 20% to a fraction, $\frac{1}{5}$, and use the formula.

$$Amount\ of\ increase = Percent\ increase \times Original\ amount$$
$$= 20\% \times \$800$$
$$= \frac{1}{5} \times \$800 = \$160$$

To find the new amount (the new selling price):

$$New\ amount = Original\ amount + Amount\ of\ increase$$
$$= \$800 + \$160 = \$960$$

On some problems, you'll need to find more than one percent or to find a percent of a percent. You can't add percents unless they are percents of the same amount.

EXAMPLE

A $100 chair is increased in price by 50 %. If the chair is then discounted by 50 % of the new price, at what price will it be offered for sale?

First, you know that the price of the chair is increased by 50%. That is the same as saying that the price becomes (100% + 50%), or 150%, of what it originally was. 150% of $100 is equal to $\frac{3}{2} \times$ $100, or $150. Then, this price is reduced by 50%. Since 50% $\times$ $150 = $75, the final price of the chair is $150 − $75 = $75.

EXPONENTIAL NOTATION; CONVERSION TO AND FROM EXPONENTIAL NOTATION

A number is said to be in scientific notation if it is expressed as the product of a number between 1 and 10 and some integral power of 10. For example, 10,000 is written in scientific notation as 1.0×10^4 or, more simply, as 10^4; 0.001 is written as 10^{-3}; $2,378 = 2.378 \times 10^3$; $0.000398 = 3.98 \times 10^{-4}$.

Since the decimal point of any number can be shifted at will to the left or to the right by multiplying by an appropriate power of 10, any number can be expressed in exponential notation. In general, x is any number; we write $x = a \times 10^z$, where a is a number between 1 and 10 and z is an integer, positive or negative.

EXAMPLE

Write 10,000 in exponential notation.

The decimal point in 10,000 is after the last zero. The first significant number is 1. Move the decimal point to the left four places (1.0000). Multiply by 10^4 to obtain the number in exponential notation: $10,000 = 1.0 \times 10^4$, or, more simply, 10^4.

EXAMPLE

Write 0.0002367 in exponential notation.

Move the decimal point to the right four places. The resulting number is $0.0002367 = 2.367 \times 10^{-4}$.

POWERS AND ROOTS

In the term $4x^2$, 4 is the *coefficient*, x is the *base*, and 2 is the *exponent*. The exponent refers to the number of times the base is multiplied by itself, or how many times the base is a factor. For instance, in 2^3, there are three factors of 2: $2 \times 2 \times 2 = 8$.

When a number is multiplied by itself twice, the result is called the *square* of that number; for example x^2 is x squared. When a number is multiplied by itself three times, the result is called the *cube* of that number; for example x^3 is x cubed.

To multiply two terms with the same base, keep the base and add the exponents.

For example: $4^3 \times 4^5 = 4^{3+5} = 4^8$

To divide two terms with the same base, keep the base and subtract the exponent of the denominator from the exponent of the numerator.

For example: $x^5 \div x^3 = \dfrac{x^5}{x^3} = x^{5-3} = x^2$

To raise a power to another power, multiply the exponents.

For example: $(5^3)^2 = 5^{2\times3} = 5^6$

Any nonzero number raised to the zero power is equal to 1: $x^0 = 1$ if $x \neq 0$. The quantity 0^0 is undefined.

A negative exponent indicates a reciprocal. To arrive at an equivalent expression, take the reciprocal of the base and change the sign of the exponent. $x^{-n} = \dfrac{1}{x^n}$.

For example: $3^{-4} = \dfrac{1}{3^4} = \dfrac{1}{81}$

A fractional exponent indicates a *root*: $(x)^{\left(\frac{1}{n}\right)} = \sqrt[n]{x}$ (Read as "the nth root of x." If no n is present, the radical sign signifies a square root.)

For example: $9^{\frac{1}{2}} = \sqrt{9} = 3$

Every positive number has two square roots, one positive and one negative. The positive square root of 16 is 4, since $4^2 = 16$; and the negative square root of 16 is –4, since $(-4)^2 = 16$ also.

By convention, the symbol $\sqrt{}$ (radical) means the *positive* square root only.

For example: $\sqrt{25} = +5$; $-\sqrt{25} = -5$

In performing the four basic arithmetic operations, radicals are treated in much the same way as variables.

ADDITION AND SUBTRACTION OF RADICALS

Only like radicals can be added to or subtracted from one another.

For example:
$$3\sqrt{2} - 4\sqrt{3} + 5\sqrt{2} + 2\sqrt{3} = (3\sqrt{2} + 5\sqrt{2}) + (2\sqrt{3} - 4\sqrt{3})$$
$$= 8\sqrt{2} + (-2\sqrt{3})$$
$$= 8\sqrt{2} - 2\sqrt{3}$$
$$4\sqrt{2} - \sqrt{2} + 2\sqrt{3} = (4\sqrt{2} - \sqrt{2}) + 2\sqrt{3}$$
$$= 3\sqrt{2} + 2\sqrt{3}$$

MULTIPLICATION AND DIVISION OF RADICALS

To multiply or divide one radical by another, multiply or divide the number outside the radical signs, then the numbers inside the radical signs.

For example: $3\sqrt{5} \times 4\sqrt{3} = (3 \times 4) \circ (\sqrt{5} \times \sqrt{3}) = 12\sqrt{3 \times 5} = 12\sqrt{15}$

$$9\sqrt{15} \div 3\sqrt{5} = (9 \div 3) \circ (\sqrt{15} \div \sqrt{5}) = 3\sqrt{\frac{15}{5}} = 3\sqrt{3}$$

$$\frac{6\sqrt{18}}{3\sqrt{6}} = \left(\frac{6}{3}\right)\left(\frac{\sqrt{18}}{\sqrt{6}}\right) = 2\sqrt{\frac{18}{6}} = 2\sqrt{3}$$

If the number inside the radical is a multiple of a perfect square, the expression can be simplified by factoring out the perfect square.

For example: $\sqrt{48} = \sqrt{16 \times 3} = \sqrt{16} \times \sqrt{3} = 4\sqrt{3}$

THE TWO COMMON SYSTEMS OF MEASUREMENT

The DAT candidate is expected to understand and operate in either the metric system of measurement or the system of common British units. You may be required to perform conversions from one system to the other.

The Common British System

You should know the following equivalences and abbreviations:

1 yard (yd.) = 3 feet (ft.) = 36 inches (in.)
1 foot = 12 inches
1 mile (mi.) = 5,280 feet = 1,760 yards
1 pound (lb.) = 16 ounces (oz.)
1 ton (T.) = 2,000 pounds
1 gallon (gal.) = 4 quarts (qt.) = 8 pints (pt.)
1 quart = 2 pints
1 pint = 16 fluid ounces

This table of equivalencies permits conversions within the British system.

EXAMPLE

How many ounces are there in 2 tons?

$$2 \text{ tons} \times \frac{2{,}000 \text{ lb.}}{\text{ton}} \times \frac{16 \text{ oz.}}{\text{lb.}}.$$

$2 \times 2{,}000 \times 16 \text{ oz.} = 64{,}000 \text{ oz.}$

Note that the names of units that appear once in the numerator and once in the denominator are canceled. For example, *lb.* ÷ *lb.* = 1. This cancellation leaves only the name of the unit, *oz.*, in which the answer is expressed.

The Metric System

The basic units for the metric system are as follows:

length: meters (m)
volume: liters (L)
mass: grams (g)

The following prefixes are attached to the names of the basic units to denote other units whose size equals the basic unit multiplied or divided by a power of 10:

pico- (p) $= 10^{-12}$
nano- (n) $= 10^{-9}$
micro- (μ) $= 10^{-6}$
milli- (m) $= 10^{-3}$
centi- (c) $= 10^{-2}$
deci- (d) $= 10^{-1}$
kilo- (k) $= 10^{3}$
mega- (M) $= 10^{6}$

Thus, a kilometer (km) is 10^3 or 1,000 times as large as a meter. A centimeter (cm) is 10^{-2} times a meter or $\frac{1}{100}$ the size of a meter. A milligram (mg) is 10^{-3} times the size of a gram or $\frac{1}{1000}$ the size of a gram.

ALGEBRAIC EQUATIONS

A *term* is a numerical constant or the product (or quotient) of a numerical constant and one or more variables.

For example: $5x$, $3abc$, $\frac{2x}{y}$

An *algebraic* expression is a combination of one or more terms. The terms in an expression are separated by either $+$ or $-$ signs.

For example: $5xy$, $3ab + 2cd$.

In the term $5xy$, the numerical constant 5 is called a coefficient. In a simple term such as z, 1 is the coefficient.

A number without any variables is called a *constant term*. An expression with one term, such as $5xy$, is called a *monomial;* one with two terms, such as $6a - 2b$, is a *binomial.* The general name for expressions with more than one term is *polynomial.*

Substitution is a method used to evaluate an algebraic expression or to express an algebraic expression in terms of other variables.

EXAMPLE

Evaluate $x^2 + 3x + 3$ when $x = -3$.

Replace every x in the expression with -3, and then carry out the designated operations.

$x^2 + 3x + 3 = (-3)^2 + 3(-3) + 3 = 9 + (-9) + 3 = 3$

EXAMPLE

Express $\dfrac{a + b}{2a}$ in terms of x and y if $a = 2x$ and $b = 3y$.

Replace every a with $2x$ and every b with $3y$:

$$\frac{a + b}{2a} = \frac{2x + 3y}{2(2x)} = \frac{2x + 3y}{4x}$$

Linear Equations

An *equation* is an algebraic sentence that says two expressions are equal to each other. The two expressions may consist of numbers, variables, and arithmetic operations to be performed on these numbers and variables. To solve for some variable, manipulate the equation until that variable is isolated on one side of the equal sign, leaving any numbers or other variables on the other side. Of course, you must be careful to manipulate the equation only in accordance with the *equality postulate:* Whenever an operation is performed on one side of the equation, the same operation must be performed on the other side. Otherwise, the two sides of the equation will no longer be equal.

A *linear* or *first-degree equation* is an equation in which all the variables are raised to the first power. To solve such an equation, perform operations on both sides of the equation in order to get the variable for which you are solving alone on one side. The operations you can perform without upsetting the balance of the equation are addition and subtraction, and multiplication or division by a number other than zero. Typically, at each step in the process, you will need to use the reverse of the operation that is being applied to the variable in order to isolate the variable.

EXAMPLE

If $3x - 8 = x + 6$, what is x?

1. To get all the terms with the variable on one side of the equation, first add $-x$ to each side. Then combine the terms.

$$3x - 8 = x + 6$$
$$3x - x - 8 = x - x + 6$$
$$2x - 8 = 6$$

2. To get the constant terms on the other side of the equation, add $+8$ to each side.

$$2x - 8 + 8 = 6 + 8$$
$$2x = 14$$

3. Isolate the variable by dividing both sides by its coefficient.

$$\frac{2x}{2} = \frac{14}{2}$$
$$x = 7$$

You can easily check your work when solving this kind of equation. The answer you arrive at represents the value of the variable that makes the equation hold true. Therefore, to check that your answer is correct, just substitute this value for the variable in the original equation. If the equation holds true, you've found the correct answer.

Equations with fractional coefficients can be a little more tricky. They can be solved using the same approach, although this often leads to rather involved calculations. Instead, an equation of this type can be transformed into an equivalent equation that does not involve fractional coefficients.

EXAMPLE

Solve for x : $\dfrac{5x + 7}{2} = 8 + x$.

1. Multiply both sides of the equation by the lowest common denominator (LCD). Here the LCD is 2.

$$2\left(\frac{5x + 7}{2}\right) = 2\left(\frac{8 + x}{1}\right)$$

2. Clear the parentheses using the distributive property.

$$5x + 7 = 2(8 + x)$$
$$5x + 7 = 16 + 2x$$

3. Get all the terms with the variable on one side. Combine like terms.

$$5x - 2x = 16 - 7$$
$$3x = 9$$

4. Isolate the variable by dividing both sides by its coefficient.

$$x = \frac{9}{3} = 3$$

Inequalities

An *inequality* is a statement that two quantities are not equal.

INEQUALITY SYMBOLS

The following symbols are used to denote inequality:

- $>$ greater than
- $<$ less than
- $\geq$ greater than or equal to
- $\leq$ less than or equal to

SOLVING INEQUALITIES

The same methods are used to solve inequalities as are used in solving equations, with one exception: If the inequality is multiplied or divided by a negative number, the direction of the inequality is reversed. Thus, if the inequality $-5x < 10$ is multiplied by -1, the resulting inequality is $5x > -10$.

EXAMPLE

Solve for x: $3x - 16 > 4x + 12$.

$$3x - 4x - 16 > 4x - 4x + 12$$
$$-x - 16 + 16 > 12 + 16$$
$$-x > 28$$
$$x < 28$$

Simultaneous Equations

Two different equations with two variables (that is, *simultaneous equations*) can be combined to obtain a unique solution set. Isolate the variable in one equation, then plug that expression into the other equation.

EXAMPLE

Find the values for x and y if $x = 9 - 2y$ and $2x - 3y = 4$.

1. You know that $x = 9 - 2y$.
   Substitute $9 - 2y$ for x
   in the second equation.

$$2x - 3y = 4$$
$$2(9 - 2y) - 3y = 4$$
$$18 - 4y - 3y = 4$$

2. Solve for y.

$$-7y = -14$$
$$y = 2$$

3. To find the value of x,
   substitute 2 for y in the
   first equation and solve.

$$x = 9 - 2y$$
$$= 9 - 2(2)$$
$$= 5$$

PROBABILITY AND STATISTICS CONCEPTS

Here is the classic definition of probability: The probability of event A equals the number of favorable outcomes of A divided by the total number of outcomes.

$$P(A) = \frac{Favorable\ outcomes}{Total\ outcomes}$$

To use this definition, we must be dealing with equally likely, mutually exclusive events. When two or more outcomes of an experiment cannot occur at the same time, the outcomes are said to be *mutually exclusive.* If no outcome is any more likely to occur than any other, the outcomes are said to be *equally likely.*

For instance, consider an ordinary deck of playing cards. If an experiment consists of drawing one card at random from the well-shuffled deck, then there are 52 equally likely outcomes because any one of the 52 cards may be drawn. It is logical to decide that the outcomes are equally likely because, if the deck is well shuffled and a card is drawn at random, there is no reason to expect any card to be more likely to be drawn than any other. Moreover, on any draw of a single card, just one card and no other will be picked, so the outcomes are mutually exclusive.

EXAMPLE

Find the probability of drawing a black card in a single random draw from a well-shuffled deck of ordinary playing cards.

There are 52 cards; hence the experiment has 52 outcomes. We reason that each of these 52 outcomes is equally likely. Also, only one card can be drawn on any draw, so the outcomes are mutually exclusive. The "event" in which we are interested is drawing a black card. There are 26 black cards in the deck, so the number of favorable outcomes of the event is 26. Thus, we have

$$P(\text{drawing a black card}) = \frac{\text{Favorable outcomes}}{\text{Total outcomes}} = \frac{26}{52} = \frac{1}{2}$$

EXAMPLE

Find the probability of drawing an ace from a deck of cards on a single draw.

There are four aces in the deck. Hence, four of the 52 possible outcomes of the experiment correspond to the event of drawing an ace. Therefore, we have

$$P(\text{drawing a black card}) = \frac{\text{Favorable outcomes}}{\text{Total outcomes}} = \frac{4}{52} = \frac{1}{13}$$

There are numerous other "ideal" situations involving dice, coins, balls of different colors, and so on that can be used to illustrate the finding of the probability of elementary events by application of the classical definition of probability.

Measures of Location

THE MIDRANGE

The midrange is the number halfway between the smallest and the largest observation. By definition:

$$\text{Midrange} = \frac{\text{Smallest observation} + \text{Largest observation}}{2}$$

EXAMPLE

A sample consists of the observations 51, 47, 62, 54, 58, 65, 48, 41. The smallest observation is 41, and the largest is 65. Thus we have

$$Midrange = \frac{41 + 65}{2} = \frac{106}{2} = 53$$

THE MODE

The mode is defined as the observation in the sample that occurs most frequently. If each observation occurs the same number of times, there is no mode. If two or more observations occur the same number of times, there is more than one mode, and the sample is said to be *multimodal*. For example: If the sample is 14, 19, 16, 21, 18, 19, 24, 15, 19, the mode is 19. If the sample is 6, 7, 7, 3, 8, 5, 3, 9, there are two modes, 3 and 7.

THE MEDIAN

If the sample observations are arranged in order from smallest to largest, the median is defined as the middle observation if the number of observations is *odd,* and as the number halfway between the two middle observations if the number of observations is *even.*

EXAMPLE

Given the observations 34, 29, 26, 37, 31. Arranging the observations in order, we have 26, 29, 31, 34, and 37. The number of observations is odd; the median is 31.

Given the observations 34, 29, 26, 37, 31, 34. Arranging the observations in order, we have 26, 29, 31, 34, 34, 37. The number of observations is even. The median is halfway between the third and fourth observations. Thus the median is 32.5.

THE ARITHMETIC MEAN

A commonly used quantitative measurement is the arithmetic mean or average. The definition is simple:

$$Mean = \frac{Sum\ of\ observations}{Number\ of\ observations}$$

The number of observations is usually denoted as *n*. Also, the first observation is denoted as x_1, the second observation as x_2, the third as x_3, and so on, with the last observation denoted as x_n. The mean of the sample is denoted by the symbol $\bar{x}$. Thus the definition can be rewritten as:

$$\bar{x} = \frac{x_1 + x_2 + x_3 + \cdots + x_n}{n}$$

EXAMPLE

If a sample consists of the observations 8, 7, 11, 8, 12, 14, what is the mean?

$$Mean = \bar{x} = \frac{8 + 7 + 11 + 8 + 12 + 14}{6} = \frac{60}{6} = 10$$

Measures of Variation

The variance and the standard deviation are measures of the spread of a set of measurements.

SAMPLE VARIANCE

The variance, like the mean, takes into account each value in a set of data. It is calculated by taking the average value of the squares of the deviation for each point from the mean. The sample variance formula is used when you have sample data and you are trying to estimate the population variance.

The variance (s^2) of a set of measurements $x_1, x_2, \ldots, x_n$ is defined as follows:

$$s^2 = \frac{\sum(x - \bar{x})^2}{n - 1}$$
$$= \frac{(x_1 - \bar{x})^2 + (x_2 - \bar{x})^2 + \cdots + (x_n - \bar{x})^2}{n - 1}$$

where $\bar{x}$ is the sample mean.

STANDARD DEVIATION

The variance and the standard deviation are intimately related. The standard deviation(s) is the square root of the variance.

$$s = \sqrt{s^2}$$

EXAMPLE

The number of kilometers, denoted as x_1, x_2, and x_3, that three cars traveled were 931, 972, and 935, respectively. Find the variance and the standard deviation for these data.

First, find the sample mean ($\bar{x}$):

$$\bar{x} = \frac{x_1 + x_2 + x_3 + \cdots + x_n}{n} = \frac{931 + 972 + 935}{3} = 946$$

Now find the sample variance:

$$s^2 = \frac{\sum(x - \bar{x})^2}{n - 1}$$
$$= \frac{(x_1 - \bar{x})^2 + (x_2 - \bar{x})^2 + \cdots + (x_n - \bar{x})^2}{n - 1}$$
$$= \frac{(931 - 946)^2 + (972 - 946)^2 + (935 - 946)^2}{3 - 1}$$
$$= \frac{225 + 676 + 121}{2} = \frac{1022}{2} = 511$$

Finally, use the sample variance to find the sample standard deviation:

$$s = \sqrt{s^2} = \sqrt{511} = 22.6$$

PLANE GEOMETRY CONCEPTS

Angles

An *angle* is formed by two lines or line segments intersecting at a point. The point of intersection is called the *vertex* of the angle. Angles are measured in degrees (°) or radians.

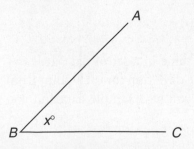

An *acute angle* is an angle whose degree measure is between 0° and 90°. A *right angle* is an angle whose degree measure is exactly 90°. An *obtuse angle* is an angle whose degree measure is between 90° and 180°. A *straight angle* is an angle whose degree measure is exactly 180°.

Two angles are *complementary* if together they make up a right angle (i.e., if the sum of their measures is 90°). Two angles are *supplementary* if together they make up a straight angle (i.e., if the sum of their measures is 180°).

Triangles

A *triangle* is a closed figure with three angles and three straight sides. The sum of the interior angles of any triangle is 180°.

The *altitude* (or height) of a triangle is the perpendicular distance from a vertex to the side opposite the vertex. The altitude may fall inside the triangle, outside the triangle, or on one of the sides.

The *perimeter* of a triangle is the distance around the triangle. In other words, the perimeter is equal to the sum of the lengths of the sides.

The *area* of a triangle can be found by using this formula:

$$Area = \frac{1}{2} Base \times height$$

$$A = \frac{1}{2} bh$$

SIMILAR AND CONGRUENT TRIANGLES

Triangles are *similar* if they have the same shape, that is, if corresponding angles have the same measure. For instance, any two triangles whose angles measure 30°, 60°, and 90° are similar. In similar triangles, corresponding sides are in the same ratio.

Triangles are *congruent* if corresponding angles have the same measure and corresponding sides have the same length.

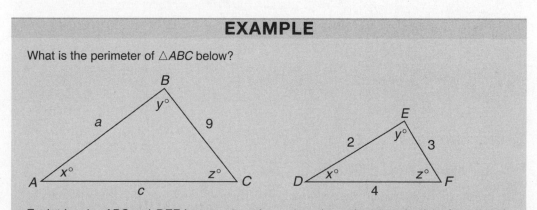

EXAMPLE

What is the perimeter of △*ABC* below?

Each triangle, *ABC* and *DEF*, has an x° angle, a y° angle, and a z° angle; therefore, the triangles are similar, and corresponding sides are in the same ratio. *BC* and *EF* are corresponding sides; each is opposite the x° angle. Since *BC* is three times the length of *EF*, each side of △*ABC* will be three times the length of the corresponding side of △*DEF*. Therefore *AB* = 3(*DF*) or 6, and *AC* = 3(*DF*) or 12. The perimeter of △*ABC* is 6 + 12 + 9 = 27.

The ratio of the *areas* of two similar triangles is the *square* of the ratio of corresponding lengths. For instance, in the example above, since each side of $\triangle ABC$ is three times the length of the corresponding side of $\triangle DEF$, $\triangle ABC$ must have 3^2 or 9 times the area of $\triangle DEF$.

RIGHT TRIANGLES

A right triangle has one interior angle of 90°. The longest side, which lies opposite the right triangle, is called the *hypotenuse.* The other two sides are the *legs.*

The *Pythagorean theorem,* which holds for all right triangles, states that the square of the length of the hypotenuse is equal to the sum of the squares of the length of the legs.

$$(Leg_1)^2 + (Leg_2)^2 = (Hypotenuse)^2$$

Some sets of integers happen to satisfy the Pythagorean theorem and are commonly referred to as *Pythagorean triplets.* One very common set that you might remember is 3, 4, and 5. Since $3^2 + 4^2 = 5^2$, you can have a right triangle with legs of lengths 3 and 4 and hypotenuse of length 5. In addition, any multiple of these lengths makes another Pythagorean triplet; for instance, $6^2 + 8^2 = 10^2$, so 6, 8, and 10 also make a right triangle. One other triplet that appears occasionally is 5, 12, and 13.

The Pythagorean theorem is very useful whenever you are given the lengths of two sides of a right triangle; you can find the length of the third side with the Pythagorean theorem.

EXAMPLE

What is the length of the hypotenuse of a right triangle with legs of lengths 6 and 7?

Use the Pythagorean theorem: The square of the length of the hypotenuse equals the sum of the squares of the lengths of the legs. Here the legs are 6 and 7, so

$$\begin{aligned} \text{Hypotenuse}^2 &= 6^2 + 7^2 \\ &= 36 + 49 \\ &= 85 \\ &= \sqrt{85} \end{aligned}$$

Quadrilaterals

RECTANGLES AND SQUARES

The most important quadrilaterals to know for the DAT are the rectangle and the square.

A *rectangle* is a quadrilateral with four equal angles, each a right angle. The opposite sides of a rectangle are equal in length. Also, the diagonals of a rectangle have equal lengths.

A *square* is a rectangle with four equal sides.

AREAS OF QUADRILATERALS

To find the *area of a rectangle*, multiply the lengths of any two adjacent sides, called the length and width:

Area of rectangle = Length × Width
$$A = lw$$

To find the *area of a square*, since the length and width are equal, square the length of the side:

Area of square = (side)²
$$A = s^2$$

Circles

A circle is the set of all points in a plane at the same distance from a certain point. This point is called the *center* of the circle.

The *diameter* is a line segment that connects two points on the circle and passes through the center of the circle.

The *radius* is a line segment from the center of the circle to any point on the circle. The length of the radius of a circle is one-half the length of the diameter.

The *circumference* is the distance around the circle. The number π (pi) is the ratio of a circle's circumference to its diameter. The value of π is 3.1415926..., usually approximated as 3.14.

Since π equals the ratio of the circumference to the diameter, a formula for the circumference is:

Circumference = π(diameter)   or   *Circumference = 2π(radius)*
$$C = \pi d \qquad\qquad\qquad\qquad C = 2\pi r$$

The *area of a circle* is given by the formula:

Area = π(radius)²
$$A = \pi r^2$$

TRIGONOMETRY

The Cartesian Coordinate System

In trigonometry, you will frequently find it necessary to describe the position of a point in a plane. You'll use the *Cartesian* or *rectangular* coordinate system to do this. For a point (x, y) in the Cartesian plane, the first, or x, coordinate determines the location of that point with respect to the horizontal, or x, axis, and the second, or y, coordinate determines the location of that point with respect to the vertical or y axis. The origin of the Cartesian coordinate system is point $(0, 0)$.

THE DISTANCE FORMULA

If $A(x_1, y_1)$ and $B(x_2, y_2)$ are two points in a Cartesian plane, the *distance* between them, d_{AB}, is the length of the straight line segment joining the two points.

$$d_{AB} = \sqrt{(x_2 - x_1)^2 + (y_2 - y_1)^2}$$

EXAMPLE

Find the distance between points $(-2, 3)$ and $(2, -3)$.

$$d = \sqrt{(-2-2)^2 + (3-(-3))^2} = \sqrt{(-4)^2 + 6^2} = \sqrt{52} = 7.21$$

EXAMPLE

Find the lengths of the sides of the triangle whose vertices are at $A(9,4)$, $B(3,8)$, and $C(0,1)$.

$$d_{AB} = \sqrt{(9-3)^2 + (4-8)^2} = \sqrt{6^2 + (-4)^2} = \sqrt{52} = 7.21$$

$$d_{AC} = \sqrt{(9-0)^2 + (4-1)^2} = \sqrt{9^2 + 3^2} = \sqrt{90} = 9.49$$

$$d_{BC} = \sqrt{(3-0)^2 + (8-1)^2} = \sqrt{3^2 + 7^2} = \sqrt{58} = 7.62$$

APPLICATION OF THE DISTANCE FORMULA TO CIRCLES

If (x, y) is a point on a circle with the center at the origin and radius r, the distance between (x, y) and $(0, 0)$ is r.

Applying the distance formula to (x, y) and $(0, 0)$ gives:

$$\sqrt{(x-0)^2 + (y-0)^2} = r$$

Simplifying and squaring both sides of the equation leads to the equation of a circle with radius r centered at the origin.

$$x^2 + y^2 = r^2$$

EXAMPLE

Find the equation for a circle with the center at the origin if $r = 2$.

Substituting into the simplified equation for a circle centered at the origin, the equation is:

$$x^2 + y^2 = 4$$

EXAMPLE

If the equation of a circle is as follows:

$$x^2 + y^2 = 25$$

What is the radius of the circle?

$$r^2 = 25$$
$$r = \sqrt{25} = 5$$

Trigonometry of the Right Triangle

A *right triangle* contains one 90° angle and two acute angles (less than 90°). By definition, y is the length of the leg opposite θ, x is the length of the leg adjacent to θ, where θ is one of the acute angles. The hypotenuse is the terminal side of θ, and its length is designated as h.

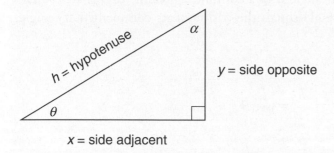

The Trigonometric Functions

The six trigonometric functions are the *sine, cosine, tangent, cosecant, secant,* and *cotangent* of an angle θ. They are defined as follows:

$$\sin \theta = \frac{\text{side opposite } \theta}{\text{hypotenuse}} = \frac{y}{h} \qquad \csc \theta = \frac{\text{hypotenuse}}{\text{side opposite } \theta} = \frac{h}{y}$$

$$\cos \theta = \frac{\text{side adjacent } \theta}{\text{hypotenuse}} = \frac{x}{h} \qquad \sec \theta = \frac{\text{hypotenuse}}{\text{side adjacent } \theta} = \frac{h}{x}$$

$$\tan \theta = \frac{\text{side opposite } \theta}{\text{side adjacent } \theta} = \frac{y}{x} \qquad \cot \theta = \frac{\text{side adjacent } \theta}{\text{side opposite } \theta} = \frac{x}{y}$$

EXAMPLE

Use the right triangle to find the six trigonometric functions of angle θ.

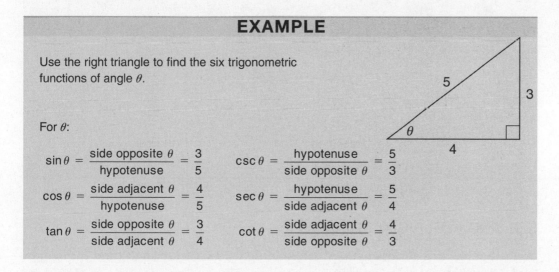

For θ:

$$\sin \theta = \frac{\text{side opposite } \theta}{\text{hypotenuse}} = \frac{3}{5} \qquad \csc \theta = \frac{\text{hypotenuse}}{\text{side opposite } \theta} = \frac{5}{3}$$

$$\cos \theta = \frac{\text{side adjacent } \theta}{\text{hypotenuse}} = \frac{4}{5} \qquad \sec \theta = \frac{\text{hypotenuse}}{\text{side adjacent } \theta} = \frac{5}{4}$$

$$\tan \theta = \frac{\text{side opposite } \theta}{\text{side adjacent } \theta} = \frac{3}{4} \qquad \cot \theta = \frac{\text{side adjacent } \theta}{\text{side opposite } \theta} = \frac{4}{3}$$

NUMERICAL RANGE OF THE TRIGONOMETRIC FUNCTIONS

The length of the hypotenuse of any right angle is never less than the length of either of the other two legs; the values of the sine and cosine of an acute angle can never be greater than $+1$ or less than -1. Similarly, the values of the cosecant and secant, since they are reciprocals of the sine and cosine, can never take values between -1 and $+1$.

Because the legs of a right triangle can be in any ratio to each other, however, the values of the tangent and cotangent can vary from arbitrarily large negative numbers to arbitrarily large positive values.

COMPLEMENTARY ANGLES

The two acute angles in a right triangle with a combined measure of 90° are *complementary angles*. The sine of an angle equals the cosine of its complementary angle. If $<A + <B = \frac{1}{2}\pi$, then:

$$\sin A = \frac{y}{h} = \cos B \qquad \csc A = \frac{h}{y} = \sec B$$

$$\cos A = \frac{x}{h} = \sin B \qquad \sec A = \frac{h}{x} = \csc B$$

$$\tan A = \frac{y}{x} = \cot B \qquad \cot A = \frac{y}{x} = \tan B$$

Values of the Trigonometric Functions for Selected Acute Angles

$\theta°$	(radians)	$\sin\theta$	$\cos\theta$	$\tan\theta$	$\csc\theta$	$\sec\theta$	$\cot\theta$
0	(0)	0	1	0	Undefined	1	Undefined
30	$\left(\frac{\pi}{6}\right)$	$\frac{1}{2}$	$\frac{\sqrt{3}}{2}$	$\frac{\sqrt{3}}{3}$	2	$\frac{2\sqrt{3}}{3}$	$\sqrt{3}$
45	$\left(\frac{\pi}{4}\right)$	$\frac{\sqrt{2}}{2}$	$\frac{\sqrt{2}}{2}$	1	$\sqrt{2}$	$\sqrt{2}$	1
60	$\left(\frac{\pi}{3}\right)$	$\frac{\sqrt{3}}{2}$	$\frac{1}{2}$	$\sqrt{3}$	$\frac{2\sqrt{3}}{3}$	2	$\frac{\sqrt{3}}{3}$
90	$\left(\frac{\pi}{2}\right)$	1	0	Undefined	1	Undefined	0

SOLVING FOR RIGHT TRIANGLES

You can solve for right triangles by determining the two acute angles and the lengths of the three sides of the triangle. A trigonometric ratio of an acute angle involves three quantities: the length of two sides and an angle. Thus, given two of these quantities, either the length of one side and the measure of one angle, or the lengths of two sides, you can find the third.

Given the lengths of two sides of a right triangle, you can use the Pythagorean theorem to determine the length of the remaining side. You can then find any trigonometric function for either of the two unknown angles. Once you know one of the acute angles, you can find the other angle because the sum of the acute angles is 90°.

The Trigonometric Identities

The following trigonometic identities are consequences of the definitions of the six trigonometric functions given on page 338:

RECIPROCAL IDENTITIES

$$\frac{1}{\sin\theta} = \frac{1}{\dfrac{y}{h}} = \frac{h}{y} = \csc\theta \qquad \sin\theta\,\csc\theta = 1$$

$$\frac{1}{\cos\theta} = \frac{1}{\dfrac{x}{h}} = \frac{h}{x} = \sec\theta \qquad \cos\theta\,\sec\theta = 1$$

$$\frac{1}{\tan\theta} = \frac{1}{\dfrac{y}{x}} = \frac{x}{y} = \cot\theta \qquad \tan\theta\,\cot\theta = 1$$

PYTHAGOREAN IDENTITIES

$$\cos^2\theta + \sin^2\theta = 1$$
$$1 + \tan^2\theta = \sec^2\theta$$
$$1 + \cot^2\theta = \csc^2\theta$$

RATIO IDENTITIES

$$\tan\theta = \frac{y}{k} = \frac{\dfrac{y}{h}}{\dfrac{x}{h}} = \frac{\sin\theta}{\cos\theta}$$

$$\cot\theta = \frac{x}{y} = \frac{\dfrac{x}{h}}{\dfrac{y}{h}} = \frac{\cos\theta}{\sin\theta}$$

VERIFYING TRIGONOMETRIC IDENTITIES

By applying algebraic processes such as factorization, addition, multiplication, and simplification of fractions to the fundamental identities, you can verify trigonometric identities.

EXAMPLE

Simplify $\sin^4\theta - \cos^4\theta$.

Factor as the difference of two squares, and use $\sin^2\theta + \cos^2\theta = 1$.

$$\begin{aligned}
\sin^4\theta - \cos^4\theta &= (\sin^2\theta - \cos^2\theta)(\sin^2\theta + \cos^2\theta) \\
&= (\sin^2\theta - \cos^2\theta)(1) = (\sin^2\theta + \cos^2\theta - \cos^2\theta) - \cos^2\theta \\
&= 1 - \cos^2\theta - \cos^2\theta \\
&= 1 - 2\cos^2\theta
\end{aligned}$$

APPLIED MATHEMATICAL PROBLEMS

Many people dislike word problems and not unreasonably. Turning a word problem into a straightforward question means that you must go to the trouble of translating the problem before you start working on it, but in some ways this actually makes the problem easier. The test makers figure that they have made the problem difficult enough by adding the extra step of translating from English to math. Once you have done this, however, you will generally find that the concepts and processes involved are rather simple, so that you stand an excellent chance of being able to solve the problem.

Here are a few general tips for solving word problems:

- Read through the whole problem first, without pausing for details, to get a sense of what is involved.

- Name the variables in a way that makes it easy to remember what they stand for. For example, denote the unknown quantity John's age as j, and the unknown quantity Brian's age as b.

- Be aware that, when you are asked to find numerical values for unknown quantities, the word problem will give you enough information to set up a sufficient number of equations to solve for those quantities.

- Be careful of the order in which you translate terms. For example, consider the following common mistranslation: 3 less than $4x$ equals 9. This translates as $4x - 3 = 9$, not $3 - 4x = 9$.

Percent Word Problems

PROFIT AND LOSS

The *profit* made on an item is the selling price minus the cost to the seller. If the cost is more than the selling price, there is a *loss*, not a profit.

EXAMPLE

If a camera priced at $360 represents a potential profit of 20% to a store if sold, what was the original cost of the camera to the store?

Let C represent the cost, then set up the equation to find the cost:

$$Cost + Profit = Selling\ price$$
$$C + (20\%)C = \$360$$
$$C + \frac{1}{5}C = \$360$$
$$\frac{6}{5}C = \$360$$
$$C = \$360 \times \frac{5}{6} = \$300$$

The cost of the camera to the store was $300.

GROSS AND NET

Gross is the total amount before any deductions are made; *net* is the amount after deductions are made. For instance, gross pay is the total amount of money earned, while net pay is gross pay minus any deductions, such as taxes.

DISCOUNT

The *discount* on an item is usually a percent of a previous price for the item.

EXAMPLE

What is the percent discount on a jacket marked down from $120 to $100?

The percent discount equals the amount of discount divided by the original price. The amount of discount is $120 − $100 or $20. The original price was $120. The percent discount equals:

$$Percent\ discount = \frac{Amount\ of\ discount}{Original\ price}$$

$$= \frac{\$120 - \$100}{\$120} = \frac{\$20}{\$120} = \frac{1}{6} = 16\frac{2}{3}\%$$

Ratio and Proportion Word Problems

A *ratio* is a comparison of two quantities by division. A ratio may be written with a fraction bar $\left(\frac{x}{y}\right)$, with a colon (*x:y*), or in words (ratio of *x* to *y*). In a ratio of two numbers, the numerator is often associated with the word *of*, the denominator with the word *to*.

We frequently deal with ratios by working with a *proportion*. A proportion is simply an equation in which two ratios are set equal to one another.

EXAMPLE

There are 32 marbles in a bag containing only blue and green marbles. If there are three green marbles for every blue marble, how many blue marbles are in the bag?

Translate from English into math. "Three green marbles for every blue marble" means the ratio of green to blue = 3:1.

Set up a proportion with a part to whole ratio to find the number of blue marbles. The ratio of the number of blue marbles to the total number of marbles is 1:[1+3] or 1:4.

Using *b* for the number of blue marbles, you have the proportion:

$$\frac{1}{4} = \frac{b}{32}$$
$$4b = 32$$
$$b = 8$$

There are eight blue marbles in the bag.

Word Problems Involving Distance, Rate, and Time

The solution of distance problems is based on this formula:

$$Distance = Rate \times Time$$

EXAMPLE

A car travels 60 kilometers in 1 hour before a piston breaks, then travels at 30 kilometers per hour for the remaining 60 kilometers to its destination. What is the average speed, in kilometers per hour for the entire trip?

The average speed equals the total distance the car travels divided by the total time. You are told that the car goes 60 kilometers in 1 hour before a piston breaks, and then travels another 60 kilometers at 30 kilometers per hour. The second part of the trip must take 2 hours, so the car travels a total of 120 kilometers and covers this distance in 3 hours. Its average speed equals

$$Rate = \frac{Distance}{Time}$$

$$= \frac{120\,km}{3h} = 40km/h$$

The average speed for the entire trip is 40 kilometers per hour.

Word Problems Involving Work Rates of Two Individuals

There is a general formula, the *work formula,* that can be used to find how long a number of people working together require to complete a task. Let's say that there are three people; the first takes t_1 units of time to complete the job, the second t_2 units of time, and the third t_3 units of time. If the time required for all three working together to complete the job is T, then

$$\frac{1}{t_1} + \frac{1}{t_2} + \frac{1}{t_3} = \frac{1}{T}$$

EXAMPLE

Cathy can finish a job in 5 hours, and Steve can finish the same job in 10 hours. How many minutes will it take both of them together to finish the job?

Call the amount of time Cathy takes to finish the job t_1 and the amount of time Steve takes t_2; that is, $t_1 = 5$ hours and $t_2 = 10$ hours. Then,

$$\frac{1}{5} + \frac{1}{10} = \frac{2}{10} + \frac{1}{10} = \frac{3}{10} = \frac{1}{T}$$
$$\frac{1}{T} = \frac{3}{10}$$
$$T = \frac{10}{3}hr$$

Convert the hours to minutes:

$$\frac{10}{3}h = \frac{10}{3} \times 60\,min = 200\,min$$

Working together, Cathy and Steve will take 200 minutes to finish the job.

Word Problems Using Odd and Even Integers

Integers are real numbers. They consist of negative numbers, zero, and positive numbers. The set of integers is (…, −5, −4, −3, −2, −1, 0, 1, 2, 3, 4, 5, …). The set of even integers is (…, −4, −2, 0, 2, 4, …). The set of odd integers is (…, −3, −1, 0, 1, 3, …).

Consecutive integers are integers that are listed in consecutive order. If *n* is an even integer, three consecutive even integers are *n*, *n* + 2, *n* + 4. For example, if *n* = 2, the three consecutive even integers are 2, 4, and 6. If *n* is an odd integer, three consecutive odd integers are *n*, *n* + 2, *n* + 4. For example, if *n* = 3, the three consecutive odd integers are 3, 5, and 7.

EXAMPLE

Find five consecutive even integers that have a sum equal to 40.

Let *n* represent the smallest even integer. The four other even integers will be expressed in terms of *n*.

Let *n* = 1st even integer,
n + 2 = 2nd even integer,
n + 4 = 3rd even integer,
n + 6 = 4th even integer,
n + 8 = 5th even integer.

$$n + (n + 2) + (n + 4) + (n + 6) + (n + 8) = 40$$
$$5n + 20 = 40$$
$$5n = 40 - 20$$
$$= 20$$
$$n = 4$$

The five consecutive even integers that have a sum of 40 are 4, 6, 8, 10, and 12.

Word Problems Involving Ages

Age problems are solved by comparing ages at the present, in the future, and in the past. If the present age is represented by *x*, a future age is found by adding years to *x*, and a past age is found by subtracting years from *x*.

EXAMPLE

Philip is now five times as old as Ed was 5 years ago. If the sum of Philip's and Ed's ages is 35, in how many years will Philip be twice as old as Ed?

Let *p* = Philip's current age

and *e* = Ed's current age

Translate the first sentence to get the first equation:

Philip's current age is five times Ed's age 5 years ago.

$$p = 5(e - 5)$$

Translate the first part of the second sentence to get the second equation:

The sum of Philip's and Ed's ages is 35.

$p + e = 35$

Now you are ready to solve for the two unknowns. Solve for e in terms of p in the second equation.

$p + e = 35$

$e = 35 - p$

Now plug this value for e into the first equation and solve for p:

$$p = 5(e - 5)$$
$$= 5(35 - p - 5)$$
$$= 5(30 - p)$$
$$= 150 - 5p$$
$$6p = 150 - 5p$$
$$p = 25$$

Plug this value for p into either equation to solve for e:

$$e = 35 - p$$
$$= 35 - 25 = 10$$

Philip is currently 25 and Ed is currently 10. You still haven't answered the question asked, though; you need to set up an equation to find the number of years after which Philip will be twice as old as Ed.

Let x be the number of years from now in which Philip will be twice as old as Ed. Set up the equation and solve for x.

$$25 + x = 2(10 + x)$$
$$25 + x = 20 + 2x$$
$$x = 5$$

So Philip will be twice as old as Ed in 5 years.

Answer Sheet 1
MODEL EXAMINATION A

Survey of the Natural Sciences

1 (A) (B) (C) (D) (E)	26 (A) (B) (C) (D) (E)	51 (A) (B) (C) (D) (E)	76 (A) (B) (C) (D) (E)
2 (A) (B) (C) (D) (E)	27 (A) (B) (C) (D) (E)	52 (A) (B) (C) (D) (E)	77 (A) (B) (C) (D) (E)
3 (A) (B) (C) (D) (E)	28 (A) (B) (C) (D) (E)	53 (A) (B) (C) (D) (E)	78 (A) (B) (C) (D) (E)
4 (A) (B) (C) (D) (E)	29 (A) (B) (C) (D) (E)	54 (A) (B) (C) (D) (E)	79 (A) (B) (C) (D) (E)
5 (A) (B) (C) (D) (E)	30 (A) (B) (C) (D) (E)	55 (A) (B) (C) (D) (E)	80 (A) (B) (C) (D) (E)
6 (A) (B) (C) (D) (E)	31 (A) (B) (C) (D) (E)	56 (A) (B) (C) (D) (E)	81 (A) (B) (C) (D) (E)
7 (A) (B) (C) (D) (E)	32 (A) (B) (C) (D) (E)	57 (A) (B) (C) (D) (E)	82 (A) (B) (C) (D) (E)
8 (A) (B) (C) (D) (E)	33 (A) (B) (C) (D) (E)	58 (A) (B) (C) (D) (E)	83 (A) (B) (C) (D) (E)
9 (A) (B) (C) (D) (E)	34 (A) (B) (C) (D) (E)	59 (A) (B) (C) (D) (E)	84 (A) (B) (C) (D) (E)
10 (A) (B) (C) (D) (E)	35 (A) (B) (C) (D) (E)	60 (A) (B) (C) (D) (E)	85 (A) (B) (C) (D) (E)
11 (A) (B) (C) (D) (E)	36 (A) (B) (C) (D) (E)	61 (A) (B) (C) (D) (E)	86 (A) (B) (C) (D) (E)
12 (A) (B) (C) (D) (E)	37 (A) (B) (C) (D) (E)	62 (A) (B) (C) (D) (E)	87 (A) (B) (C) (D) (E)
13 (A) (B) (C) (D) (E)	38 (A) (B) (C) (D) (E)	63 (A) (B) (C) (D) (E)	88 (A) (B) (C) (D) (E)
14 (A) (B) (C) (D) (E)	39 (A) (B) (C) (D) (E)	64 (A) (B) (C) (D) (E)	89 (A) (B) (C) (D) (E)
15 (A) (B) (C) (D) (E)	40 (A) (B) (C) (D) (E)	65 (A) (B) (C) (D) (E)	90 (A) (B) (C) (D) (E)
16 (A) (B) (C) (D) (E)	41 (A) (B) (C) (D) (E)	66 (A) (B) (C) (D) (E)	91 (A) (B) (C) (D) (E)
17 (A) (B) (C) (D) (E)	42 (A) (B) (C) (D) (E)	67 (A) (B) (C) (D) (E)	92 (A) (B) (C) (D) (E)
18 (A) (B) (C) (D) (E)	43 (A) (B) (C) (D) (E)	68 (A) (B) (C) (D) (E)	93 (A) (B) (C) (D) (E)
19 (A) (B) (C) (D) (E)	44 (A) (B) (C) (D) (E)	69 (A) (B) (C) (D) (E)	94 (A) (B) (C) (D) (E)
20 (A) (B) (C) (D) (E)	45 (A) (B) (C) (D) (E)	70 (A) (B) (C) (D) (E)	95 (A) (B) (C) (D) (E)
21 (A) (B) (C) (D) (E)	46 (A) (B) (C) (D) (E)	71 (A) (B) (C) (D) (E)	96 (A) (B) (C) (D) (E)
22 (A) (B) (C) (D) (E)	47 (A) (B) (C) (D) (E)	72 (A) (B) (C) (D) (E)	97 (A) (B) (C) (D) (E)
23 (A) (B) (C) (D) (E)	48 (A) (B) (C) (D) (E)	73 (A) (B) (C) (D) (E)	98 (A) (B) (C) (D) (E)
24 (A) (B) (C) (D) (E)	49 (A) (B) (C) (D) (E)	74 (A) (B) (C) (D) (E)	99 (A) (B) (C) (D) (E)
25 (A) (B) (C) (D) (E)	50 (A) (B) (C) (D) (E)	75 (A) (B) (C) (D) (E)	100 (A) (B) (C) (D) (E)

The actual DAT is given in a computer test format. It is highly recommended that you obtain a copy of the DAT tutorial disk to familiarize yourself with the format.

Perceptual Ability Test

1 Ⓐ Ⓑ Ⓒ Ⓓ Ⓔ	24 Ⓐ Ⓑ Ⓒ Ⓓ Ⓔ	47 Ⓐ Ⓑ Ⓒ Ⓓ Ⓔ	70 Ⓐ Ⓑ Ⓒ Ⓓ Ⓔ
2 Ⓐ Ⓑ Ⓒ Ⓓ Ⓔ	25 Ⓐ Ⓑ Ⓒ Ⓓ Ⓔ	48 Ⓐ Ⓑ Ⓒ Ⓓ Ⓔ	71 Ⓐ Ⓑ Ⓒ Ⓓ Ⓔ
3 Ⓐ Ⓑ Ⓒ Ⓓ Ⓔ	26 Ⓐ Ⓑ Ⓒ Ⓓ Ⓔ	49 Ⓐ Ⓑ Ⓒ Ⓓ Ⓔ	72 Ⓐ Ⓑ Ⓒ Ⓓ Ⓔ
4 Ⓐ Ⓑ Ⓒ Ⓓ Ⓔ	27 Ⓐ Ⓑ Ⓒ Ⓓ Ⓔ	50 Ⓐ Ⓑ Ⓒ Ⓓ Ⓔ	73 Ⓐ Ⓑ Ⓒ Ⓓ Ⓔ
5 Ⓐ Ⓑ Ⓒ Ⓓ Ⓔ	28 Ⓐ Ⓑ Ⓒ Ⓓ Ⓔ	51 Ⓐ Ⓑ Ⓒ Ⓓ Ⓔ	74 Ⓐ Ⓑ Ⓒ Ⓓ Ⓔ
6 Ⓐ Ⓑ Ⓒ Ⓓ Ⓔ	29 Ⓐ Ⓑ Ⓒ Ⓓ Ⓔ	52 Ⓐ Ⓑ Ⓒ Ⓓ Ⓔ	75 Ⓐ Ⓑ Ⓒ Ⓓ Ⓔ
7 Ⓐ Ⓑ Ⓒ Ⓓ Ⓔ	30 Ⓐ Ⓑ Ⓒ Ⓓ Ⓔ	53 Ⓐ Ⓑ Ⓒ Ⓓ Ⓔ	76 Ⓐ Ⓑ Ⓒ Ⓓ Ⓔ
8 Ⓐ Ⓑ Ⓒ Ⓓ Ⓔ	31 Ⓐ Ⓑ Ⓒ Ⓓ Ⓔ	54 Ⓐ Ⓑ Ⓒ Ⓓ Ⓔ	77 Ⓐ Ⓑ Ⓒ Ⓓ Ⓔ
9 Ⓐ Ⓑ Ⓒ Ⓓ Ⓔ	32 Ⓐ Ⓑ Ⓒ Ⓓ Ⓔ	55 Ⓐ Ⓑ Ⓒ Ⓓ Ⓔ	78 Ⓐ Ⓑ Ⓒ Ⓓ Ⓔ
10 Ⓐ Ⓑ Ⓒ Ⓓ Ⓔ	33 Ⓐ Ⓑ Ⓒ Ⓓ Ⓔ	56 Ⓐ Ⓑ Ⓒ Ⓓ Ⓔ	79 Ⓐ Ⓑ Ⓒ Ⓓ Ⓔ
11 Ⓐ Ⓑ Ⓒ Ⓓ Ⓔ	34 Ⓐ Ⓑ Ⓒ Ⓓ Ⓔ	57 Ⓐ Ⓑ Ⓒ Ⓓ Ⓔ	80 Ⓐ Ⓑ Ⓒ Ⓓ Ⓔ
12 Ⓐ Ⓑ Ⓒ Ⓓ Ⓔ	35 Ⓐ Ⓑ Ⓒ Ⓓ Ⓔ	58 Ⓐ Ⓑ Ⓒ Ⓓ Ⓔ	81 Ⓐ Ⓑ Ⓒ Ⓓ Ⓔ
13 Ⓐ Ⓑ Ⓒ Ⓓ Ⓔ	36 Ⓐ Ⓑ Ⓒ Ⓓ Ⓔ	59 Ⓐ Ⓑ Ⓒ Ⓓ Ⓔ	82 Ⓐ Ⓑ Ⓒ Ⓓ Ⓔ
14 Ⓐ Ⓑ Ⓒ Ⓓ Ⓔ	37 Ⓐ Ⓑ Ⓒ Ⓓ Ⓔ	60 Ⓐ Ⓑ Ⓒ Ⓓ Ⓔ	83 Ⓐ Ⓑ Ⓒ Ⓓ Ⓔ
15 Ⓐ Ⓑ Ⓒ Ⓓ Ⓔ	38 Ⓐ Ⓑ Ⓒ Ⓓ Ⓔ	61 Ⓐ Ⓑ Ⓒ Ⓓ Ⓔ	84 Ⓐ Ⓑ Ⓒ Ⓓ Ⓔ
16 Ⓐ Ⓑ Ⓒ Ⓓ Ⓔ	39 Ⓐ Ⓑ Ⓒ Ⓓ Ⓔ	62 Ⓐ Ⓑ Ⓒ Ⓓ Ⓔ	85 Ⓐ Ⓑ Ⓒ Ⓓ Ⓔ
17 Ⓐ Ⓑ Ⓒ Ⓓ Ⓔ	40 Ⓐ Ⓑ Ⓒ Ⓓ Ⓔ	63 Ⓐ Ⓑ Ⓒ Ⓓ Ⓔ	86 Ⓐ Ⓑ Ⓒ Ⓓ Ⓔ
18 Ⓐ Ⓑ Ⓒ Ⓓ Ⓔ	41 Ⓐ Ⓑ Ⓒ Ⓓ Ⓔ	64 Ⓐ Ⓑ Ⓒ Ⓓ Ⓔ	87 Ⓐ Ⓑ Ⓒ Ⓓ Ⓔ
19 Ⓐ Ⓑ Ⓒ Ⓓ Ⓔ	42 Ⓐ Ⓑ Ⓒ Ⓓ Ⓔ	65 Ⓐ Ⓑ Ⓒ Ⓓ Ⓔ	88 Ⓐ Ⓑ Ⓒ Ⓓ Ⓔ
20 Ⓐ Ⓑ Ⓒ Ⓓ Ⓔ	43 Ⓐ Ⓑ Ⓒ Ⓓ Ⓔ	66 Ⓐ Ⓑ Ⓒ Ⓓ Ⓔ	89 Ⓐ Ⓑ Ⓒ Ⓓ Ⓔ
21 Ⓐ Ⓑ Ⓒ Ⓓ Ⓔ	44 Ⓐ Ⓑ Ⓒ Ⓓ Ⓔ	67 Ⓐ Ⓑ Ⓒ Ⓓ Ⓔ	90 Ⓐ Ⓑ Ⓒ Ⓓ Ⓔ
22 Ⓐ Ⓑ Ⓒ Ⓓ Ⓔ	45 Ⓐ Ⓑ Ⓒ Ⓓ Ⓔ	68 Ⓐ Ⓑ Ⓒ Ⓓ Ⓔ	
23 Ⓐ Ⓑ Ⓒ Ⓓ Ⓔ	46 Ⓐ Ⓑ Ⓒ Ⓓ Ⓔ	69 Ⓐ Ⓑ Ⓒ Ⓓ Ⓔ	

Answer Sheet 2
MODEL EXAMINATION A

Reading Comprehension Test

1 Ⓐ Ⓑ Ⓒ Ⓓ Ⓔ   14 Ⓐ Ⓑ Ⓒ Ⓓ Ⓔ   27 Ⓐ Ⓑ Ⓒ Ⓓ Ⓔ   40 Ⓐ Ⓑ Ⓒ Ⓓ Ⓔ
2 Ⓐ Ⓑ Ⓒ Ⓓ Ⓔ   15 Ⓐ Ⓑ Ⓒ Ⓓ Ⓔ   28 Ⓐ Ⓑ Ⓒ Ⓓ Ⓔ   41 Ⓐ Ⓑ Ⓒ Ⓓ Ⓔ
3 Ⓐ Ⓑ Ⓒ Ⓓ Ⓔ   16 Ⓐ Ⓑ Ⓒ Ⓓ Ⓔ   29 Ⓐ Ⓑ Ⓒ Ⓓ Ⓔ   42 Ⓐ Ⓑ Ⓒ Ⓓ Ⓔ
4 Ⓐ Ⓑ Ⓒ Ⓓ Ⓔ   17 Ⓐ Ⓑ Ⓒ Ⓓ Ⓔ   30 Ⓐ Ⓑ Ⓒ Ⓓ Ⓔ   43 Ⓐ Ⓑ Ⓒ Ⓓ Ⓔ
5 Ⓐ Ⓑ Ⓒ Ⓓ Ⓔ   18 Ⓐ Ⓑ Ⓒ Ⓓ Ⓔ   31 Ⓐ Ⓑ Ⓒ Ⓓ Ⓔ   44 Ⓐ Ⓑ Ⓒ Ⓓ Ⓔ
6 Ⓐ Ⓑ Ⓒ Ⓓ Ⓔ   19 Ⓐ Ⓑ Ⓒ Ⓓ Ⓔ   32 Ⓐ Ⓑ Ⓒ Ⓓ Ⓔ   45 Ⓐ Ⓑ Ⓒ Ⓓ Ⓔ
7 Ⓐ Ⓑ Ⓒ Ⓓ Ⓔ   20 Ⓐ Ⓑ Ⓒ Ⓓ Ⓔ   33 Ⓐ Ⓑ Ⓒ Ⓓ Ⓔ   46 Ⓐ Ⓑ Ⓒ Ⓓ Ⓔ
8 Ⓐ Ⓑ Ⓒ Ⓓ Ⓔ   21 Ⓐ Ⓑ Ⓒ Ⓓ Ⓔ   34 Ⓐ Ⓑ Ⓒ Ⓓ Ⓔ   47 Ⓐ Ⓑ Ⓒ Ⓓ Ⓔ
9 Ⓐ Ⓑ Ⓒ Ⓓ Ⓔ   22 Ⓐ Ⓑ Ⓒ Ⓓ Ⓔ   35 Ⓐ Ⓑ Ⓒ Ⓓ Ⓔ   48 Ⓐ Ⓑ Ⓒ Ⓓ Ⓔ
10 Ⓐ Ⓑ Ⓒ Ⓓ Ⓔ   23 Ⓐ Ⓑ Ⓒ Ⓓ Ⓔ   36 Ⓐ Ⓑ Ⓒ Ⓓ Ⓔ   49 Ⓐ Ⓑ Ⓒ Ⓓ Ⓔ
11 Ⓐ Ⓑ Ⓒ Ⓓ Ⓔ   24 Ⓐ Ⓑ Ⓒ Ⓓ Ⓔ   37 Ⓐ Ⓑ Ⓒ Ⓓ Ⓔ   50 Ⓐ Ⓑ Ⓒ Ⓓ Ⓔ
12 Ⓐ Ⓑ Ⓒ Ⓓ Ⓔ   25 Ⓐ Ⓑ Ⓒ Ⓓ Ⓔ   38 Ⓐ Ⓑ Ⓒ Ⓓ Ⓔ
13 Ⓐ Ⓑ Ⓒ Ⓓ Ⓔ   26 Ⓐ Ⓑ Ⓒ Ⓓ Ⓔ   39 Ⓐ Ⓑ Ⓒ Ⓓ Ⓔ

Quantitative Reasoning Test

1 Ⓐ Ⓑ Ⓒ Ⓓ Ⓔ   11 Ⓐ Ⓑ Ⓒ Ⓓ Ⓔ   21 Ⓐ Ⓑ Ⓒ Ⓓ Ⓔ   31 Ⓐ Ⓑ Ⓒ Ⓓ Ⓔ
2 Ⓐ Ⓑ Ⓒ Ⓓ Ⓔ   12 Ⓐ Ⓑ Ⓒ Ⓓ Ⓔ   22 Ⓐ Ⓑ Ⓒ Ⓓ Ⓔ   32 Ⓐ Ⓑ Ⓒ Ⓓ Ⓔ
3 Ⓐ Ⓑ Ⓒ Ⓓ Ⓔ   13 Ⓐ Ⓑ Ⓒ Ⓓ Ⓔ   23 Ⓐ Ⓑ Ⓒ Ⓓ Ⓔ   33 Ⓐ Ⓑ Ⓒ Ⓓ Ⓔ
4 Ⓐ Ⓑ Ⓒ Ⓓ Ⓔ   14 Ⓐ Ⓑ Ⓒ Ⓓ Ⓔ   24 Ⓐ Ⓑ Ⓒ Ⓓ Ⓔ   34 Ⓐ Ⓑ Ⓒ Ⓓ Ⓔ
5 Ⓐ Ⓑ Ⓒ Ⓓ Ⓔ   15 Ⓐ Ⓑ Ⓒ Ⓓ Ⓔ   25 Ⓐ Ⓑ Ⓒ Ⓓ Ⓔ   35 Ⓐ Ⓑ Ⓒ Ⓓ Ⓔ
6 Ⓐ Ⓑ Ⓒ Ⓓ Ⓔ   16 Ⓐ Ⓑ Ⓒ Ⓓ Ⓔ   26 Ⓐ Ⓑ Ⓒ Ⓓ Ⓔ   36 Ⓐ Ⓑ Ⓒ Ⓓ Ⓔ
7 Ⓐ Ⓑ Ⓒ Ⓓ Ⓔ   17 Ⓐ Ⓑ Ⓒ Ⓓ Ⓔ   27 Ⓐ Ⓑ Ⓒ Ⓓ Ⓔ   37 Ⓐ Ⓑ Ⓒ Ⓓ Ⓔ
8 Ⓐ Ⓑ Ⓒ Ⓓ Ⓔ   18 Ⓐ Ⓑ Ⓒ Ⓓ Ⓔ   28 Ⓐ Ⓑ Ⓒ Ⓓ Ⓔ   38 Ⓐ Ⓑ Ⓒ Ⓓ Ⓔ
9 Ⓐ Ⓑ Ⓒ Ⓓ Ⓔ   19 Ⓐ Ⓑ Ⓒ Ⓓ Ⓔ   29 Ⓐ Ⓑ Ⓒ Ⓓ Ⓔ   39 Ⓐ Ⓑ Ⓒ Ⓓ Ⓔ
10 Ⓐ Ⓑ Ⓒ Ⓓ Ⓔ   20 Ⓐ Ⓑ Ⓒ Ⓓ Ⓔ   30 Ⓐ Ⓑ Ⓒ Ⓓ Ⓔ   40 Ⓐ Ⓑ Ⓒ Ⓓ Ⓔ

Model Examination A

SURVEY OF THE NATURAL SCIENCES   TIME: 90 MINUTES

The following items are questions or incomplete statements. Read each item carefully, then choose the best answer. Blacken the corresponding space on the answer sheet.

1. In the process of exocytosis, the plasma membrane and the membrane of which organelle come together?

    A. mitochondria
    B. peroxisome
    C. nucleus
    D. secretory vesicle
    E. ribosome

2. In comparison to the passage of polar solvents through a cell membrane, the passage of nonpolar solvents through a cell membrane occurs much more rapidly. This is indicative of

    A. the presence of more than a single layer of cells in the membrane
    B. the random distribution of the molecules of the membrane
    C. the "fluidity" of the membrane under normal conditions
    D. a significant proportion of lipid in the composition of the membrane
    E. an organized and layered arrangement of molecules within the membrane

3. When energy is expended to move molecules up a concentration gradient, the process is termed

    A. passive transport
    B. active transport
    C. simple diffusion
    D. facilitated diffusion
    E. osmosis

4. Which of the following organelles is NOT encapsulated within a membrane?

    A. nucleus
    B. mitochondrion
    C. Golgi apparatus
    D. peroxisome
    E. centriole

5. The addition of an enzyme to a solution yields glucose. The enzyme may have acted on which of the following components of the original solution to produce the glucose?

    A. lipids
    B. RNA
    C. DNA
    D. glycogen
    E. albumin

6. NAD and FAD are important to biochemical pathways because of their role as

    A. oxidation-reduction coenzymes
    B. regulators of O_2 levels
    C. enzymes to reduce the activation energy needed for essential reactions
    D. glycolytic ATP
    E. regulators of acetyl Co-A levels

7. Organisms that use respiration in conjunction with glycolysis are _____ organisms that use anaerobic means of obtaining energy from the degradation of food.

   A. half as efficient as
   B. twice as efficient as
   C. many more times as efficient as
   D. equally as efficient as
   E. not as efficient as

8. The accessory pigments involved in photosynthesis, chlorophyll *b*, xanthophylls, anthocyanins, and carotenoids, have importance because they

   A. can go from a ground state to an excited state without any form of electromagnetic radiation
   B. absorb different wavelengths and pass them on to chlorophyll *a*
   C. receive photons from chlorophyll *a*
   D. are responsible for the absorption of O_2 and nutrients
   E. are primarily responsible for the absorption of X rays and gamma rays

9. Which of the following invertebrates share the most similarities with primitive vertebrates?

   A. Arthropoda
   B. Annelida
   C. Cnidaria
   D. Nematoda
   E. Echinodermata

10. Of the following, which is (are) considered to be a true cell (true cells)?

    I.   Erythrocytes
    II. Leukocytes
    III. Platelets

    A. I only
    B. II only
    C. III only
    D. I and II
    E. I and III

11. When referring to the propagation of an impulse within the heart, the _____ is referred to as the "pacemaker" because it has the _____ rate of spontaneous depolarization.

    A. atrioventricular node; slowest
    B. atrioventricular node; fastest
    C. sinoatrial node; fastest
    D. sinoatrial node; slowest
    E. moderator band; fastest

12. A coma may result from an excessive amount of insulin. This coma is due to

    A. a depletion of norepinephrine
    B. a depletion of epinephrine
    C. a depletion of blood sugar
    D. an excessivly high blood sugar level
    E. an exceesively high level of both norepinephrine and epinephrine

13. Which of the following are globular proteins?

    I.   Antibodies
    II. Actin and myosin
    III. Collagen
    IV. Hemoglobin

    A. I and IV
    B. II and III
    C. I and III
    D. II and IV
    E. I, II, and III

14. Tropomyosin

    A. blocks the binding sites on actin, preventing myosin cross-bridge attachment at low Ca^{2+} levels
    B. blocks the binding sites on myosin preventing actin cross-bridge attachment at high Ca^{2+} levels
    C. blocks the binding sites on actin preventing myosin cross-bridge attachment at high Ca^{2+} levels
    D. blocks the binding sites on myosin preventing actin cross-bridge attachment at low Ca^{2+} levels
    E. assists the binding of actin to myosin at low Ca^{2+} levels

15. A cell undergoing mitosis that has lost its nuclear membrane and in which chromosomes are aligned before separation and migration to opposite poles is in which stage?

   A. Anaphase
   B. Prophase
   C. Telophase
   D. Metaphase
   E. Between anaphase and telophase

16. In contrast to electrical synapses, chemical synapses are

   A. the site of bidirectional communication between neurons
   B. the site of unidirectional communication between neurons
   C. gap junctions that contain protein channels
   D. far more common in embryonic nervous tissue
   E. more abundant in cardiac muscle fibers to permit rhythmic excitation

17. Assuming independent assortment, the possible number of different gamete types from three homologous pairs is

   A. 3
   B. 4
   C. 8
   D. 9
   E. 16

18. The final electron acceptor in the electron transport chain is

   A. FAD
   B. NAD+
   C. molecular oxygen
   D. pyruvate
   E. oxaloacetate

19. Unequal distribution of cytoplasm from the germ cell is found in

   A. oogenesis
   B. spermatogenesis
   C. both oogenesis and spermatogenesis during the primary cytokinesis
   D. both oogenesis and spermatogenesis during the secondary cytokinesis
   E. neither oogenesis nor spermatogenesis

20. Gastrulation refers to

   A. the formation of the cardiac, fundic, and pyloric divisions of the stomach
   B. the body's natural defense to parasitic attack on the musculature of the digestive system
   C. the formation of gastrin and HCL
   D. the division of the gastrointestinal tract into regions with specialized tasks of digestion
   E. the developmental process that produces the three primary germ layers

21. A "zinger" denotes an abnormal phenotype. When zingers are interbred, a phenotypic ratio of two zingers to one normal occurs; $\frac{1}{4}$ of the offspring die. When a zinger is crossed with a mate having a normal phenotype, the phenotype ratio is one zinger to one normal, and none die. The most probable explanation is that zingers

   A. have recessive traits that are lethal when homozygous
   B. have dominant traits that are lethal when homozygous
   C. are recessive traits that are lethal when heterozygous
   D. are dominant traits that are lethal when heterozygous
   E. have weak immune systems when young

22. _____ polymerizes to form the fibrous portion of a clot.

    A. Fibrinogen
    B. Prothrombin
    C. Fibrin
    D. Thrombin
    E. Platelets

23. Which of the following vessels carries oxygenated blood?

    A. Pulmonary artery
    B. Umbilical artery
    C. Thoracic duct
    D. Umbilical vein
    E. Hepatic vein

24. Tooth enamel is the hardest substance in the body. It is derived from which of the following germ layers?

    A. Morula
    B. Blastula
    C. Ectoderm
    D. Mesoderm
    E. Endoderm

25. Most homeostatic control mechanisms function via

    A. biological control centers that respond primarily to changes in blood pH
    B. positive feedback causing an increase in the original stimulus
    C. negative feedback causing an increase in the original stimulus
    D. positive feedback causing an increase in the original stimulus
    E. negative feedback causing a decrease in the original stimulus

26. When members of two species live in close existence and one is benefited but the other is neither helped nor harmed, the relationship is termed

    A. parasitism
    B. mutualism
    C. commensalism
    D. behavioral adaptation
    E. symbiosis

27. Of the following, the level of taxonomic classification that includes the greatest number of organisms is the

    A. genus
    B. class
    C. order
    D. species
    E. family

28. Meat is cured with large amounts of salt to retard spoilage. The salt causes the cells of bacteria and fungi to

    A. hemolyze
    B. crenate
    C. form ionic bonds with the myofilaments
    D. form ionic bonds with each other
    E. reach an isotonic state

29. DNA is comprised of all of the following nitrogenous bases EXCEPT:

    A. adenine
    B. cytosine
    C. guanine
    D. thymine
    E. uracil

30. The primary difference between eukaryotes and prokaryotes is that prokaryotes lack

    A. a nuclear envelope
    B. a cell wall
    C. a plasma membrane
    D. cytoplasm
    E. chlorophyll

31. A cell is found to have ribosomes, lysosomes, and chromosomes, but no cell wall. This cell is from

    A. an animal, but not a protozoan
    B. either an animal or protozoan
    C. a plant
    D. a protozoan
    E. a plant or a protozoan

32. Two different DNA molecules are described below.

    DNA molecule #1 has a greater proportion of adenine-thyamine (A–T) bonds than guaninc-cytosine (G–C) bonds. DNA molecule #2 has a greater proportion of guanine-cytosine (G–C) bonds than adenine-thyamine (A–T) bonds. It can be concluded that

    A. DNA #1 will be more stable
    B. DNA #2 will be more stable
    C. DNA #1 and #2 will exhibit equal stability
    D. DNA #1 will be altered during mitosis
    E. DNA #2 will be altered during meiosis

33. Bat wings, bird wings, and bee wings arose through _____ evolution. They are said to be _____ structures.

    A. convergent, homologous
    B. convergent, analogous
    C. divergent, homologous
    D. divergent, analogous
    E. homologous, analogous

34. If yellow peas are wrinkled 90% of the time, it can be assumed that the genes for color and wrinkling are not assorted independently. Instead, they are

    A. chiasmatic
    B. linked
    C. codependent
    D. incompletely dominant
    E. joined

35. During transcription

    A. the information contained within RNA is transferred to a polypeptide
    B. the information contained within the polypeptide sequence is transferred to RNA
    C. information from nucleic acids is moved to proteins
    D. RNA molecules are formed from DNA templates by a process not unlike DNA replication
    E. tRNA functions as an important interpreter

36. Which of the following statements is FALSE regarding the process of protein synthesis?

    A. The A site holds the tRNA attached to the growing polypeptide chain, while the P site holds the next amino acid to be added.
    B. If the reading frame is shifted, a completely different set of amino acids will result.
    C. The start codon is usually AUG.
    D. There are three steps: chain initiation, chain elongation, and chain termination.
    E. Peptidyl transferase is the enzyme involved in the formation of the peptide bond between the polypeptide in the P site and the amino acid in the A site.

37. Which of the statements below is (are) true in regard to the following pedigree?

    The father has the genotype *rr* and the mother has the genotype *Rr*.

    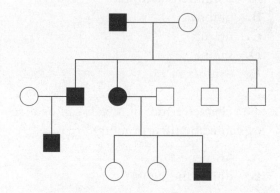

    I. The recessive homozygotes are phenotypically normal.
    II. The genotype for the male grandchildren is *rr*.
    III. The probability that the first generation will be affected is $\frac{1}{2}$.
    A. I
    B. II
    C. II and III
    D. I and II
    E. I and III

38. Which of the following hormones is secreted in the posterior pituitary?

    A. Prolactin
    B. Leutinizing hormone
    C. Growth hormone
    D. Corticosteroid hormone
    E. Oxytocin

39. A pathogenic bacteria is challenged by an antibiotic. Some of the bacteria mutate, developing resistance to the antibiotic, and are able to flourish more than the bacteria that do not have the mutation. This is an example of

    A. allopatric speciation
    B. sympatric speciation
    C. kin selection
    D. natural selection
    E. altruism

40. Fertilization of the human egg must occur within 24 hours of being released from the ovary. Fertilization occurs in the

    A. seminiferous tubules
    B. fimbriea
    C. uterus
    D. vagina
    E. oviduct

41. The characteristics of metals can be best explained by their property of

    A. brittleness
    B. dipole moments
    C. molecular crystals
    D. highly mobile electrons
    E. ionic bonding

42. Which of the following is expected to be tetrahedral?

    A. H_2O
    B. NH_3+
    C. HCN
    D. NH_4+
    E. CO_3

43. The diffusion rate of methane gas compared to that of helium is

    A. twice as fast
    B. 4 times as slow
    C. 4 times as fast
    D. half as fast
    E. 12 times as fast

44. Which of the following shows atoms and ions in order of decreasing size?

    A. $Ar > Cl^- > S^{2-} > K^+$
    B. $K^+ > S^{2-} > Cl^- > Ar$
    C. $S^{2-} > Cl^- > Ar > K^+$
    D. $S^{2-} > Ar > Cl^- > K^+$
    E. $K^+ > Ar > S^{2-} > Cl^-$

45. Which ion is isoelectronic with Ba^{2+}?

    A. Xe
    B. Cs
    C. Rb
    D. Hf
    E. I

46. What is the mass, in grams, of 245 milliliters of SO_2 at STP?

    A. 7.01
    B. 0.701
    C. 0.651
    D. 0.732
    E. 6.51

47. In the following reaction,

    $$N_2 \text{ (g)} + 3 H_2 \text{ (g)} \leftrightarrow 2 NH_3 \text{ (g)},$$

    an increase in pressure would cause the reaction to

    A. shift to the right
    B. shift to the left
    C. shut down
    D. do nothing, it is at equilibrium
    E. Not enough information is given.

48. Which of the following is NOT a colligative property?

   A. Freezing point depression
   B. Osmotic pressure
   C. Melting point depression
   D. Boiling point elevation
   E. Vapor pressure lowering

49. Which of the following will produce an increase in the entropy of a system?

   I. Increase in temperature
   II. Formation of gaseous products from solid reactants
   III. Formation of a precipitate in a liquid solution
   IV. Increase in the volume of a system
   V. Formation of a solid from a gas

   A. I, II, III
   B. I, V
   C. I, II, IV, V
   D. I, II, IV
   E. I, II, III, IV

50. To balance the following equation:
$$ZnS + HCl \rightarrow ZnCl_2 + H_2S$$
the correct order of coefficients is

   A. 1, 2, 2, 1
   B. 1, 2, 1, 1
   C. 1, 1, 2, 2
   D. 2, 4, 2, 2
   E. 1, 4, 2, 1

51. How many mole(s) of sulfur are in 1 mole of As_2S_3?

   A. 3
   B. 2.4
   C. 1
   D. 0.1
   E. 5

52. How many mole(s) are in 50 grams of aluminum?

   A. 0.669
   B. 2.3
   C. 1.85
   D. 2.43
   E. 1.2

53. For the reaction $A + 2B \rightarrow C$, the rate of formation of C is given by the formula
$$\text{Rate} = k[A][B]^2.$$

Doubling the concentration of A will

   A. quadruple the initial rate
   B. double the initial rate
   C. have no effect on the initial rate
   D. reduce the rate to $\frac{1}{4}$ of its value
   E. reduce the rate to $\frac{1}{2}$ of its value

54. In which reaction is H_2O acting like an acid?

   A. $Zn(s) + 2H_3O^+ \rightarrow Zn^{++} + H_2O\,(g) + 2H_2O$
   B. $HCl\,(g) + H_2O \rightarrow H_3O^+ + Cl-$
   C. $HC_2H_3O_2 + H_2O \leftrightarrow H_3O^+ + C_2H_3O_2^-$
   D. $NH_3 + H_2O \leftrightarrow NH_4^+ + OH^-$
   E. $NH_3 + H_2O^+ \leftrightarrow NH_4^+ + H_2O$

55. Catalysts have which of the following effects on a chemical reaction?

   A. They lower the activation energy.
   B. They increase the free energy.
   C. They cause the reaction to proceed spontaneously.
   D. They change the equilibrium so that product formation is increased.
   E. They change the equilibrium so the reverse reaction proceeds more easily.

56. Which of the following has the LOWEST percent of carbon by mass?

   A. CH_4
   B. C_2H_4
   C. $Na_2C_2O_2$
   D. $C_6H_{12}O_6$
   E. CH_3CO_2H

57. What is the equilibrium constant for the following reaction?

$$2A + 2B \leftrightarrow 3C + D$$

    A. $[A]^2[B]^2/[C]^3[D]$
    B. $[C]^3[D]/[A]^2[B]^2$
    C. $[A]^2[B]^2$
    D. $[C]^3[D]$
    E. $[A][B]/[C][D]$

58. If 14 grams of NaF are dissolved in 400 milligrams of water, what is the resulting molality of the solution?

    A. 0.4 m
    B. 0.83 m
    C. 0.93 m
    D. 0.54 m
    E. 0.32 m

59. How much 4 M $Ca(OH)_2$ is needed to neutralize 300 milliliters of 3 M HNO_3?

    A. 234 mL
    B. 655 mL
    C. 623 mL
    D. 723 mL
    E. 112.5 mL

60. How many atoms of carbon are in 4.00×10^{-8} grams of C_3H_8?

    A. 1.64×10^{15}
    B. 2.34×10^{11}
    C. 1.89×10^{14}
    D. 4.66×10^2
    E. 4.00×10^4

61. In an experiment, 3.4 grams of a carbon-oxygen containing compound was obtained in a test tube. The weight of oxygen was found to be 0.65 gram. What was the percentage of carbon in the compound?

    A. $(1 - 0.65/3.4)(100)$
    B. $((1 + 0.65)/3.4)(100)$
    C. $(0.65)(1/100 \times 3.4)$
    D. $(3.4/0.65)(100)$
    E. $(3.4 \times 0.65)(100)$

62. An alloy contains atoms of

    A. one element and has the properties of a metal
    B. more than one element and has the properties of a nonmetal
    C. one element and has the properties of a nonmetal
    D. more than one element and has the properties of a metal
    E. one element and has the properties of a semiconductor

63. Which of the following is the definition of an Arrhenius base?

    A. A substance that donates a proton to another substance
    B. A substance that accepts a proton from another substance
    C. A substance that produces a hydroxy ion in the presence of an aqueous solution
    D. A substance that donates a pair of electrons
    E. A substance that donates a hydrogen ion in the presence of an aqueous solution

64. Which of the following, if any, is FALSE?

Chemical reactions are accelerated by . . .

    A. increasing the concentrations of reactants
    B. adding a catalyst
    C. decreasing the surface area available for the reaction
    D. increasing the temperature
    E. All of the above are correct.

65. If all of the chloride in a 5.0-gram sample of an unknown metal chloride is precipitated as AgCl with 70.9 milliliters of 0.201 M $AgNO_3$, what is the percentage of chloride in the sample?

    A. 50.55%
    B. 20.22%
    C. 1.43%
    D. 10.10%
    E. None of the above

66. For reaction A→B, if ΔG is negative, and $\Delta H = 0$, then ΔS is

    A. negative
    B. positive
    C. equal to 0
    D. positive or negative depending on the equilibrium constant
    E. positive or negative depending on the rate of the reaction

67. As one moves across the periodic table in a leftward and descending direction, which of the following properties increases?

    A. Ionization energy
    B. Electron affinity
    C. Electronegativity
    D. Electron withdrawal
    E. Atomic radius

68. Which of the following is an example of a halogen?

    A. F
    B. Ba
    C. O
    D. C
    E. He

69. The geometric configuration of CO_2 is

    A. linear
    B. bent
    C. tetrahedral
    D. trigonal planar
    E. trigonal pyramidal

70. Isotopes have

    A. the same number of protons and electrons
    B. the same atomic number and equal numbers of protons
    C. the same mass number and equal numbers of protons
    D. the same atomic number and equal numbers of neutrons
    E. the same mass number and equal numbers of neutrons

71. The breaking of an O—H bond in water is an example of _____ cleavage. The breaking of the O—O bond in hydrogen peroxide is an example of _____ cleavage.

    A. homolytic, heterolytic
    B. heterolytic, homolytic
    C. homolytic, homolytic
    D. heterolytic, heterolytic
    E. None of the above

72. The orientation of the bond between the two sp^2 hybridized carbons in the molecule ethene can best be described as _____ in relation to the orientation of its pi bond.

    A. parallel
    B. perpendicular
    C. at a 109.5° angle
    D. at a 120° angle
    E. at a 180° angle

73. The correct name for the following compound is

$$CH_3 - CH - \overset{\overset{\displaystyle O}{\|}}{C} - CH - CH_2 - CH_3$$
$$\underset{\displaystyle CH_3}{|} \qquad \underset{\displaystyle CH_3}{|}$$

    A. 3,5-dimethyl-4-hexanone
    B. 2,4-dione-3-hexane
    C. 2-ethyl-4-methyl-3-pentanone
    D. 2-methyl-4-ethyl-3-pentanone
    E. 2,4-dimethyl-3-hexanone

74. Which of the following compounds is NOT aromatic?

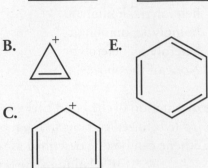

A.

D.

B.

E.

C.

75. Which of the following will be produced when an oxidizing agent reacts with a 2° alcohol?

A. Esters
B. Ethers
C. Aldehydes
D. Ketones
E. Caroxylic acids

76. Which is the best description of the propagation step in free-radical halogenation?

A. Two radicals bond to create a nonradical.
B. Two radicals react to form a third radical.
C. A halogen radical is formed from the presence of light or heat.
D. A radical causes the homolytic cleavage of an alkane. The reaction proceeds with an alkyl radical that splits an X_2.
E. None of the above

77. Which of the following has an effect on the strength of an acid?

A. The number of resonance forms possible for the conjugate base
B. The electronegativity of the conjugate base
C. Inductive effects that cause a shift in electron density
D. All of the above
E. None of the above

78. All of the following are oxidizing agents EXCEPT

A. $KMnO_4$
B. CrO_3
C. $LiAlH_4$
D. H_2CrO_4
E. OsO_4

79. Of the following, the most stable radical is

A.

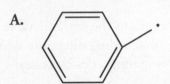

B. $\cdot CH_3$

C.

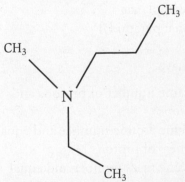

D.

E. $CH_3 - C\dot{H}_2$

80. Which is the most basic?

A. $C_6H_5NH_2$
B. $BrCH_2NH_2$
C. FCH_2NH_2
D. CH_3NH_2
E. $ClCH_2NH_2$

81. The correct IUPAC name for the following compound is

A. N-propyl-N-ethyl-1-methanamine
B. N-ethyl-N-methyl-1-propanamine
C. N,N-propylethylamine
D. N,N,N-propylethylmethylamine
E. N-ethyl-N-propyl-1-methanamine

82. The correct ranking of the following in order of increasing acid strength is

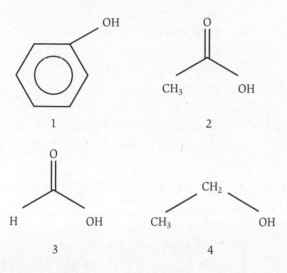

1

2

3

4

A. 1, 2, 4, 3
B. 4, 1, 2, 3
C. 4, 3, 1, 2
D. 1, 2, 3, 4
E. 3, 2, 4, 1

83. What will be produced if acetaldehyde is added to a Grignard reagent?

A. A secondary alcohol
B. A primary alcohol
C. An alkene
D. An alkyne
E. An alkane

84. All of the following are characteristics of which nucleophilic reaction(s)?
One step;
bimolecular-second order;
prefers smaller, less sterically hindered reactants;
results in an inversion of configuration;
nucleophile replaces leaving group.

A. S_N1
B. S_N2
C. $E1$
D. $E2$
E. B and D

85. The following NMR and IR spectroscopy information is characteristic of which group?

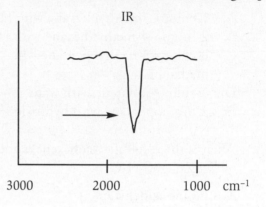

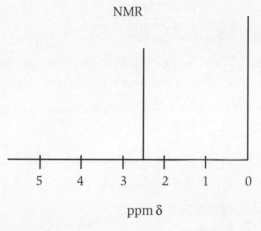

A. Alcohol
B. Phenyl
C. Double bond
D. Ketone
E. Aldehyde

86. What is the IUPAC name of the following compound?

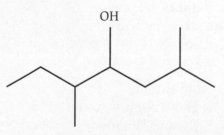

A. 4-hydroxy-2,5-dimethylheptane
B. 2-ethyl-3-hydroxy-5-methylhexane
C. 4-hydroxy-3,6-dimethylheptane
D. 5-ethyl-4-hydroxy-2-methylhexane
E. either A or C

87. Which of the following reactions is most likely to proceed by a S_N1 mechanism?

    A. 1-chloro-3-methyl hexane with HBr
    B. 2-bromo-4-methyl hexane with HCl
    C. 3-chloro-3-methyl pentane with methanol
    D. 1-chloro-2-butene with water
    E. 2-bromopentane with hydroxide

88. What is the result if cyclohexene is added to O_3, Zn, and H_2O?

    A. Propionaldehyde
    B. Propionic acid
    C. A diketone
    D. A dicarboxylic acid
    E. A dialdehyde

89. Which of the following compounds is(are) needed to produce a hemiacetal under acidic conditions?

    I. A ketone
    II. An aldehyde
    III. An alcohol
    IV. A carboxylic acid

    A. only I
    B. only II
    C. I and III
    D. II and III
    E. I and IV

90. Which of the following is (are) considered terminal functional groups?

    I. Aldehydes
    II. Ketones
    III. Carboxylic acids
    IV. Alcohols

    A. III only
    B. I and III only
    C. II and III only
    D. I, III, and IV only
    E. I, II, III, and IV

91. Which of the following is true concerning the isoelectric point (pI) of glutamic acid?

    A. pI = 7
    B. pI is between 6 and 7
    C. pI > 7
    D. pI is between 5 and 6
    E. pI < 5

92. Which of the following reactions is an example of a free-radical chain termination step?

    A. $Cl\bullet + CH_4 \rightarrow HCl + CH_3\bullet$
    B. $Cl_2 \rightarrow 2Cl\bullet$
    C. $Cl\bullet + CH_3\bullet \rightarrow CH_3Cl$
    D. $\dot{C}H_3\bullet + Cl_2 \rightarrow CH_3Cl + Cl\bullet$
    E. $Cl\bullet + CH_2 = CH_2 \rightarrow CH_2Cl–CH_2\bullet$

93. Which of the following conformations of cyclohexane is (are) most stable?

    I.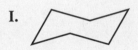

    II.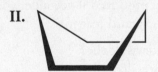

    III.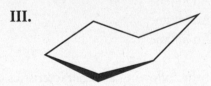

    A. I
    B. II
    C. III
    D. I and II exhibit identical stability.
    E. II and III exhibit identical stability.

94. Which of the following conformations of butane is (are) most stable?

A.

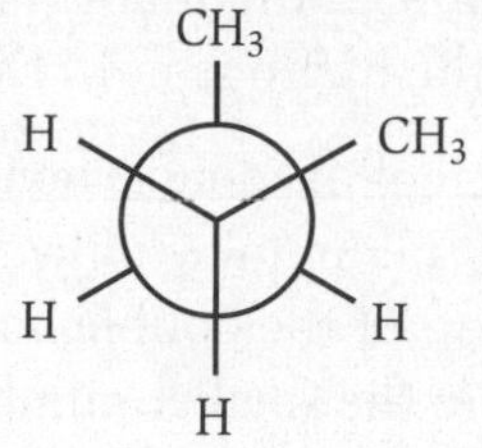

B.

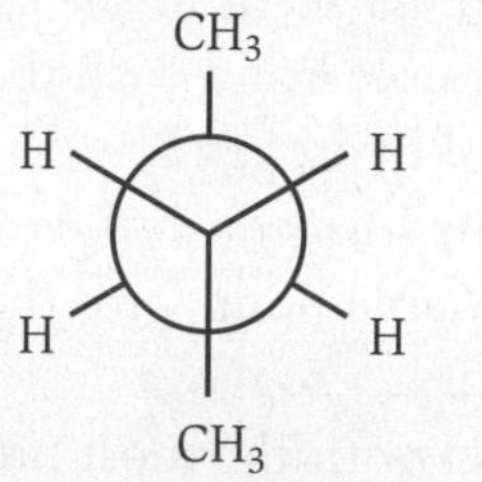

C.

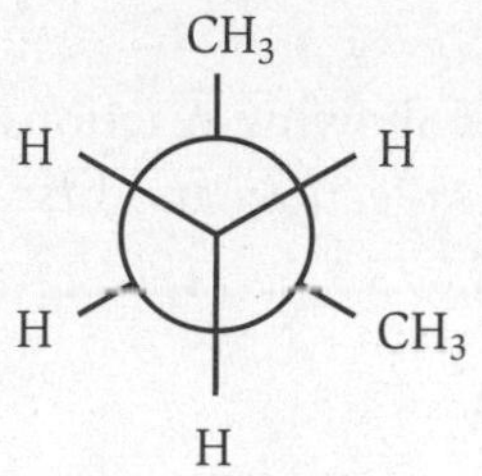

D.

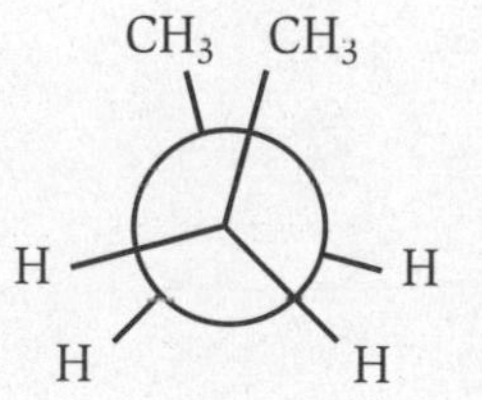

E. A and B are equally stable.

95. Which of the following compounds, if any, is NOT optically active?

A.

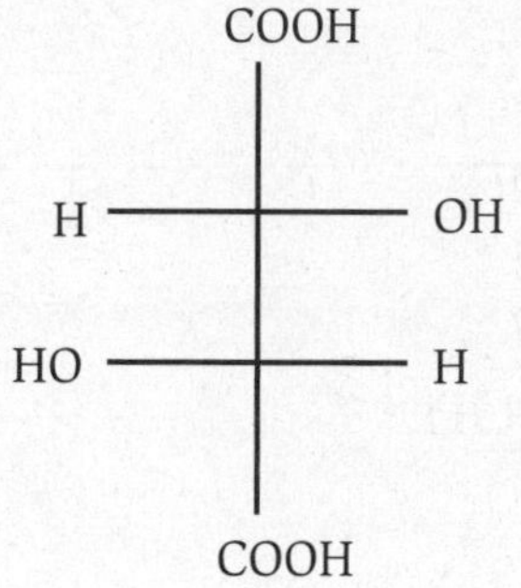

B.

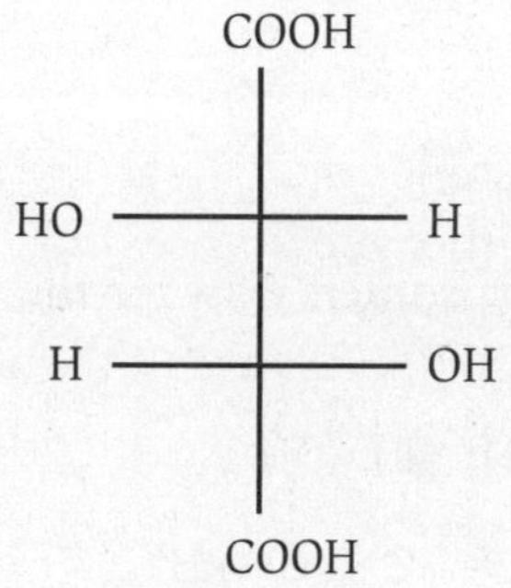

C.

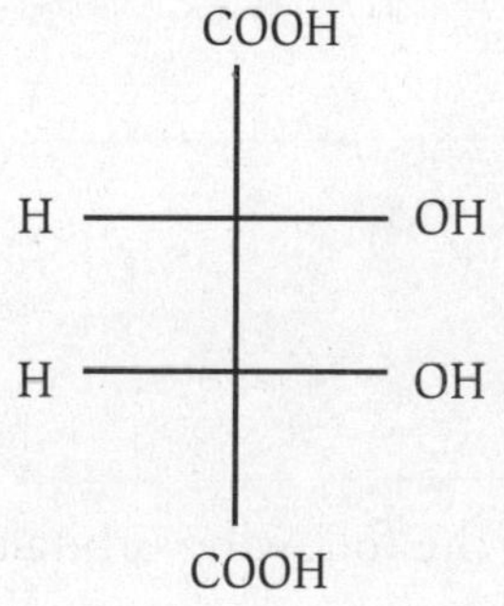

D.

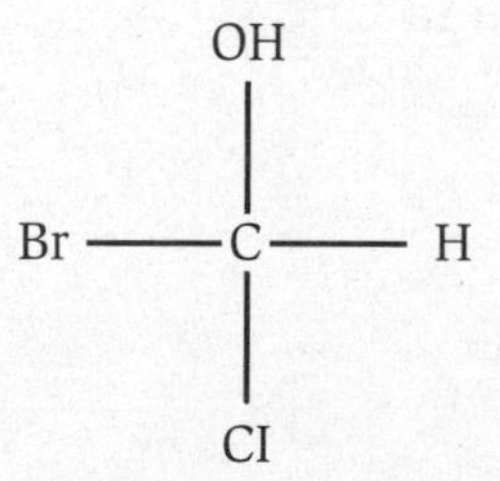

E. All of the above compounds contain chiral centers; hence, all are optically active.

96. What is the number of asymmetric or chiral carbons in the molecule below?

$$
\begin{array}{c}
\text{CHO} \\
\text{HO} - \text{H} \\
\text{H} - \text{OH} \\
\text{HO} - \text{H} \\
\text{HO} - \text{H} \\
\text{CH}_2\text{OH}
\end{array}
$$

- **A.** 1
- **B.** 2
- **C.** 3
- **D.** 4
- **E.** 5

97. How many isomers exist for the following aldehyde?

$$
\underset{O}{\overset{H}{\diagdown}}C - \underset{H}{\overset{OH}{\underset{|}{C}}} - \underset{H}{\overset{OH}{\underset{|}{C}}} - \underset{H}{\overset{OH}{\underset{|}{C}}} - H
$$

- **A.** 2
- **B.** 3
- **C.** 4
- **D.** 8
- **E.** 16

98. Which of the following orbitals is (are) contained in the outer energy level of the carbon atom in CH_4?

- **I.** s
- **II.** p
- **III.** sp
- **IV.** sp^2
- **V.** sp^3

- **A.** I, II, and V only
- **B.** I, II, and IV only
- **C.** I and II only
- **D.** II and V only
- **E.** V only

99. Markovnikov's rule applies to the addition of HX (where X is a halide) to an unsymmetrical carbon-carbon double bond. In this addition the hydrogen of HX goes to

- **A.** that carbon of the double bond that carries the greater number of hydrogens.
- **B.** that carbon of the double bond that carries the smaller number of hydrogens.
- **C.** the carbon adjacent to the carbon-carbon double bond with the most number of hydrogens.
- **D.** the carbon adjacent to the carbon-carbon double bond with the least number of hydrogens.
- **E.** the carbon with the most number of halides attached.

100. Which of the following reactions is(are) two step, unimolecular, and first-order?

- **I.** S_N1
- **II.** S_N2
- **III.** E 1
- **IV.** E 2

- **A.** I only
- **B.** II only
- **C.** III only
- **D.** I and III
- **E.** II and IV

PERCEPTUAL ABILITY TEST   TIME LIMIT: 60 MINUTES

Part 1: Aperture Passing

For questions 1 through 15:

This section of the exam consists of 15 items similar to the example below. In each item, a three-dimensional object is shown on the left, followed by outlines of five apertures to its right.

The task is the same for each item. Conceptualize how the three-dimensional object looks from each possible side (in addition to the side shown). Then, pick the outline in which the three-dimensional object could pass if the proper side were inserted. Choose the letter corresponding to the correct aperture.

Here are rules for Part 1, the aperture section:

1. The irregular solid three-dimensional object on the left can be rotated in any direction prior to passing through the aperture.
2. The object may not be twisted or rotated in any way once it has started to be passed through the aperture. The correct answer is the exact representation of the external outline of the object viewed from the appropriate side.
3. The objects and the outlines are drawn to the same scale.
4. There are no irregularities in hidden portions of the objects. If the figure has symmetric indentations, it is assumed that the hidden portion is symmetric with the portion shown.
5. There is only one correct answer.

EXAMPLE

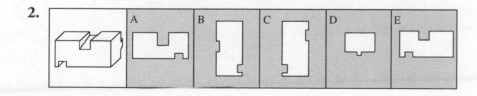

The correct answer is C.

1.

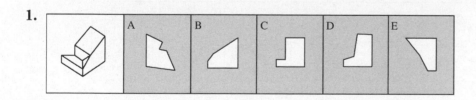

2.

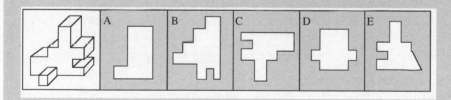

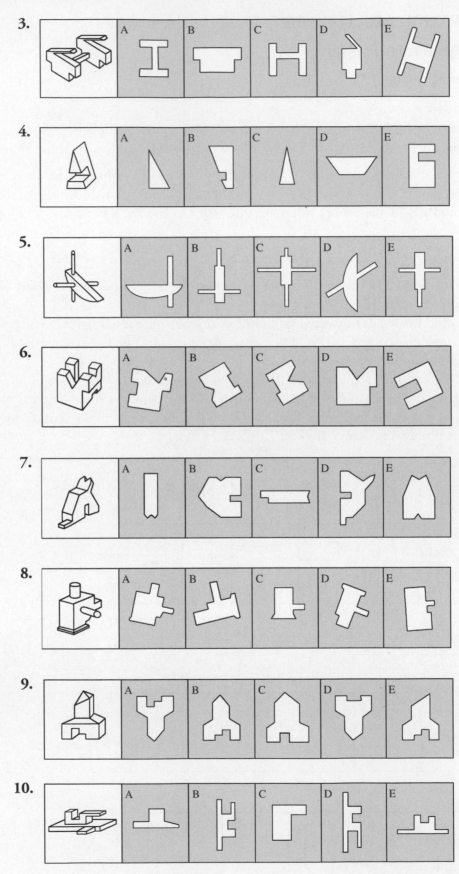

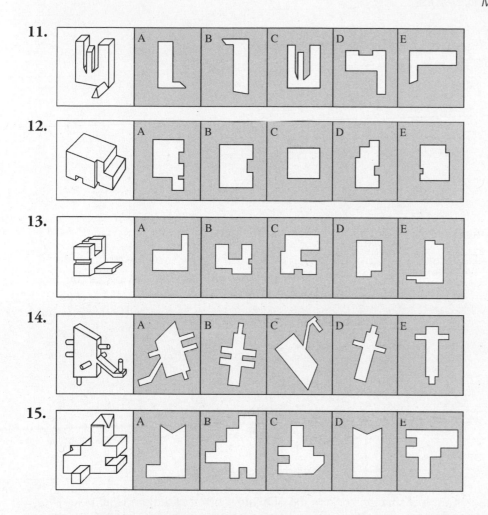

11.
12.
13.
14.
15.

Part 2: Orthographic Projections

For questions 16 through 30:

The pictures that follow are representations of solid objects from three different views: top, front, and end views. The pictures are views drawn without perspective: the surface viewed is along parallel lines of vision. The projection that is labeled TOP VIEW is shown looking DOWN on its top surface and is pictured in the upper-left corner. The projection labeled FRONT VIEW is shown looking at the object from the FRONT and is pictured in the lower-left corner. The projection labeled END VIEW is shown looking at the object from the END (or side) and is pictured in the lower-right corner. These three views are always in their respective corners and labeled accordingly.

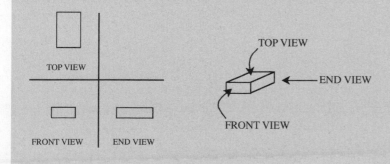

If there were a hole in the figure, it would be represented like this:

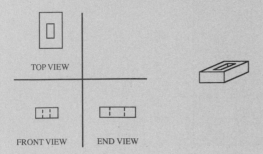

DOTTED lines indicate lines that exist but cannot be seen in the perspective shown.

In the following problems, TWO of the previous three views discussed will be shown with four alternatives to the right. Choose the correct letter that represents the correct view that completes the set.

EXAMPLE

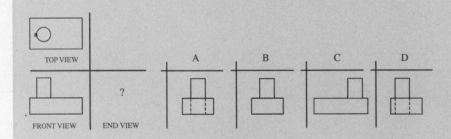

The FRONT VIEW shows that there is a smaller block on top of a larger block and there is no hole. The TOP VIEW shows that the top block is round and is centered on a rectangular block. From this information gathered in the two views given, the correct answer must be B.

In the following problems, one of the three views will be omitted; it is not always the END VIEW as shown in the example.

16. Choose the correct FRONT VIEW.

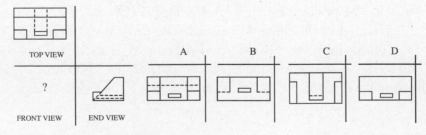

17. Choose the correct FRONT VIEW.

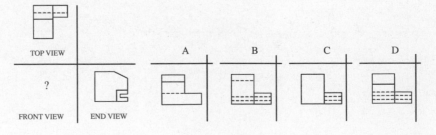

18. Choose the correct TOP VIEW.

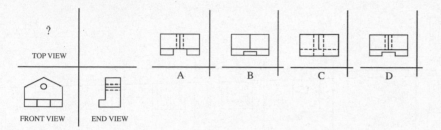

19. Choose the correct END VIEW.

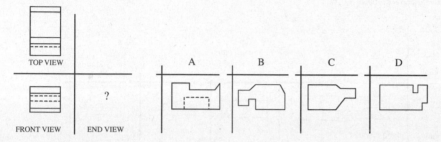

20. Choose the correct FRONT VIEW.

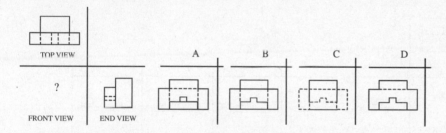

21. Choose the correct END VIEW.

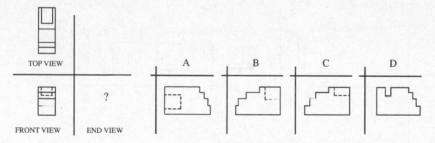

22. Choose the correct TOP VIEW.

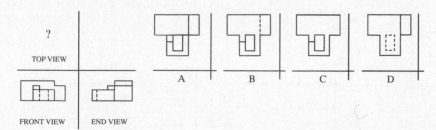

23. Choose the correct END VIEW.

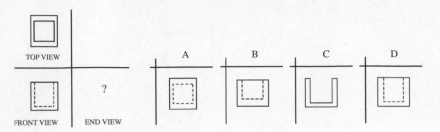

24. Choose the correct FRONT VIEW.

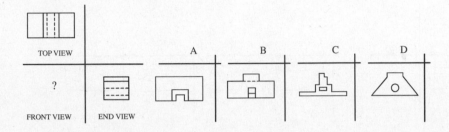

25. Choose the correct FRONT VIEW.

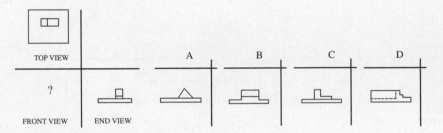

26. Choose the correct TOP VIEW.

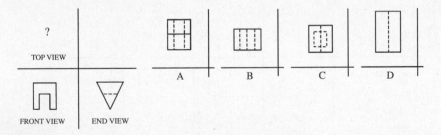

27. Choose the correct END VIEW.

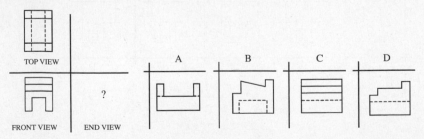

28. Choose the correct END VIEW.

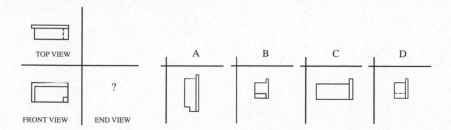

29. Choose the correct TOP VIEW.

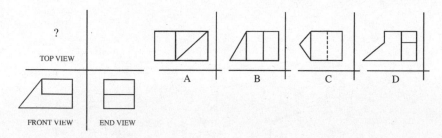

30. Choose the correct TOP VIEW.

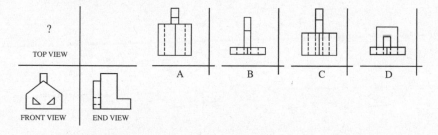

Part 3: Angle Discrimination

For questions 31 through 45:

Examine the INTERNAL ANGLES and rank them in terms of degrees from SMALL to LARGE. Select the alternative that represents the correct ranking.

EXAMPLE

A. 1 – 2 – 4 – 3
B. 2 – 1 – 4 – 3
C. 3 – 4 – 2 – 1
D. 3 – 4 – 1 – 2

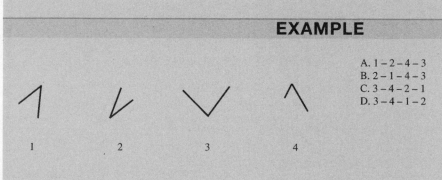

The correct ranking is 2–1–4–3. Therefore, the correct answer is B.

31.

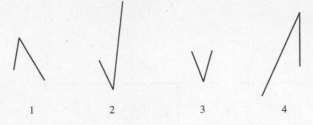

A. 2 – 4 – 3 – 1
B. 4 – 2 – 3 – 1
C. 4 – 2 – 1 – 3
D. 2 – 3 – 4 – 1

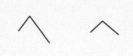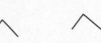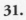

1   2   3   4

32.

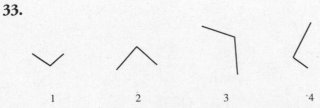

A. 3 – 4 – 1 – 2
B. 1 – 3 – 2 – 4
C. 3 – 1 – 4 – 2
D. 1 – 3 – 4 – 2

1   2   3   4

33.

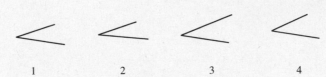

A. 1 – 2 – 4 – 3
B. 2 – 4 – 1 – 3
C. 4 – 1 – 2 – 3
D. 1 – 4 – 2 – 3

1   2   3   '4

34.

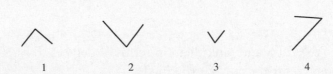

A. 2 – 1 – 3 – 4
B. 2 – 1 – 4 – 3
C. 2 – 4 – 1 – 3
D. 2 – 4 – 3 – 1

1   2   3   4

35.

A. 2 – 3 – 4 – 1
B. 1 – 3 – 4 – 2
C. 4 – 3 – 2 – 1
D. 3 – 4 – 1 – 2

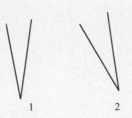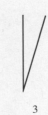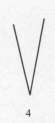

1   2   3   4

36.

A. 3 – 2 – 1 – 4
B. 4 – 3 – 2 – 1
C. 3 – 1 – 2 – 4
D. 2 – 3 – 1 – 4

1   2   3   4

37.

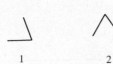

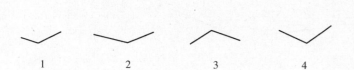

A. 4 – 2 – 1 – 3
B. 2 – 1 – 3 – 4
C. 3 – 1 – 2 – 4
D. 1 – 2 – 4 – 3

38.

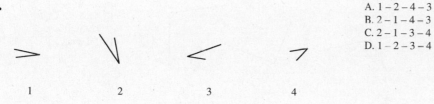

A. 4 – 3 – 1 – 2
B. 3 – 4 – 2 – 1
C. 1 – 3 – 4 – 2
D. 3 – 2 – 4 – 1

39.

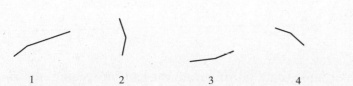

A. 1 – 2 – 4 – 3
B. 2 – 1 – 4 – 3
C. 2 – 1 – 3 – 4
D. 1 – 2 – 3 – 4

40.

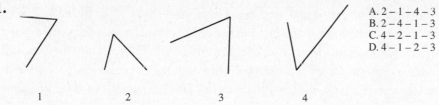

A. 1 – 2 – 3 – 4
B. 2 – 1 – 4 – 3
C. 4 – 2 – 3 – 1
D. 2 – 4 – 1 – 3

41.

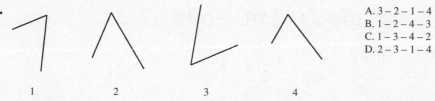

A. 2 – 1 – 4 – 3
B. 2 – 4 – 1 – 3
C. 4 – 2 – 1 – 3
D. 4 – 1 – 2 – 3

42.

A. 3 – 2 – 1 – 4
B. 1 – 2 – 4 – 3
C. 1 – 3 – 4 – 2
D. 2 – 3 – 1 – 4

43.

A. 1 – 2 – 4 – 3
B. 2 – 1 – 3 – 4
C. 1 – 2 – 3 – 4
D. 1 – 2 – 4 – 3

44.

A. 4 – 1 – 2 – 3
B. 2 – 4 – 3 – 1
C. 4 – 1 – 3 – 2
D. 4 – 2 – 3 – 1

45.

A. 3 – 2 – 4 – 1
B. 4 – 3 – 2 – 1
C. 4 – 3 – 1 – 2
D. 3 – 4 – 2 – 1

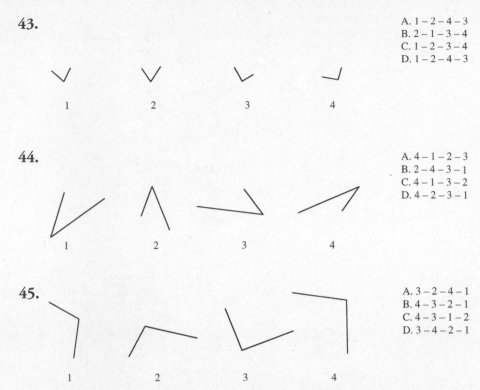

Part 4: Paper Folding

For questions 46 through 60:

A flat, square piece of paper is folded one or more times starting from the left, proceeding stepwise, to the illustrations to the right. The original position of the paper is represented by broken lines. The solid line indicates edges of the folded paper. The piece of paper is never twisted or turned and always remains within the outline of the original square. There may be ONE FOLD, TWO FOLDS, or THREE FOLDS in each item. After the last fold, a hole is punched in the paper. Your task is to unfold the paper in your mind and determine the placement of the holes on the original flat, square piece of paper. There is only one correct pattern of hole punches for each item. The black circles indicate hole punches. Choose the pattern that indicates the correct pattern of hole punches in the unfolded paper.

PRACTICE ILLUSTRATIONS

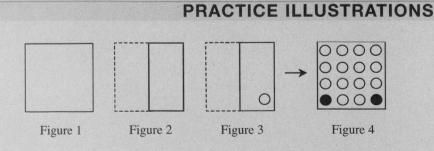

Figure 1   Figure 2   Figure 3   Figure 4

In this example Figure 1 shows the original flat, square piece of paper. Figure 2 shows the first fold. Figure 3 shows the location of the hole punch in the folded paper. The black circles in Figure 4 show the pattern of the hole punches on the unfolded paper. The answer has two holes since the paper was two layers thick in the position where the hole was punched.

EXAMPLE

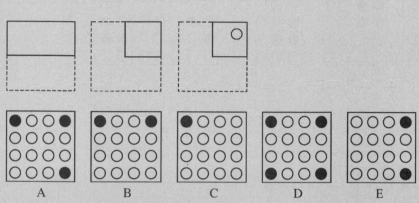

The correct answer is D. The paper was four thicknesses and therefore has four hole punches. The punch was made in the corner, so the four hole punches in the four corners are shown in black in the correct pattern.

46.

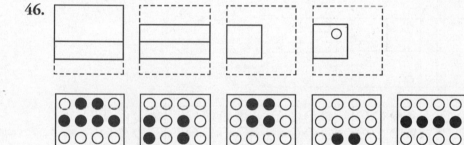

47.

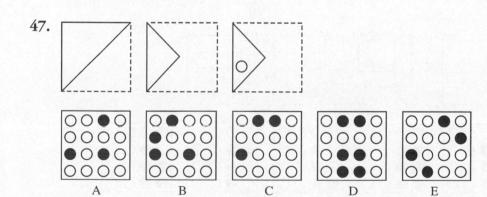

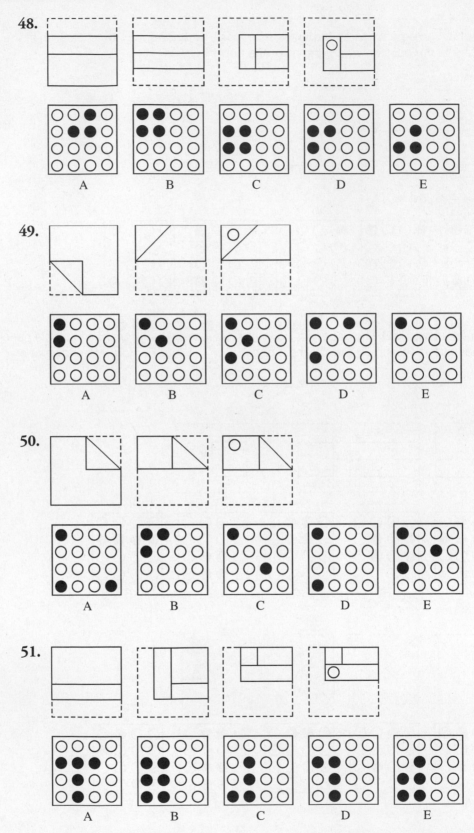

52.

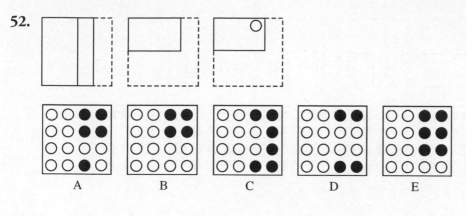

53.

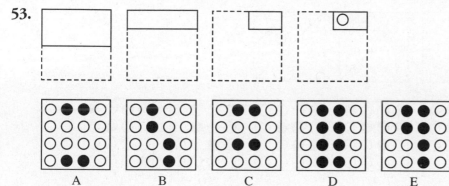

54.

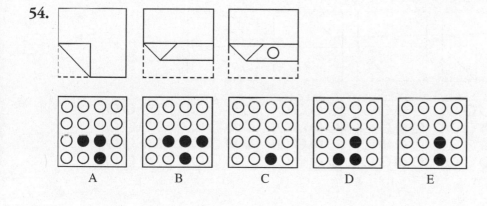

55.

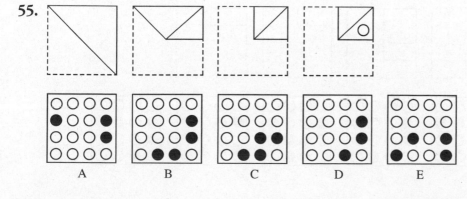

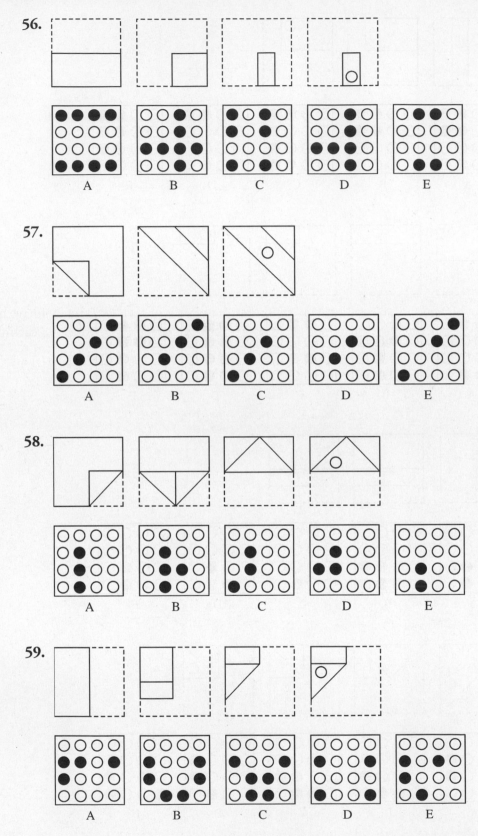

60.

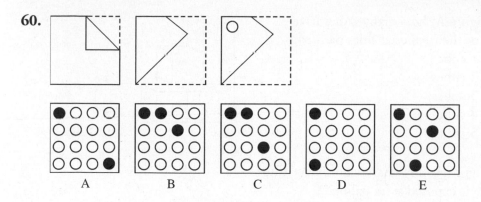

Part 5: Cubes

For questions 61 through 75:

Each of the figures in this section is representative of cubes of the same size that have been cemented together. After the cubes were cemented, the group of cubes were painted on each of the exposed sides WITH EXCEPTION TO THE BOTTOM SIDE ON WHICH THE FIGURE IS RESTING. Some illustrations contain hidden cubes. The only hidden cubes are cubes that are necessary to support other cubes.

In each item you are to determine how many cubes have

- ONE side painted,
- TWO sides painted,
- THREE sides painted,
- FOUR sides painted, or
- FIVE sides painted.

There are no problems that will ask for the number of cubes that have none (zero) of their sides painted.

EXAMPLE

In Figure A, how many cubes have two of their sides painted?

A. 1 cube
B. 2 cubes
C. 3 cubes
D. 4 cubes
E. 5 cubes

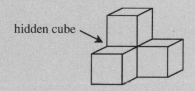

FIGURE A

There are four cubes in Figure A (one is hidden supporting the top cube). The top cube has five sides painted. The hidden cube supporting it has two sides painted. The two cubes in the foreground each have four sides painted. Therefore, there is only one cube that has just two sides painted and the correct answer is A.

Choose the letter that corresponds to the correct number of cubes with the given number of sides painted. Remember that THE BOTTOM OF THE CUBE IS NOT PAINTED.

61. In Figure A, how many cubes have two of their exposed sides painted?
    A. 1 cube
    B. 2 cubes
    C. 3 cubes
    D. 4 cubes
    E. 5 cubes

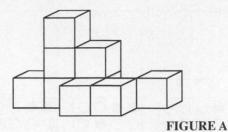

FIGURE A

62. In Figure A, how many cubes have three of their exposed sides painted?
    A. 1 cube
    B. 2 cubes
    C. 3 cubes
    D. 4 cubes
    E. 5 cubes

63. In Figure A, how many cubes have four of their exposed sides painted?
    A. 1 cube
    B. 2 cubes
    C. 3 cubes
    D. 4 cubes
    E. 5 cubes

64. In Figure A, how many cubes have five of their exposed sides painted?
    A. 1 cube
    B. 2 cubes
    C. 3 cubes
    D. 4 cubes
    E. 5 cubes

65. In Figure B, how many cubes have two of their exposed sides painted?
    A. 1 cube
    B. 2 cubes
    C. 3 cubes
    D. 4 cubes
    E. 5 cubes

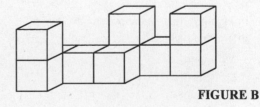

FIGURE B

66. In Figure B, how many cubes have five of their exposed sides painted?
    A. 1 cube
    B. 2 cubes
    C. 3 cubes
    D. 4 cubes
    E. 5 cubes

67. In Figure C, how many cubes have
two of their exposed sides painted?
A. 1 cube
B. 2 cubes
C. 3 cubes
D. 4 cubes
E. 5 cubes

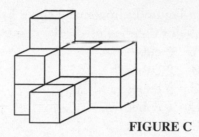

FIGURE C

68. In Figure C, how many cubes have three
of their exposed sides painted?
A. 1 cube
B. 2 cubes
C. 3 cubes
D. 4 cubes
E. 5 cubes

69. In Figure C, how many cubes have five
of their exposed sides painted?
A. 1 cube
B. 2 cubes
C. 3 cubes
D. 4 cubes
E. 5 cubes

70. In Figure D, how many cubes have
two of their exposed sides painted?
A. 1 cube
B. 2 cubes
C. 3 cubes
D. 4 cubes
E. 5 cubes

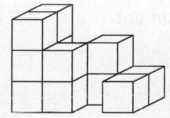

FIGURE D

71. In Figure D, how many cubes have three
of their exposed sides painted?
A. 1 cube
B. 2 cubes
C. 3 cubes
D. 4 cubes
E. 5 cubes

72. In Figure D, how many cubes have four of their exposed sides painted?
A. 1 cube
B. 2 cubes
C. 3 cubes
D. 4 cubes
E. 5 cubes

73. In Figure E, how many cubes have one of their exposed sides painted?
    A. 1 cube
    B. 2 cubes
    C. 3 cubes
    D. 4 cubes
    E. 5 cubes

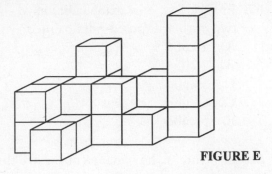

FIGURE E

74. In Figure E, how many cubes have two of their exposed sides painted?
    A. 2 cubes
    B. 3 cubes
    C. 4 cubes
    D. 5 cubes
    E. 6 cubes

75. In Figure E, how many cubes have four of their exposed sides painted?
    A. 1 cube
    B. 2 cubes
    C. 3 cubes
    D. 4 cubes
    E. 5 cubes

Part 6: Form Development

For questions 76 through 90:

A flat pattern will be presented in the box to the left. Your task is to mentally fold this pattern into a three-dimensional figure and choose the correct representation from the choices to the right. There is only one correct choice for each item.

EXAMPLE

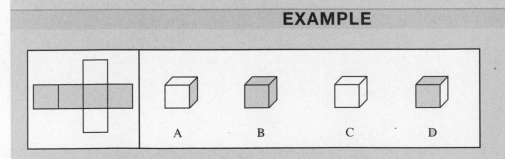

Folding the pattern in the left-most box can form only one of the figures to the right. The only figure that accurately represents the shaded areas once the pattern is folded is D.

Choose the letter that represents the three-dimensional object that correctly represents the folded pattern.

76.

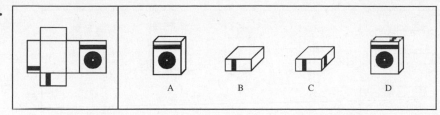

77.

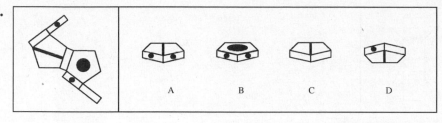

78.

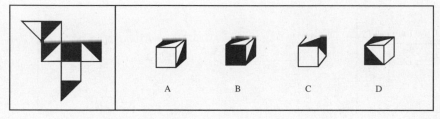

79.

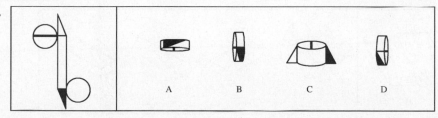

80.

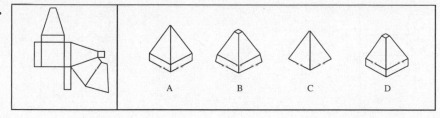

81.

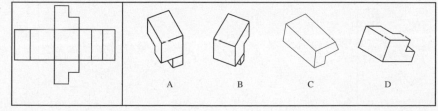

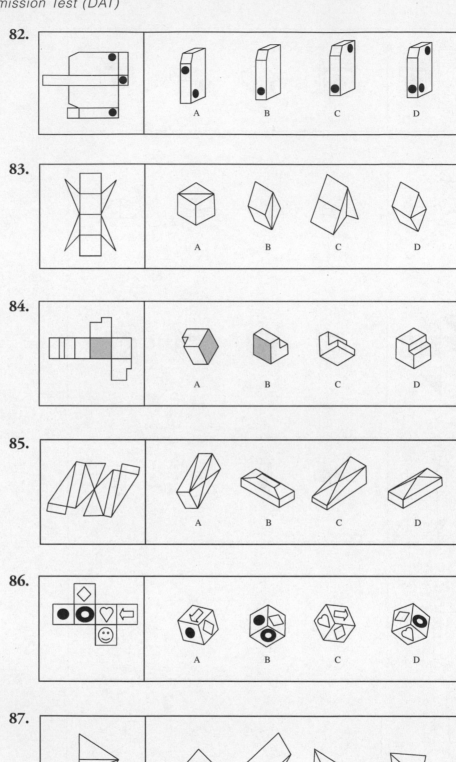

82.

83.

84.

85.

86.

87.

88.

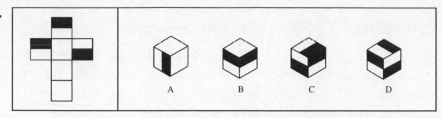

89.

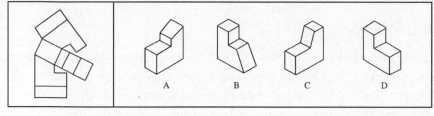

90.

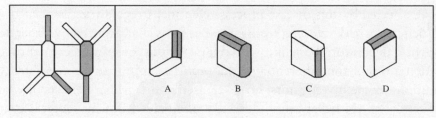

READING COMPREHENSION TEST   TIME LIMIT: 60 MINUTES

This section consists of three passages, with questions and/or incomplete statements following each passage. Read each passage; then read the questions and/or incomplete statements and answer choices carefully. For each question and/or incomplete statement choose the best answer and blacken the corresponding space on the answer sheet. This section contains 50 items.

Vitamin A Deficiency

Although tissues of ectodermal origin—that is, the epidermis—are primarily affected in vitamin A deficiency, bones and teeth also record this deficiency. Vitaminosis A is evinced by marked metaplasia of the enamel organ, which results in defective enamel and dentin formation. Likewise, bone is laid down in abnormal locations, and its remodeling sequences seem to be affected. Both osteoclasts and osteoblasts have been shown to be affected by this disease process. Dentinal irregularities associated with vitamin A deficiency in developing teeth appear as areas characterized by either excessive osteodentin deposition (bonelike, with cell inclusions) or insufficient dentin depositions. Alterations of the differentiated odontoblasts appear to be associated with these conditions. Some investigators, however, ascribe the primary effects of vitamin A deficiency to oral epithelial cells. This view originates from histological changes seen initially in the oral mucosa and extending to the degeneration of the epithelial-derived ameloblasts, which results in a hypoplastic enamel matrix. If the vitamin A deficiency is severe, ameloblast cells will become completely atrophied, resulting in an absence of enamel formation. In less severe cases, the columnar ameloblasts apparently shorten, and adjacent enamel exhibits hypoplasia. Several authors have described bone defects due to vitamin A deficiency. Most have noted that the defects are attributable to impaired endochondral ossification and faulty bone modeling. The normal appositional rhythm of dentin deposition may be altered. Vascular inclusions sometimes are seen in the dentin. If the vitamin A deficiency is relieved during subsequent tooth development, normal dentin and enamel are produced, although defective tissue is not repaired.

Vitamin C Deficiency

Ascorbic acid deficiency has been described in guinea pigs, monkeys, and humans. Because none of these species synthesizes vitamin C, they must depend on a dietary supply to maintain health. Scurvy, the disease resulting from vitamin C deficiency, causes bone, dentin, and cementum deposition to cease and formative cells to atrophy, if severe. Vitamin C is required for collagen formation. It is necessary for the hydroxylation of the amino acids proline and lysine; an absence or deficiency of vitamin C during dentinogenesis results in defective dentinal tissue development. Dentinal tubules become irregular and reduced in number, vascular inclusions become apparent, and those odontoblasts present are short, with some taking on a spindle-shaped, fibroblast-like appearance. Embryologically, vitamin C is essential for proper development of all mesenchymally derived structures, including bone, dentin, and cementum. Clinically, vitamin C deficiency is manifested by gingival bleeding and loosening of the teeth due to bone resorption. Weakness, anemia, and susceptibility to hemorrhage also may be evident. Administration of vitamin C results in rapid elimination of the symptoms associated with this deficiency.

Tetracycline and Fluoride

Tetracycline and fluoride, if available during the mineralization phases, may be incorporated in dentin, enamel, cementum, and bone. They are very different compounds. Fluoride is a binary compound of fluorine useful as an anticaries substance. Tetracycline, on the other hand, is used as an antibacterial agent. Both are deposited along with minerals in developing hard tissues. Tetracycline is derived from a yellow-gold fungus whose color is maintained in the purified antibiotic and transferred to the hard tissues in which it is incorporated. On prolonged exposure to light, tetracycline-stained dental tissue will change in color to brown and then to gray (i.e., these shades of discoloration are eventually seen in the teeth). Other effects of tetracyclines include hypoplasia or absence of enamel. Staining is most notable in the dentin, especially in the first-formed dentin at the dentinoenamel junction. Notable staining of the crown results primarily from discolored dentin being seen through the translucent and relatively unaffected enamel. Tetracycline staining is more notable under ultraviolet (UV) light. The amount of damage is directly related to the magnitude and duration of the dosage; any defects caused by the tetracycline may be compounded by the effects of the illness for which it was prescribed. The precise mechanism of tetracycline incorporation into mineralizing tissue is not yet known, but it is believed that a chelate of calcium and tetracycline forms. At higher concentrations, cells may be altered. In both ameloblasts and odontoblasts, the cisternae of the endoplasmic reticulum become dilated, and protein synthesis is impaired. This, in turn, will result in hypoplasia of the enamel and dentin matrix.

Tetracycline and, to a limited extent, sodium fluoride cross the placental barrier and are available to the human fetus. If a pregnant female consumes fluoridated water during mineralization of the fetal teeth, the teeth will incorporate this compound. Such teeth exhibit higher resistance to dental caries. Compared with fluoride blood levels in the maternal circulation, fluoride blood levels in the fetus are relatively low. If, on the other hand, tetracycline antibiotics are administered to the mother during the period of tooth mineralization, the deciduous teeth may later be stained. Tetracycline staining of teeth is permanent; staining of bone is not permanent because bone is remodeled continuously. The period marked by mineralization of crowns extends from approximately 5 months in utero to 12 years of age and includes the mineralization of both primary and permanent dentitions. Sodium fluoride when taken into the body in concentrations of 5 parts per million (ppm) (which occurs in some naturally fluoridated areas in this country) is anticariogenic but often causes mottled enamel. The mottled areas may or may not be mineralized. The enamel rods follow an irregular course through these areas. Despite their unsightly appearance, these teeth are completely free of caries. Fluoride is most beneficial to the teeth in concentrations of approximately 0.5 to 1 ppm of water. Concentrations of 0.5 ppm may not prevent caries. Higher concentrations, such as 5 ppm, cause mottling and hypoplasia of the enamel and hypomineralized dentin, with increased interglobular spaces.

As hydroxyapatite crystals form, they may incorporate fluoride either by an exchange with the hydroxyl groups or by simple adsorption. The hydroxyl group exchange is slower and less reversible than adsorption. In the latter process, the fluoride may be adsorbed to the surface of hydroxyapatite crystals. This adsorptive process involves weak electrostatic bonding. Adsorption is believed to be rapid although reversible. It is believed that fluoride found in inner enamel is taken up mainly during the secretory stage of amelogenesis and that fluoride found in the outer 30 to 50 μm of enamel is deposited during the maturative stage. Because the latter stage lasts longer, there is time for more fluoride to be deposited in the outer enamel. The maturative stage lasts from 1 to 2 years in primary teeth and from 4 to 5 years in permanent teeth. This may be the reason why less fluoride is found in primary teeth than in permanent teeth.

When histological examination is conducted on teeth from areas of high fluoride concentration, the enamel is found to be altered more than is the dentin. Enamel rod formation is affected, and zones of hypoplasia are commonly found. Tetracycline was first discovered to be present in human teeth and bones when traces were detected in bones being viewed under UV light. This observation provided a new method of marking bones and teeth in order to follow their development. Tetracycline compound initially is deposited in the predentin as it mineralizes into dentin. Evidence of this marking is demonstrated in the increasing distance between new predentin formed and the area of fluorescent dentin. Because the therapeutic dosage level and visual tissue-labeling levels coincide, tetracycline has been widely used to visually record growth in experimental animals. The daily deposition rate of dentin can thus be recorded by measuring the width of dentin between each two fluorescent dines. Some tetracycline is deposited in the dentinal tubules. Tetracycline may be used also to evaluate tooth movement by revealing bone and dentin formation.

1. What will happen if ascorbic acid is withheld during dentinogenesis?

   A. Dentinal tissue formation will not be affected.
   B. Enamel will be metaplastic.
   C. Scurvy will result.
   D. Enamel tissue development will be defective.
   E. Dentinal tissue development will be affected.

2. When does mineralization of the crowns take place?

   A. 5 months to 12 years of age
   B. 5 years to 12 years of age
   C. 5 months to 12 months of age
   D. 5 days in utero to 12 years of age
   E. 5 months in utero to 12 years of age

3. Which of the following is an antibacterial agent?

   A. Fluoride
   B. Ascorbic acid
   C. Tetracycline
   D. Vitamin A
   E. Ameloblast

4. What may be seen with severe vitamin A deficiency?

   A. Atrophy of ameloblast cells
   B. Thinning of enamel
   C. Vitamin C deficiency
   D. Tetracycline staining
   E. Excessive enamel deposition

5. Vitamin C is essential for which of the following?

   A. Development of bone
   B. Development of dentin
   C. Hydroxylation of lysine
   D. Development of cementum
   E. All of the above

6. Marked metaplasia of enamel may be due to which of the following?

   A. Ascorbic acid deficiency
   B. High fluoride levels
   C. Vitaminosis A
   D. Fluoride deficiency
   E. High levels of vitamin A

7. What experimental function does tetracycline serve?

   A. To mark the boundary between dentin and enamel
   B. To measure pulp growth
   C. To record the deposition rate of dentin
   D. To record the deposition rate of enamel
   E. Tetracycline is not used experimentally because of its toxicity.

8. Where is tetracycline staining most evident?

   A. In the dentin at the dentinoenamel junction
   B. In the enamel at the dentinoenamel junction
   C. In the pulp
   D. Tetracycline does not stain teeth.
   E. Tetracycline stains the whole tooth evenly.

9. Vitamin A deficiency may result in which of the following?

   A. Excessive osteodentin deposition
   B. Excessive enamel deposition
   C. Insufficient dentin deposition
   D. B and C
   E. A and C

10. Fluoride has the greatest effect on which of the following?

    A. Dentin
    B. Pulp
    C. Dentinoenamel junction
    D. Enamel
    E. Root

11. Why would monkeys be used to study vitamin C deficiency?

    A. Monkeys can synthesize vitamin C.
    B. The effects are seen soon after the withdrawal of vitamin C.
    C. The effects are pronounced.
    D. Monkeys do not synthesize vitamin C.
    E. Only guinea pigs are used for this purpose.

12. Vitamin C is necessary for which of the following?

    A. Hydroxylation of lysine
    B. Collagen formation
    C. Hydroxylation of purine
    D. The onset of scurvy
    E. All of the above

13. Tetracycline forms a chelate with what substance?

    A. Fluoride
    B. Sodium fluoride
    C. Calcium
    D. Vitamin A
    E. Ascorbic acid

14. When is the fluoride found in the inner enamel introduced?

    A. Throughout enamel formation
    B. During dentin formation
    C. During pulp formation
    D. In the maturative stage of amelogenesis
    E. In the secretory stage of amelogenesis

15. What will happen if vitamin A deficiency is relieved during tooth development?

A. Defective tissue will be repaired.

B. Normal dentin and enamel will be produced.

C. Normal dentin will be produced, but enamel will still be defective.

D. Normal enamel will be produced, but dentin will still be defective.

E. A and B

16. At what concentration is fluoride most beneficial to teeth?

A. 5 ppm

B. 0.5–1 ppm

C. 1–5 ppm

D. 0.1–0.5 ppm

E. 30–50 ppm

17. Scurvy is a result of what?

A. Ascorbic acid deficiency

B. Vitamin A deficiency

C. Tetracycline deficiency

D. Fluoride deficiency

E. Excessive fluoride intake

Effect of Organic Peroxide Additives on Wear Resistance of Composite Resin

Composite resin plays a major role in the esthetic restoration of anterior teeth. Caries preparations for Classes III, IV, and V are routinely restored with this type of agent. However, composite resin is used much less often in posterior teeth. The problems associated with posterior composite resins commonly relate to technique sensitivity, time required for placement, and inadequate wear resistance. Although manipulation techniques remain complex and relatively difficult to master, the problem of wear has been reduced appreciably with several newer composite resin systems.

Recent clinical studies at the University of Alabama have identified a number of formulations that exhibit annual wear values slightly better than those for amalgam. Although wear rates of earlier composite systems have an annual average ranging from 40 μm to 50 μm, the values for most current formulations are 10 μm or less.

Almost all composite resin manufacturers currently require the use of visible-light energy to cause polymerization. One exception is the Marathon® system. Although this system can be light-cured, it can also be converted into a dual-cure type of system by adding Marathon® Initiator with Infinite Cure®. This organic peroxide not only permits autocuring but also extends the depth of cure to all areas of the restoration, regardless of how the composite resin is polymerized.

In the last several years, an in vitro wear-testing device has been developed that generates wear rates closely resembling those obtained with clinical restorations. Designed as a three-body wear system, the device is capable of predicting 3-year clinical wear rates in fewer than 100 hours of in vitro testing. Such a test has great potential for manufacturers who may be considering several formulations for clinical trial.

The purpose of the in vitro study at the University of Alabama was to determine the potential for increasing the wear resistance of a composite resin by using a special organic peroxide additive, Marathon® Infinite Cure®. Another purpose was to evaluate the wear rate.

Materials and Methods

The in vitro device used in this study measures the wear of posterior composite resins. It can best be described as a three-body wear system. All the restorative systems evaluated are presented. They included Marathon® and TrueVitality™, with and without organic peroxide (Marathon® Infinite Cure® paste). Three other proprietary posterior composite resins were included for the purpose of comparison: P-50™ Posterior Restorative, Heliomolar®, and Tetric®. An amalgam, Dispersalloy®, was used as a control.

Sample Preparation

Sound, caries-free, extracted human molars were selected and mounted in a brass specimen holder. The occlusal surface was ground flat within enamel, using a series of metallographic papers to a 600 grit. After surfacing, a well-defined cylindrical-shaped cavity preparation was developed in the center of the tooth specimen. The preparation was 4 mm in diameter and 3 mm in depth. All cavosurface margins were carefully finished with a sharp No. 245 carbide bun. The taper of the preparation closely resembled that of the cutting instrument.

Next, the entire preparation was acid-conditioned, and an enamel or dentin bonding agent was placed according to the manufacturer's recommendations. For the Marathon® composite resin, the entire cavity was etched with Etch-N-Seal™ (37% phosphoric acid) for 20 seconds, rinsed thoroughly with tap water, and then gently air-dried. Then, Tenure® Quick™ with fluoride bonding agent was applied to the entire cavity three times and air-dispersed. For specimens without organic peroxide, Marathon® shade paste was used directly. The composite was inserted in three segments. Each increment was photo-cured for 40 seconds. The last segment, however, was cured for 60 seconds.

For specimens to which the additive was included, an equal amount of Marathon® Infinite Cure® paste was hand-mixed with the Marathon® Shade paste. The composite paste was bulk-filled into the cavity with a Centrix™ syringe and light-cured for 60 seconds.

The surface of the tooth/restoration specimen was ground carefully to a flat plane using a series of silicon carbide papers, and the final surface was completed with a 600-grit paper. This was all accomplished by using a special hand-held device to ensure that the flat occlusal surface was parallel to the flat surface of the energy-generating stylus.

For the inlay preparation, the walls of the cavity were tapered slightly to the occlusal margin. The inlay restoration was first prepared directly as an inlay. This was accomplished by generating the inlay in the cavity preparation after applying a separating medium. The composite resin was light-cured in the same manner as the direct restoration. The inlay restoration was removed and then heat-treated in a specially made tubular at 110°C for 10 minutes (as recommended by the manufacturer). At this point, the inlay was cemented into the preparation using a composite resin luting agent (Infinity® cement). Cementation was performed in strict accordance with the manufacturer's instruction. Equal amounts of base and catalyst paste were mixed thoroughly for 30 seconds and applied to the inlay, as well as to the walls of the preparation. The luting cement was light-cured for 60 seconds and maintained at room temperature for 30 minutes to achieve maximum polymerization. The tooth/restoration specimen was resurfaced with a 600-grit metallographic paper.

Specimens for the other composite materials were fabricated according to their respective manufacturers' instructions. All specimens for both the direct and indirect restorations were stored in 37°C water for 24 hours before wear testing.

In Vitro Wear Test

Using a specially designed aligning device, the mounted specimen was inserted in the wear-testing apparatus. The mounted tooth was then surrounded by a tight-fitting cylinder or ring. Next, a water slurry of unplasticized polymethylmethacrylate (PMMA) beads, averaging 44 μm, was poured on the surface of the restored teeth. The small acrylic resin beads served as an artificial food bolus. This assembly, along with a bank of three other specimens, was submerged in a water bath at room temperature. A flat-planed stylus, machined from polyacetal, was then positioned over the restored area. The diameter of the flat stylus, approximately 8 mm, was appropriately centered so that it covered the entire restoration, as well as 2 mm beyond the margins. At a rate of 1.2 times per second, the stylus was vertically loaded on the restored surface under a load of 17 lbs. or 75.6 Newtons (N). As the stylus initiated contact with the particles of PMMA lying over the restored surface, it automatically began to rotate clockwise 30 degrees. After counterrotating, the stylus moved upward vertically to its original position. The entire cycling procedure was repeated 400,000 times and took approximately 90 hours. After the wear test, the surface was replicated twice with a polyvinylsiloxane impression (Reprosil® light body). The first impression was discarded because it served to debride the surface. The second one was converted into epoxy replicas with an epoxy die model (Epoxy Die) and used for wear determinations using a profilometric stylus (Surfanalyzer®). Procedurally, the profilometric stylus was traversed across the specimen surface in single planes, each 45 degrees away from the next. This procedure produced eight different wear-measurement readings. Five different specimens were tested for each experiment. The vertical distance between the cavo-surface margin and the worn occlusal surface of the composite resin was used to express the amount of material loss or wear in microns. This procedure generated eight readings, which were averaged to express the wear value for each resin composite. The accuracy of the profilometer was 0.15 μm, and the data were statistically analyzed by analysis of variance.

Results

The Marathon® formulation without the organic peroxide additive exhibited the highest wear among the materials tested. Also, it was significantly different ($p < .05$) from the other materials. The addition of the peroxide modifier to Marathon® increased the wear resistance dramatically. The wear value of the modified material dropped from 17.2 μm to 8.6 μm, nearly a 50% reduction. There were no statistically significant differences among the values for Marathon® with Infinite Cure®, Tetric®, P-50™ Posterior Restorative, and Heliomolar®.

The heat-treated composite inlay (TrueVitality™) had minimal wear values compared to the other composite resins tested. A comparison of the values for the two groups of inlays with and without the Marathon® Infinite Cure® demonstrated again that the peroxide additive resulted in a lower wear rate. Specifically, the wear rate for the Marathon® Infinite Cure®-free TrueVitality™ averaged 4.9 μm, whereas TrueVitality™ with the additive revealed a 1.8 μm rate. (The differences between the two values are statistically significant.) Interestingly, this heat-treated composite inlay system with the peroxide additive exhibited a wear value that was significantly lower than the amalgam control wear value (1.8 μm vs. 3 μm).

18. Before wear testing, all specimens were

    A. stored in 37°K water for 24 hr
    B. stored in 37°C water for 24 days
    C. stored in 47°C water for 24 hr
    D. stored in 37°C water for 24 hr
    E. stored in 37°C water for 24 min

19. The resulting wear values in this experiment are

    A. averages of 5 readings
    B. averages of 5 specimens
    C. averages of 8 readings
    D. averages of 8 readings on 5 specimens
    E. approximately 0.15 μm

20. What is meant by surfacing?

    A. finishing of cavo-surface margins
    B. tapering the preparation
    C. formation of a cylindrical-shaped cavity preparation
    D. placing acid on the preparation
    E. grinding down the occlusal surface

21. Recent studies show that composite resins may be better than amalgam because of

    A. lower annual wear values for composites
    B. the fact that composites are visible-light-cured
    C. an annual wear of 40–50 μm for amalgam
    D. the inability to use amalgam for Classes III, IV, and V
    E. the Marathon® system

22. What type of inlay, based on the experiment, will most likely last the longest?

    A. True Vitality™ with peroxide
    B. True Vitality™ without peroxide
    C. amalgam
    D. P-50
    E. light-cured composite

23. How was the composite with organic peroxide placed?

    A. In three segments
    B. In two segments
    C. In bulk
    D. In four segments
    E. This information is not provided in the passage.

24. What was the purpose of using PMMA beads?

    A. To aid in polymerization
    B. To simulate a food bolus
    C. To surface the tooth
    D. To cure the composite resin
    E. To aid in storage

25. How many restorative materials were included in the trial?

    A. 3
    B. 4
    C. 5
    D. 6
    E. 7

26. How long did the actual wear test take?

    A. 90 min
    B. 100 hr
    C. 100 min
    D. 45 hr
    E. 90 hr

27. Based on the results, which composite resin would the experimenter be LEAST likely to endorse?

    A. Tetric®
    B. Marathon® with peroxide additive
    C. Heliomolar®
    D. Marathon® without Infinite Cure®
    E. All are basically the same.

28. The passage suggests that autocuring may be better than light curing because

    A. light curing takes longer
    B. autocuring is more reliable
    C. autocuring extends the cure depth to all areas of the preparation
    D. autocuring allows the composite resin to polymerize
    E. all of the above

29. The polyacetal stylus was used to

    A. load the restoration
    B. pack the restoration
    C. place the composite resin
    D. place the inlay
    E. cure the composite resin

30. What was done after each of the first two segments of composite resin was placed?

    A. Marathon® shade paste was added.
    B. The specimen was light-cured for 40 sec.
    C. Etch-N-Seal™ was added.
    D. The specimen was light-cured for 60 sec.
    E. The specimen was air-dried.

31. The purpose(s) of taking two impressions after the wear test was (were)

    A. to ensure at least one accurate impression
    B. to determine wear
    C. to debride the surface
    D. to make it possible to run two tests simultaneously
    E. B and C

32. Why is the new wear-testing device such an important advancement?

    A. It allows composite resin durability to be tested.
    B. It allows amalgam durability to be tested.
    C. It is more accurate than previous devices.
    D. Long-term results can be determined in a matter of days.
    E. A and C

33. Composite resin luting agent was used to

    A. cement the inlay to the restoration
    B. prepare the restoration for the inlay
    C. surface the tooth
    D. cure the composite resin
    E. test wear on the composite

34. Composite resin is generally used for_____

    A. Class III
    B. Class V
    C. Class VI
    D. Posterior teeth
    E. A and B

Bone Implant Interfaces

In 1952, Branemark embarked on studies that resulted in the introduction of a treatment concept and implant design in the early 1980s after an extensive examination of cylindrical, threaded endosteal implants. A variety of implant models and surgical techniques have led to the development of our present concepts of fibro-osseous integration, osseointegration, and biointegration. Fibro-osseous integration is defined as a connective tissue-encapsulated implant within bone. This type of integration was an early histological finding in implant development and resulted from early types of implant materials, possibly because of a lack of primary stability, premature loading of the implant, and/or a traumatic surgical procedure causing heat-induced bone necrosis. A long-term clinical study has demonstrated a success rate of approximately 50% over a 10-year period for this type of implant integration. Materials that stimulate this type of reaction are nonprecious metals, acrylates, polymers, and vitreous carbon. With the newer materials, fibro-osseous integration makes up a much smaller percentage of the interface to the implant, while osseointegration or biointegration comprises the majority of the interface.

Osseointegration was defined by Branemark as a direct structural and functional connection between ordered, living bone and the surface of a load-carrying implant without soft tissue intervention at the light microscopic level. This type of integration has been shown to yield the most predictable success for long-term implant stability. Factors that enhance osseointegration include (1) atraumatic surgical procedures with minimal heat generated, and (2) close fit of the implant fixture to the formed socket. Present implant surgical research indicates that the best result is achieved with a low drilling speed (under 800 rpm) and abundant irrigation with chilled saline, which minimizes bone tissue injury. Use of a precision drilling system increases the initial implant-bone contact. The implant materials, surface characteristics of the implant, and type of recipient bone are factors that help determine the final implant-tissue interface. In addition, the appropriate timing of placing the implant in function supporting a prosthesis is an essential element in maintaining osseointegration.

Biointegration is a form of implant interface that is achieved with bioactive materials such as hydroxylapatite (HA) and bioglass that bond directly to bone, similar to ankylosis of natural teeth. The bone matrix is deposited on the HA layer as the result of a physiochemical interaction between the collagen of bone and the HA crystals of the implant. HA-coated implants appear to develop bone contact faster than do noncoated implants. However, after a year, there seems to be little difference in bone contact between coated and noncoated implants. The HA-coated implants continue to be improved in their purity and manufacturing processes. Dental implants differ significantly from natural teeth in their interface with the alveolar bone and connective tissue fibers. The junctional epithelium, however, appears to have the same interface characteristics with implants as with natural teeth. Because implants do not have a cemental surface for the insertion of the periodontal ligament and gingival connective tissue fibers, successful implants depend on direct contact with the alveolar bone and connective tissue adhesion coronal to the alveolar housing. A histologically successful implant would be defined as having 35 to 90% direct bone contact, a connective tissue adhesion above the bone, and an intact noninflamed junctional epithelium. Clinically, the implant should be nonmobile and free of discomfort in function. An implant can be considered successful if (1) mucosal health is substantiated by clinical parameters such as a lack of redness, of bleeding on probing, or of suppuration. Soft tissue inflammation, when present, should be amenable to treatment; (2) there is no significant or progressive loss of supporting bone; (3) there is no persistent infection; (4) the implant functions in the absence of discomfort; (5) there is no increasing mobility of the implant on evaluation when the prosthesis is removed; and (6) the implant is prosthetically useful.

Bone is a specialized, calcified connective tissue. Alveolar bone is a combination of both cortical and cancellous bone. Both forms of bone have been shown to osseointegrate with the implant surface. In addition, blood vessels within the bone have been shown to proliferate in contact with the implant surface. To date, the implant materials that have demonstrated the most rapid ability for osseointegration are titanium (commercially pure, alloy, and plasma-sprayed) and the calcium phosphate ceramic material, HA. The biologically active surface on titanium is a dense protective oxide layer 15 to 50 μm thick. This layer forms quickly after processing and is relatively resistant to further corrosion by proteolytic enzymes or chemical attack. Titanium plasma-spraying of the implant increases the surface area for osseointegration almost sixfold. The HA-coated implants appear to osseointegrate more rapidly and to have a higher percentage of bone contact than titanium. However, within a year's time, the difference does not appear to be clinically significant. The HA coating is used because it is manufactured with a commercially pure material that has proved to be nontoxic and has a resemblance to the inorganic phase of the human skeleton. The percentage of cortical bone in contact with implants appears to increase because of the remodeling of the bone associated with functional adaptation.

Epithelium Tissue Interface

The interface of epithelium with an implant is similar to that found with the natural tooth. The sulcus and the junctional epithelium are both in contact with the implant. The healthy sulcus consists of a 5- to 15-cell layer of nonkeratinized epithelium with wide intercellular spaces. The junctional epithelium is approximately 2 mm in length and 2 to 5 cell layers thick, with basal and suprabasal cells in direct contact with the implant surface. These cells are attached to the implant surface by a basal lamina and hemidesmosomes. The epithelial interface is similar to that with the natural tooth, whereas the connective tissue interface is significantly different.

Connective Tissue Interface

The initial success of dental implants is determined by the ability of the implant material to integrate with the alveolar bone. With the placement of the implant abutment through the oral mucosa, the long-term success is dependent on the "transmucosal seal" that forms between the implant abutment's polished or machined surface and the mucosa's connective tissue and epithelium. In the peri-implant tissue, the vast majority of large collagen fiber bundles are attached to the marginal alveolar bone and insert into the marginal gingiva, not onto the titanium. These fiber bundles are highly organized and are oriented parallel to the surface of the machined titanium surface. The connective tissues adjacent to a tooth above the crestal bone are normally arranged into three different fiber groups: (1) dentogingival fibers extending from their insertion into cementum to the marginal connective tissue; (2) dentoperiosteal fibers extending from the cementum to the alveolar bone crest; and (3) circular fibers present in the connective tissue of the marginal gingiva and supra-alveolar connective tissue. All these fiber groups are functionally oriented (perpendicular) to the tooth. One research group has observed collagen fibers appearing to insert into the neck of a plasma-sprayed implant surface in monkeys. These collagen fibers were arranged in a perpendicular arrangement similar to the connective tissue fibers in cementum, as in a normal functioning tooth. The results of this research are not well understood. The width of supracrestal connective tissue around the neck of a healthy implant is approximately 1 to 1.5 mm. This width may vary based on the initial thickness of the mucosa and the degree of adaptation of the mucosa at the time the transmucosal abutment is placed. If the direct bone-implant contact is broken, connective tissue will fill the space between the alveolar crest and implant. These fiber bundles run parallel to the implant surface. Both the connective tissue and the epithelial interfaces have proved to provide adequate resistance to oral function and marginal irritation.

35. Why might biointegration be preferable to osseointegration?

   A. With biointegration more bone is deposited.
   B. With biointegration bone contact occurs more rapidly.
   C. With biointegration less connective tissue is deposited.
   D. With biointegration the bone-implant interface is stronger.
   E. With biointegration higher drill speeds can be used.

36. Over the long term the success of an implant depends on

   A. the epithelium tissue interface
   B. the amount of osseointegration
   C. the ability of the implant to integrate with alveolar bone
   D. the transmucosal seal
   E. all of the above

37. What term describes an implant that is within bone and encapsulated by connective tissue?

   A. Fibro-osseous integration
   B. Biointegration
   C. Osseointegration
   D. Bone-implant interface
   E. Implant fixture

38. For rapid osseointegration to occur, what type of material should be used?

   A. Vitreous carbon
   B. Acrylates
   C. Titanium
   D. Polymer
   E. Nonprecious metal

39. The width of supracrestal connective tissue around the neck of a healthy implant

   A. May vary based on initial mucosal thickness
   B. Is approximately 1–1.5 μm
   C. Is approximately 1–1.5 cm
   D. May vary with time
   E. A and B

40. If vitreous carbon implants are used, what percent can be expected to fail?

   A. 40%
   B. 35%
   C. 60%
   D. 50%
   E. This information is not provided in the passage.

41. After 1 year what difference can be noted between a plasma-sprayed titanium implant and an HA-coated implant?

    A. Little to no difference is apparent.
    B. The plasma-sprayed implant has a six-fold increase in osseointegration.
    C. The HA-coated implant has a higher percentage of bone contact.
    D. The HA-coated implant has less bone contact.
    E. The plasma-sprayed implant has less bone contact.

42. An implant coated with bioglass will result in

    A. osseointegration
    B. fibro-osseous integration
    C. reduced bone deposition
    D. biointegration
    E. C and D

43. Alveolar bone is made up of

    A. fibrous connective tissue
    B. cancellous bone
    C. cortical bone
    D. junctional epithelium
    E. B and C

44. What reason is (reasons are) given to explain why fibro-osseous integration occurs?

    A. Premature loading of the implant
    B. Heat-induced bone necrosis
    C. Lack of primary stability
    D. A and B
    E. All of the above

45. Suprabasal cells are attached to the implant by

    A. junctional epithelium
    B. nonkeratinized epithelium
    C. hemidesmosomes
    D. connective tissue
    E. transmucosal seal

46. The best results are achieved with osseointegration when

    A. space is left around the implant for bone growth
    B. heat is kept to a minimum
    C. drill speed is kept above 800 rpm
    D. warm saline is used
    E. A and B

47. What biologically active surface is added to titanium implants?

    A. Oxide layer 25–30 μm thick
    B. Oxide layer 15–50 μm thick
    C. Peroxide layer 15–50 μm thick
    D. Plasma
    E. None

48. Osseointegration differs from fibro-osseous integration in that with osseointegration

    A. soft tissue intervenes at the micro-scopic level
    B. bone contacts the implant except at the microscopic level
    C. bone directly contacts the implant
    D. the implant ankyloses to the bone
    E. the implant is encapsulated in connective tissue

49. In peri-implant tissue most large collagen fiber bundles are attached at the

    A. marginal gingiva
    B. marginal alveolar bone
    C. titanium
    D. HA
    E. A and B

50. For an implant to be deemed histologically successful what requirement must be met?

    A. 35–90% connective tissue adhesion
    B. No connective tissue adhesion
    C. Connective tissue adhesion within the bone
    D. Biointegration
    E. 35–90% direct bone contact

QUANTITATIVE REASONING TEST TIME LIMIT: 45 MINUTES

The following items are questions or incomplete statements. Read each item carefully, then choose the best answer or completion. Blacken the corresponding space on the answer sheet. This section contains 40 items.

1. Since 1 meter = 3.28 feet, $\frac{2}{3}$ foot equals approximately what fraction of a meter?

   A. $\frac{1}{5}$

   B. $\frac{1}{4}$

   C. $\frac{1}{3}$

   D. $\frac{1}{2}$

   E. $\frac{3}{4}$

2. If $y = \frac{x+4}{x-1}$, which of the following represents x?

   A. $\frac{3y}{y+1}$

   B. $\frac{3y+2}{y-1}$

   C. $\frac{3y+2}{y}$

   D. $\frac{4+y}{y-1}$

   E. $\frac{4y-2}{y-1}$

3. E. $\sqrt{6+\frac{1}{x}} = 8$, $x = ?$

   A. $\frac{1}{2}$

   B. 2

   C. 58

   D. $\sqrt{\frac{1}{28}}$

   E. $\frac{1}{58}$

4. A train covers 150 yards in 12.5 seconds. What is the average speed, in feet per second, of the train?

   A. 18
   B. 34
   C. 24
   D. 36
   E. 12

5. If $4x - 6 > 5x + 4$, which of the following must be true?

   A. $x > -10$
   B. $x > \frac{4}{5}$
   C. $x < -4$
   D. $x < 10$
   E. $x < -10$

6. Evaluate the expression $(4 \times 10^{-5}) \times (2 \times 10^{8})$.

   A. 6×10^{-3}
   B. 8×10^{3}
   C. 8×10^{13}
   D. 8×10^{-3}
   E. 6×10^{3}

7. The perimeter of a square is 40. Which of the following represents the area?

   A. 100
   B. 10
   C. 40
   D. 80
   E. 20

8. If $F(x) = 4x^2 - 5x$, then $F(-1)$ equals which of the following?

   A. −9
   B. −1
   C. 9
   D. 1
   E. 6

9. A salesperson receives a 15% commission on all sales. If he receives $300 in commissions in a week, what is the value of his sales?

   A. $45
   B. $20
   C. $4,500
   D. $20,000
   E. $2,000

10. The slope of the line $10 - 2y = -4x$ is

    A. −5
    B. −2
    C. 2
    D. 5
    E. 4

11. The value of sec t is equal to

    A. $\dfrac{1}{\cos t}$
    B. $\dfrac{1}{\tan t}$
    C. $\dfrac{\cos t}{\sin t}$
    D. $\dfrac{1}{\sin t}$
    E. $\dfrac{\sin t}{\cos t}$

12. If the side length of a square is increased by 50%, the area increases by what percent?

    A. 125
    B. 225
    C. 25
    D. 50
    E. 75

13. Which of the following is the largest?

    A. $\dfrac{23}{25}$
    B. $\dfrac{27}{30}$
    C. $\dfrac{15}{16}$
    D. $\dfrac{14}{15}$
    E. $\dfrac{7}{8}$

14. Which line is parallel to the y-axis?

    A. $x = 4y$
    B. $x = (\dfrac{2}{y°})b$
    C. $x = y + 6$
    D. $xy = 2$
    E. $xy = 2 + 4y^{-1}$

15. A fly sits at the edge of a 12-inch-diameter phonograph record that is playing at $33\frac{1}{3}$ revolutions per minute. Approximately how fast, in feet per minute, is the fly moving?

    A. 3
    B. 33
    C. 50
    D. 100
    E. 396

16. Rich is $\dfrac{1}{6}$ of his father's age. In 20 years he will be $\dfrac{1}{2}$ of his father's age at that time. How old is his father now?

    A. 24 yr.
    B. 36 yr.
    C. 30 yr.
    D. 42 yr.
    E. 38 yr.

17. If $3x + y = 5$ and $5x + y = 6$, then $y = ?$

    A. 1

    B. 3.5

    C. $\dfrac{5}{6}$

    D. 2

    E. 3

18. What is the distance on a two-dimensional graph between points $(7, 6)$ and $(2, -6)$?

    A. 9

    B. 5

    C. 17

    D. 13

    E. $\sqrt{153}$

19. Kate has six different books. Assuming the order of selection doesn't matter, how many ways can Kate select, from these six books, two different books?

    A. 18

    B. 15

    C. 30

    D. 36

    E. 12

20. If $z = 2$, $y = \dfrac{1}{2}$, and $\dfrac{1}{x} = 1$, what is the value of $x + \dfrac{1y}{z}$?

    A. $\dfrac{5}{4}$

    B. 2

    C. 7

    D. $1\dfrac{1}{2}$

    E. $1\dfrac{2}{3}$

21. Sales reductions force a factory to cut back its output by 20%. By what percentage must the reduced sales be increased to allow production to be brought back to normal?

    A. 40

    B. 30

    C. 35

    D. 20

    E. 25

22. The current sales price of a power drill is $117.00. This is $30.00 more than half the list price. At what discount is the drill being sold?

    A. 32.8%

    B. 25.6%

    C. 74.4%

    D. 67.2%

    E. 48.7%

23. The set of numbers (1, 2, 3, 6) has an arithmetic mean (average) of 3 and a variance of 3.5. What are the arithmetic mean and the variance of the set of numbers (2, 8, 10, 16)?

    A. 12; 7.5

    B. 9; 25

    C. 6; 9

    D. 6; 25

    E. 9; 10.5

24. A bowl contains 7 blue and 3 red marbles. What is the probability that 2 marbles selected at random from this bowl without replacement are both red?

    A. $\dfrac{9}{100}$

    B. $\dfrac{1}{15}$

    C. $\dfrac{6}{10}$

    D. $\dfrac{47}{90}$

    E. $\dfrac{21}{100}$

25. Which of the following represents 5% of 2% of 0.6?

    A. 6
    B. 0.06
    C. 0.006
    D. 0.0006
    E. 0.00006

26. One pump can fill a pool in 10 minutes. Another pump can fill the pool in 15 minutes. How many minutes are required to fill the pool if both pumps are operating at the same time?

    A. 12
    B. 12.5
    C. 6
    D. 25
    E. $\dfrac{1}{6}$

27. If Bob must have a mark of 70% to pass a test of 30 items, the number of items he may miss and still pass the test is

    A. 8
    B. 10
    C. 9
    D. 28
    E. 21

28. A 25-foot ladder is placed against a building at a point 20 feet from the ground. The distance from the base of the building to the base of the ladder is

    A. 12 ft.
    B. 25 ft.
    C. 18 ft.
    D. 30 ft.
    E. 15 ft.

29. Two committees are formed with seven people on one committee and eight on the other. If three people are in both groups, how many people belong to only one group?

    A. 7
    B. 9
    C. 12
    D. 8
    E. 6

30. If $5 - 2x = 13$, what is the value of y if $10 - y = x^2$?

    A. −6
    B. 30
    C. 2
    D. 22
    E. 4

31. Right triangle ABC has the right angle at C, and $AB = 12$, $BC = 6$. Find AC.

    A. 3
    B. $3\sqrt{3}$
    C. 6
    D. 12
    E. $6\sqrt{3}$

32. 20 is to $4y$ as $25x$ is to which of the following?

    A. $\dfrac{5x}{y}$
    B. $5x$
    C. $\dfrac{5y}{x}$
    D. $5xy$
    E. $\dfrac{x}{5y}$

33. If 0.04 is 25% of x, x is

    A. 0.01
    B. 0.16
    C. 0.1
    D. 1.0
    E. 1.6

34. If $(a^3 b^{-2})^{-2}$ is simplified to a form in which the exponents are positive, the result is

A. $\dfrac{a^6}{b^4}$

B. $a^2 b$

C. $\dfrac{a}{b_4}$

D. $\dfrac{b^4}{a_6}$

E. $\dfrac{1}{a^2 b}$

35. The distance a train travels varies directly according to its rate times the time it takes to complete the trip. If the rate and one time are both quadrupled, the distance

A. becomes 16 times greater
B. becomes 8 times greater
C. stays the same
D. is doubled
E. is quadrupled

36. If $x = 4$, $y = \dfrac{1}{8}$, and $z = 2\dfrac{2}{3}$,

then $\dfrac{1}{x} + \dfrac{1}{y} - \dfrac{1}{z} = ?$

A. 0

B. $7\dfrac{7}{8}$

C. $\dfrac{35}{24}$

D. $\dfrac{7}{8}$

E. $8\dfrac{5}{8}$

37. David weighs $1\dfrac{1}{4}$ times what Mark weighs and twice what Susan weighs. If Mark weighs 176 pounds, how much does Susan weigh?

A. 110 lb.
B. 70 lb.
C. 88 lb.
D. 141 lb.
E. 220 lb.

38. A gift of \$180 is to be shared by Brett and Andrew in such a way that Andrew gets 25% more than Brett. How much does Brett get?

A. \$100
B. \$72
C. \$108
D. \$144
E. \$80

39. Which of the following is the equation of the line that contains point $(3, -1)$ and is perpendicular to the line $y = 3x + 3$?

A. $y = \left(\dfrac{-1}{3}\right) x$

B. $y = 3x - 10$

C. $y = 3 - 8$

D. $y = \left(\dfrac{-1}{3}\right) x + 2$

E. $y = \left(\dfrac{-1}{3}\right) x - 2$

40. Simplify: $\dfrac{-7}{8} + \dfrac{1}{6} - \dfrac{3}{4}$

A. $\dfrac{1}{4}$

B. $1\dfrac{11}{24}$

C. $\dfrac{5}{12}$

D. $\dfrac{-5}{12}$

E. $-1\dfrac{11}{24}$

Answer Key
MODEL EXAMINATION A

Survey of the Natural Sciences

1. D	14. A	27. B	40. E	53. B	65. D	77. D	89. D
2. D	15. D	28. B	41. D	54. D	66. B	78. C	90. B
3. B	16. B	29. E	42. D	55. A	67. E	79. A	91. E
4. E	17. C	30. A	43. D	56. C	68. A	80. D	92. C
5. D	18. C	31. B	44. B	57. B	69. A	81. B	93. A
6. A	19. A	32. B	45. A	58. B	70. B	82. B	94. B
7. C	20. E	33. B	46. B	59. E	71. B	83. A	95. C
8. B	21. A	34. B	47. A	60. A	72. A	84. B	96. D
9. E	22. C	35. D	48. C	61. A	73. E	85. D	97. C
10. D	23. D	36. A	49. D	62. D	74. C	86. A	98. E
11. C	24. C	37. C	50. B	63. C	75. D	87. C	99. A
12. C	25. E	38. E	51. A	64. C	76. D	88. E	100. D
13. A	26. C	39. D	52. C				

Perceptual Ability Test

1. C	13. A	25. C	36. C	47. E	58. C	69. A	80. D
2. B	14. D	26. C	37. B	48. B	59. C	70. B	81. C
3. C	15. E	27. D	38. A	49. E	60. A	71. E	82. B
4. E	16. D	28. B	39. D	50. D	61. B	72. D	83. B
5. E	17. B	29. A	40. D	51. B	62. B	73. A	84. A
6. A	18. A	30. B	41. C	52. D	63. C	74. E	85. D
7. A	19. B	31. B	42. D	53. D	64. B	75. D	86. B
8. B	20. B	32. D	43. B	54. E	65. A	76. B	87. A
9. B	21. C	33. B	44. A	55. B	66. C	77. C	88. A
10. D	22. A	34. A	45. D	56. A	67. D	78. C	89. B
11. E	23. D	35. C	46. C	57. C	68. B	79. D	90. A
12. C	24. D						

Reading Comprehension Test

1. E	8. A	15. B	21. A	27. D	33. A	39. E	45. C
2. E	9. E	16. B	22. A	28. C	34. E	40. D	46. B
3. C	10. D	17. A	23. C	29. A	35. B	41. A	47. E
4. A	11. D	18. D	24. B	30. B	36. D	42. D	48. C
5. E	12. B	19. C	25. D	31. E	37. A	43. E	49. B
6. C	13. C	20. E	26. E	32. D	38. C	44. E	50. E
7. C	14. E						

Quantitative Reasoning Test

1. A	6. B	11. A	16. C	21. E	26. C	31. E	36. B
2. D	7. A	12. A	17. B	22. A	27. C	32. D	37. A
3. E	8. C	13. C	18. D	23. A	28. E	33. B	38. E
4. D	9. E	14. B	19. B	24. B	29. B	34. D	39. A
5. E	10. C	15. D	20. A	25. D	30. A	35. A	40. E

Answers Explained

SURVEY OF THE NATURAL SCIENCES

1. **D** The secretory vesicle transports proteins destined for extracellular release via exocytosis.

2. **D** Polar molecules are transported across membranes via pores or gated protein channels. Nonpolar molecules and solvents can travel more freely through the uncharged lipid bilayer.

3. **B** Active transport requires energy in the form of ATP to move molecules against the concentration gradient. Osmosis and simple diffusion are forms of passive transport.

4. **E** Centrioles are microtubular organelles that are not membrane bound.

5. **D** Glycogen is the polymerized form of glucose that is stored in the liver. When blood sugar levels become low, glucose molecules are cleaved off of glycogen in a process called glycogenolysis.

6. **A** NAD and FAD are electron acceptors and transporters in glycolysis, photosynthesis, and other key cellular processes.

7. **C** Glycolysis alone yields 2 net ATP, while the Krebs cycle and electron transport chain yield 36 ATP.

8. **B** A variety of pigments absorb different wavelengths of sunlight; photons are passed on from one pigment molecule to the next until they reach cholorophyll *a*, beginning the light reactions of photosynthesis.

9. **E** Larval stages of echinodermata are similar to those of chordates, suggesting a close evolutionary relationship.

10. **D** Platelets are cell fragments, erythrocytes are red blood cells, and leukocytes are white blood cells.

11. **C** The sonoatrial (SA) node sets the heart's pace by initiating contraction of the right and left atria. The impulse is then transmitted to the atrioventricular (AV) node, with the subsequent contraction of the ventricles.

12. **C** Insulin stimulates the uptake of blood glucose by the liver and body cells, thereby lowering the levels of sugar in the blood. Excessive insulin can lead to blood sugar levels that are too low, called hypoglycemia. In extreme hypoglycemia, coma can result.

13. **A** Antibodies, also known as immunoglobulins, hemoglobin, and actin are globular proteins. Collagen is fibrous. Myosin is mostly fibrous with globular heads.

14. **A** When Ca^{2+} levels are sufficiently high, Ca^{2+} binds tropenin, releasing tropomyosin from actin, thereby allowing myosin to bind actin.

15. **D** In metaphase, chromosomes line up at the metaphase plate in the midline of the cell.

16. B Electrical synapses allow for bidirectional communication, while chemical synapses involve unidirectional communication.

17. C In independent assortment, the number of possible gametes can be determined by the formula 2^n where n = haploid number. In this case, $2^3 = 8$.

18. C FAD and NAD are electron transporters, but the final electron acceptor is molecular oxygen, O_2, yielding water (H_2O).

19. A Unequal distribution of cytoplasm in meiosis I and II of oogenesis leads to only one viable gamete.

20. E Gastrulation involves the differentiation of cells into ectoderm, mesoderm, and endoderm tissue layers.

21. A Recessive traits are only expressed when they are homozygous. Zingers are heterozygous carriers of a lethal allele, but so long as they have a dominant allele as well, they will live.

22. C Thrombin catalyzes the conversion of fibrinogen to fibrin. Fibrin forms the fibrous portion of the clot, while platelets form the initial plug.

23. D Pulmonary and umbilical arteries carry deoxygenated blood. All other arteries carry oxygenated blood away from the heart.

24. C Ectoderm gives rise to tooth enamel as well as skin epithelium, hair follicles, sweat glands, cornea and lens of the eye, nails, nervous system, and epithelial lining of the mouth and rectum.

25. E In the endocrine system and beyond, most biochemical pathways are regulated by negative feedback.

26. C Symbiosis describes a close relationship between two species in a community. In parasitism, one is hurt, and one is helped; in mutualism, both species benefit; in commensalisms, one benefits, while the other is neither helped nor harmed.

27. B Taxonomic classification, in order from broadest to narrowest, is domain, kingdom, phylum, class, order, family, genus, and species.

28. B When cells are placed in a hypertonic environment, they lose water and crenate.

29. E Thymine, cytosine, adenine, and guanine are found in DNA. In RNA, uracil replaces thymine such that the adenine of a DNA template strand pairs with uracil of the mRNA during transcription.

30. A Eukaryotic cells contain membrane-bound organelles; prokaryotic cells do not. In eukaryotic cells, genetic information is enclosed in a nucleus. In prokaryotic cells, a mass of DNA called the nucleoid contains the genetic information.

31. B Protozoans are protists; animal cells and most protists lack cell walls.

32. B Three hydrogen bonds form between cytosine and guanine; two hydrogen bonds form between adenine and thymine. DNA #2 will be more stable because it has more bonds holding it together.

33. B Wings of bats, birds, and bees arose independently in evolution, making them analogous structures. Similar structures arising independently are said to be evolutionarily convergent.

34. B Genes that are frequently inherited together and do not follow the laws of Mendelian independent assortment are said to be linked.

35. D In transcription, DNA is used as a template to create a complementary mRNA molecule. In translation, the mRNA molecule is interpreted by tRNA molecules to form a polypeptide chain.

36. A The P site holds the tRNA that is actively adding an amino acid to the growing polypeptide chain; the A site holds tRNA that contains the next-in-line amino acid to be joined to the polypeptide chain.

37. C The father is the homozygous recessive individual that is affected. All offspring that are affected are also homozygous recessive.

38. E Oxytocin and antidiuretic hormone (ADH) are produced in the hypothalamus, but stored in and secreted by the posterior pituitary gland.

39. D Natural selection allows for the mutated bacteria with an added advantage to flourish. No new species are formed.

40. E In a normal fertilization, the sperm swims through the uterus and fertilizes the ovum in the oviduct, also called the fallopian tube.

41. D Metals have a large number of positive ions blended with a large number of electrons.

42. D NH_4^+ is the only molecule of the choices that could be tetrahedral since it has a central atom bound to four other atoms.

43. D Dalton's law says the diffusion rate of one gas to another is inversely proportional to the square roots of the molecular weights of the gases. In this case, methane has a MW = 16 and He has a MW = 4, so $\sqrt{4/16} = 1/2$.

44. B Atomic radii increase on the periodic table as you move down and to the left. Also, cations of atoms are smaller than the neutral atoms, and anions are larger than their neutral atoms.

45. A Ba^{2+} has 54 electrons, as does Xe.

46. B At STP, 22.4 liters is equivalent to a mole of gas. To solve this problem, divide 245 mL by 22.4 L and multiple by the MW of SO_2 to get the answer.

47. A Following Le Chatelier's principle in this case, pressure will cause an equilibrium shift to the side of the reaction with the lesser number of moles of gas.

48. C Melting point depression is not classified as a colligative property.

49. D Formation of a gas, increase in temperature, and an increase in volume will all increase entropy in a system.

50. B There are two atoms of Cl and two atoms of H on the right side of the equation, but not on the left. Having 2 HCl on the left side of the equation will balance both H and Cl.

51. A The subscript of 3 following S in As_2S_3 indicates the number of moles of S released after breakup of As_2S_3.

52. C Dividing 50 g by 26.98 g/mole = 1.85 moles.

53. B Since the rate is dependent upon the concentration of A to the first power, doubling the concentration of A will double the rate of the reaction.

54. D Only in answer D does H_2O donate a proton as an acid.

55. A A catalyst accelerates a reaction by lowering the activation energy of the reaction.

56. C The percent of C in $Na_2C_2O_2$ is less than 25%. The percent of C in all other compounds is 40% or greater.

57. B The equilibrium constant for $aA + bB \leftrightarrows cC + dD$ is equal to $[C]^c[D]^d/[A]^a[B]^b$.

58. B Fourteen grams of NaF (MW = 42 g) = 1/3 mole. If dissolved in 400 mL, the (1/3)/0.4 L = 5/6 M = 0.83 M.

59. E (3 M (of H^+) × 300 mL) / 8 M (of OH^-) = 112.5 mL.

60. A $(4 \times 10^{-8}$ g/44 g/mole) × 3 moles C/mole C_3H_8 × 6.02 × 10^{23} atoms/mole = 1.64 × 10^{15} atoms.

61. A If the percent of oxygen is (0.65/3.4)100, then the percent of carbon is 100 − (0.65/3.4)100 = (1 − 0.65/3.4)100.

62. D An alloy has metallic properties and is composed of two or more elements.

63. C The Arrhenius base produces hydroxide ions.

64. C For a solid or liquid reactant, the greater the surface area per unit volume, the more contact it makes with the other reactant(s), and the faster the chemical reaction will occur.

65. D Grams of Cl = 70.9 mL/1000 mL/L × 0.201 M × 35.45 g/mole Cl. Divide the grams of Cl by 5 grams to get the percentage of chloride in the sample.

66. B $\Delta G = \Delta H - T\Delta S$. If ΔG is negative and $\Delta H = 0$, and T is always positive, then ΔS must be positive.

67. E Atomic radii generally increase in a group from top to bottom and generally increase in a period from right to left.

68. A The halogens are Group 7A in the periodic table and include fluorine (F).

69. A Carbon forms a double bond with both oxygen atoms, so the structure is linear.

70. B Isotopes have the same number of electrons and protons but differ in the number of neutrons.

71. B Heterolytic cleavage occurs when both electrons remain together after the reaction. In the case of a radical reaction, the reaction is homolytic because the electrons are split between the products.

72. **A** Pi bonds run parallel on top and below the sigma bonds in a double bond configuration.

73. **E** The molecule has a ketone group with six carbons in the chain. This makes the molecule a hexanone. The system of assigning the lowest number for the hexanone makes answer E correct.

74. **C** Answer C does not obey Huckel's rule for aromaticity ($4n + 2$ pi electrons).

75. **D** A secondary alcohol has carbon groups on either side of the alcohol group, so when the alcohol group is oxidized to a carbonyl group, the result will be a ketone.

76. **D** Propagation occurs when a radical + reactant form a product and another radical.

77. **D** Answers A, B, and C all affect the strength of an acid.

78. **C** $LiAlH_4$ is a very powerful reducing agent.

79. **A** In addition to being the most substituted radical, molecule A also has resonance stabilization.

80. **D** The resonance in molecule A will be disrupted if it binds to a proton. Molecules B, C, and E have halogen attachments that will incur inductive effects to decrease basicity.

81. **B** The longest carbon chain is three carbons long and is bound to an amine group, so the molecule must be a propamine.

82. **B** Carboxylic acids are stronger acids than alcohols. Phenol is a better acid than ethanol because the phenolic anion has resonance stabilization. Acetic acid is not as good an acid as formic acid because the methyl group of acetic acid stabilizes the carboxyl group before it donates a proton.

83. **A** A Grignard reagent will reduce an aldehyde to an alcohol. Further, in this reduction process, there is addition of an alkane to the carbonyl carbon of the aldehyde that will produce a secondary alcohol.

84. **B** The fact that a "nucleophile replaces leaving group" makes for a nucleophilic reaction. Since the reaction is one-step and bimolecular-second order, it cannot be an S_N1 reaction.

85. **D** The IR spectrum indicates a C=O bond (1700–1750 cm^{-1}), and an aldehyde would have two peaks on the NMR spectrum (instead of a single peak for a ketone).

86. **A** The longest carbon chain is 7, making this a heptane. The IUPAC rules dictate the lowest numbering system, so answer C is not correct.

87. **C** 3-chloro-3-methyl pentane is most likely to form a carbocation when Cl^- detaches from the molecule. The carbocation then reacts with methanol.

88. **E** Ozonolysis oxidizes both carbons in a double bond to carbonyl groups. In this case, both carbons are oxidized to aldehydes at the opposite ends of the chain.

89. **D** Both an alcohol and an aldehyde are needed to produce a hemiacetal under acidic conditions.

90. **B** Aldehydes and carboxylic acids must be at a terminal end of a molecule, since either group could not be in the middle of a molecule and still fit the functional group definition.

91. **E** Glutamic acid has two carboxyl groups and one amino group. The *pK*s for most carboxyl groups are between 2 and 5. Since the *pI* lies halfway between the two carboxyl group *pK*s of glutamic acid, the *pI* must be lower than 5.

92. **C** A chain termination step occurs when two radicals come together to form a non-radical product.

93. **A** The chair form is the most stable form for cyclohexanes.

94. **B** The staggered form for Newman structures is the most stable.

95. **C** Compound C is a meso compound, where half of the molecule is structurally identical to the other half. This internal symmetry results in no optical activity.

96. **D** Carbons 2, 3, 4, and 5 are asymmetrical or chiral since they each bond to four different groups.

97. **C** There are two asymmetric carbons, so there are $2^n = 4$ isomers (where *n* is the number of asymmetric carbons).

98. **E** All four bonds in methane are identical and are sp^3 hybridized.

99. **A** Answer A completes the occurrence in what is known as Markovnikov's rule.

100. **D** Both S_N1 and $E1$ mechanisms have all three characteristics.

PERCEPTUAL ABILITY TEST

1. **C** Entry-1, top/bottom, as viewed in the diagram.

2. **B** Entry-2, after object rotated 90 degrees to counterclockwise.

3. **C** Entry-2, after object rotated 180 degrees clockwise.

4. **E** Entry-3, after object rotated 180 degrees clockwise.

5. **E** Entry-3, as seen in diagram, after object rotated 180 degrees clockwise.

6. **A** Entry-2, toward right, as viewed.

7. **A** Entry-2, after object rotated 180 degrees clockwise.

8. **B** Entry-2, after object rotated 90 degrees counterclockwise.

9. **B** Entry-2, after object rotated 180 degrees.

10. **D** Entry-2, after object rotated 90 degrees clockwise.

11. **E** Entry-2, after object rotated 90 degrees. Note object proportions.

12. **C** Entry-3, toward right, as viewed.

13. **A** Entry-2, after object rotated 90 degrees counterclockwise.

14. **D** Entry-3, after object rotated 180 degrees clockwise.

15. **E** Entry-2, after object rotated 180 degrees counterclockwise.

16. **D** Note front view (6 solid lines), side view (4 solid lines), lower hidden.

17. **B** Note end view, 6 total lines (2 hidden) on lower edge, 1 hidden to upper.

18. **A** Note front view, 7 total lines (2 hidden), end view-3 solid lines (2 hidden).

19. **B** Note 6 lines from all views.

20. **B** Note top view, 6 lines (4 hidden), end view, (2 hidden).

21. **C** Note top view, 6 lines (none hidden), front view, hidden box at top.

22. **A** Note front view, 6 lines, end view 5 lines (2 hidden). Note small projection.

23. **D** Front view shows a hidden box open to top (hidden lines). Note proportions.

24. **D** Note top view, 6 lines (2 hidden), 2 hidden lines at lower front to back.

25. **C** Note top and side view positions of 5 lines.

26. **C** Note side view, 3 lines (1 hidden), front view, 4 lines (2 hidden).

27. **D** Note top view, position of 2 solid lines and 2 hidden.

28. **B** Note all proportions and all solid lines from the front view.

29. **A** Note front view, vertical, 3 solid lines.

30. **B** Note front view, 7 lines and 4 hidden.

31. **B** 4 appears smallest (omit A, D), 3 appears smaller than 1 (omit C).

32. **D** 2 appears largest (omit B, C), 2 appears larger than 4 (omit A).

33. **B** 2 appears smallest (omit A, C, D).

34. **A** 4 appears largest (omit B, C, D).

35. **C** 4 appears smallest, 1 appears largest (omit A, B, D).

36. **C** 3 appears smallest, 4 appears largest (omit A, B, D).

37. **B** 4 appears largest (omit A, D), 1 appears smaller than 3 (omit C).

38. **A** 4 appears smallest (omit B, C, D).

39. **D** 1 appears smallest (omit B, C), 3 appears smaller than 4 (omit A).

40. **D** 3 appear largest (omit A, C), 4 appears larger than 1 (omit B).

41. **C** 4 appears smallest (omit A, B), 2 appears smaller than 1 (omit D).

42. **D** 2 appears smallest (omit A, B, C).

43. **B** 4 appears largest (omit A, D), 1 appears smaller than 3 (omit C).

44. **A** 4 appears smallest (omit B), 3 appears largest (omit C, D).

45. **D** 3 appears smaller (omit B, C), 4 appears smaller than 2 (omit A).

46. C 4 folds at final position (omit A, B), 1 unfold identifies E.

47. E 4 folds at final position (omit A, C, D), 1 unfold identifies E.

48. B 4 folds at final position (omit A, D, E), 2 unfolds identifies B.

49. E 1 fold at final position (omit A, B, C, D).

50. D 2 folds at final position (omit A, B, E), 1 unfold identifies D.

51. B 6 folds at final position (omit A, C, D, E).

52. D 4 folds at final position (omit A, C, E), 1 unfold identifies D.

53. D 8 folds at final position (omit A, B, C, E).

54. E 2 folds at final position (omit A, B, C, D).

55. B 4 folds at final position (omit A, D), 1 unfold identifies D.

56. A 8 folds at final position (omit E), 2 unfolds identifies A.

57. C 3 folds at final position (omit A, D), 1 unfold (omit E), 2 unfolds identifies C.

58. C 8 folds at final position (omit B, E), 1 unfold identifies C.

59. C 6 folds at final position (omit A, D, E), 1 unfold identifies C.

60. A 2 folds at final position (omit B, C, E), 1 unfold isolates A.

61. B Note 1 partially hidden cube (3 painted sides).

62. B Note 1 partially hidden cube (3 painted sides).

63. C Note 1 partially hidden cube (3 painted sides).

64. B Note 1 partially hidden cube (3 painted sides).

65. A Note 1 partially hidden cube, 1 fully hidden cube (3 & 2 painted sides).

66. C Note 1 partially hidden cube, 1 fully hidden cube (3 & 2 painted sides).

67. D Note 3 hidden cubes (1, 2, 2 painted sides).

68. B Note 3 hidden cubes (1, 2, 2 painted sides).

69. A Note 3 hidden cubes (1, 2, 2 painted sides).

70. B Note 1 hidden cube, 1 partially hidden cube (3, 3 painted sides).

71. E Note 1 hidden cube, 1 partially hidden cube (3, 3 painted sides).

72. D Note 1 hidden cube, 1 partially hidden cube (3, 3 painted sides).

73. A Note 3 hidden cubes, 1 partially hidden cube (2, 0, 3, 3 painted sides).

74. E Note 3 hidden cubes, 1 partially hidden cube (2, 0, 3, 3 painted sides).

75. D Note 3 hidden cubes, 1 partially hidden cube (2, 0, 3, 3 painted sides).

76. B Focus on the position of the circle and adjacent sides.

77. C Focus on the line and adjacent sides.

78. C Focus on solid square and adjacent sides.

79. D Focus on planes of points and positions of shaded area.

80. **D** Note size and shapes of base and top.

81. **C** Note relative positions and shapes of sides and top.

82. **B** Note relative positions of dots.

83. **B** Note shapes and positions of pointed objects.

84. **A** Note relative sizes of notches on notched sides.

85. **D** Note positions of larger triangular surfaces, note relative positions and sizes.

86. **B** Note relative positions of objects and planes.

87. **A** Note relative positions of all triangles, no rectangles.

88. **A** Focus on relative positions of clear square and shaded areas.

89. **B** Note relative size of angle surface.

90. **A** Focus on shaded areas and relative positions of extensions.

READING COMPREHENSION TEST

1. **E** Paragraph 2, sentence 5.

2. **E** Paragraph 4, sentence 7.

3. **C** Paragraph 3, sentence 4.

4. **A** Paragraph 1, sentence 9.

5. **E** Paragraph 2, sentences 5 and 7.

6. **C** Paragraph 1, sentence 2.

7. **C** Paragraph 5, sentences 7–8.

8. **A** Paragraph 3, sentence 9.

9. **E** Paragraph 1, sentence 5.

10. **D** Paragraph 5, sentence 6.

11. **D** Paragraph 2, sentences 1–2.

12. **B** Paragraph 2, sentence 4.

13. **C** Paragraph 3, sentence 13.

14. **E** Paragraph 5, sentence 6.

15. **B** Paragraph 1, last sentence.

16. **B** Paragraph 4, sentence 12.

17. **A** Paragraph 2, sentence 3.

18. **D** Paragraph 12, last sentence.

19. **C** Paragraph 13, second to last sentence. Answer D is the distracter choice. While it is stated in paragraph 13 that "5 different specimens were tested for each experiment" the wear value was estimated by averaging the 8 readings.

20. **E** Paragraph 7, sentences 2–3.

21. **A** Paragraph 2, sentence 1.

22. **A** Paragraph 15, sentences 1–2.

23. **C** Paragraph 9, sentence 2.

24. **B** Paragraph 12, sentences 3–4.

25. **D** Paragraph 6, sentences 4–6. As stated in the passage, there were 5 different types of composites tested along with 1 type of amalgam, bringing the total number of restorative materials included in the trial to 6.

26. **E** Paragraph 12, sentence 11.

27. **D** Paragraph 14, sentence 1.

28. **C** Paragraph 3, sentence 4.

29. **A** Paragraph 13, sentences 6–8.

30. **B** Paragraph 8, sentence 6.

31. **E** Paragraph 13, sentences 12–14.

32. **D** Paragraph 4. Remember that answers to most questions are explicitly found in the passage. Answer C is a distracter and might be extrapolated from the first sentence of paragraph 13. However, answer D is the best answer.

33. **A** Paragraph 11, sentence 6.

34. **E** Paragraph 1, sentence 2.

35. **B** Paragraph 3, sentences 1–3.

36. **D** Last paragraph, sentence 2.

37. **A** Paragraph 1, sentence 3.

38. **C** Paragraph 4, sentence 5.

39. **E** Last paragraph, sentences 10–11.

40. **D** Paragraph 1, sentences 5–6.

41. **A** Paragraph 4, sentences 8–10.

42. **D** Paragraph 3, sentences 1–2.

43. **E** Paragraph 4, sentence 2.

44. **E** Paragraph 1, sentences 3–4.

45. **C** Paragraph 5, sentences 4–5.

46. **B** Paragraph 2, sentences 3–4.

47. **E** Paragraph 4, sentences 5–8. Right off, we can eliminate answers A and C. Next, focus on the key word "added." The passage states that "the biologically active surface on titanium is a dense protective oxide layer 15 to 50 μm thick [and] forms quickly after processing." There is no information that this

surface is added, which allows us to eliminate answer B. Finally, the passage does not mention whether the sprayed on plasma is biologically active, which allows us to eliminate answer D. This leaves E as the most correct answer.

48. C Paragraph 2, sentence 1.

49. B Paragraph 6, sentence 3. Pay attention to "attached" versus "inserted" as they are not the same thing. "Large collagen fibers are *attached* to the marginal alveolar bone and *insert* into the marginal gingiva," which helps us to eliminate answers A and E. Answers C and D are irrelevant to the question.

50. E Paragraph 3, sentence 9.

QUANTITATIVE REASONING TEST

1. A $(2/3)/3.28 = 2/9.84$ is approximately $1/5$.

2. D Convert equation so that values of x are on one side of the equation. $y(x - 1) = x + 4$; $xy - y = x + 4$; $xy - x = y + 4$; $x(y - 1) = y + 4$; $x = (y + 4)/(y - 1)$.

3. E $(6 + 1/x)^{1/2} = 8$ means $(6 + 1/x) = 64$ so x is $1/58$.

4. D $150 \text{ yd}/12.5 \text{ sec} = 12 \text{ yd/sec} = 36 \text{ ft/sec}$.

5. E Rearranging $4x - 6 > 5x + 4$; $-x > 10$ is equivalent to $x < -10$.

6. B Rearrange $(4 \times 10^{-5}) \times (2 \times 10^{8}) = 8 \times 10^{-5} \times 10^{8} = 8 \times 10^{3}$.

7. A $4L = 40$, so $L = 10$ and $L^2 = 100$.

8. C Substituting -1 for x gives $F(-1) = 4 + 5 = 9$.

9. E If $0.15x = 300$, then $x = 300/0.15 = 2000$.

10. C If $10 - 2y = -4x$, then $-2y = -4x - 10$ and $y = 2x + 5$. So the slope $= 2$.

11. A $\cos t = 1/\sec t$ so $\sec t = 1/\cos t$.

12. A If $L = 1$ originally but increased to 1.5, then $L^2 = 1$ for the original, but $L^2 = (1.5)^2 = 2.25$ after increasing L by 50%. The percent increase is $(2.25 - 1)100 = 125\%$.

13. C Normally $n_0/(n_0 + 1)$ is the largest fraction for the largest n_0. However, $n_1/(n_1 + 2)$ is larger if n_1 is more than twice the largest n_0.

14. B By convention $y^0 = 1$, and x is a constant.

15. D $33.33\pi D$ in./min is approximately 400π in./min$=$ approximately 1200 in./min $= 100$ ft/min.

16. C If $R = (1/6)F$ and $R + 20 = 0.5(F + 20)$. By substituting for R in equation #2, $F = 30$.

17. B Subtract $3x + y = 5$ from $5x + y = 6$ to get $2x = 1$. Hence $x = 1/2$. Substitute x into either equation and $y = 3.5$.

18. D The x and y differences between $(7, 6)$ and $(2, -6)$ are 5 and 12. These lengths represent the sides of a right triangle. Using the Pythagorean theorem ($a^2 + b^2 = c^2$) or knowing about 5-12-13 right triangles, the hypotenuse has a distance of 13.

19. B This is a probability problem where the equation used is $6!/(4!2!) = 15$.

20. A Substituting for x, y, and z, $x + 1y/z = 1 + 1/(2 \times 2) = 5/4$

21. E Output reduction by 20% is akin to a decrease from 5 to 4. To return to a production of 5 from 4 is a 25% increase.

22. A If L is the listing price, $0.5L + 30 = 117$ and $L = 174$. The current price is $57 less than the listing price, so the discount is $57/174 = 32.8\%$.

23. A The average of the 4 numbers is $36/4 = 9$. Variance $= ((2-9)^2 + (8-9)^2 + (10-9)^2 + (16-9)^2)/4 = 25$.

24. B The probability of selecting a red marble first is 3/10, and the probability of selecting another red marble of the remaining 9 marbles is 2/9, so the overall probability is $3/10 \times 2/9 = 1/15$.

25. D $0.05 \times 0.02 \times 0.6 = 0.0006$.

26. C In one minute, one pump can fill 1/10 of the pool independently. The other pump can fill 1/15 of the pool independently in one minute. Together the pumps can fill $1/10 + 1/15 = 1/6$ of the pool in one minute. Hence, both pumps can fill the pool in 6 minutes.

27. C If 70% is passing, Bob can miss 30% of the items. 30 items $\times$ 30% = 9 items.

28. E The hypotenuse of this triangle is 25 ft, and one side is 20 ft. This is a right triangle and the third side can be solved by the Pythagorean theorem ($a^2 + b^2 = c^2$), or knowing that this is a multiple of a 3-4-5 right triangle. In this case the multiple is 5, and the unknown side is $3 \times 5 = 15$ ft.

29. B If 3 people are in both groups, then $7 - 3 = 4$ people are only in Group A, and $8 - 3 = 5$ people are only in Group B. Hence, there are $4 + 5 = 9$ people who are only in a single group.

30. A From equation 1, $x = -4$. Substituting -4 for x in equation 2, $y = -6$.

31. E Using the Pythagorean theorem ($a^2 + b^2 = c^2$), the unknown side is $(144 - 36)^{\frac{1}{2}} = (108)^{\frac{1}{2}} = 6\sqrt{3}$.

32. D To solve this problem, set up a proportion such that $20/4y = 25x/z$, where z is the unknown. In this case $z = 5xy$.

33. B Reset the equation so that $(\frac{1}{4})x = 0.04$ and $x = 0.16$.

34. D Simplify $(a^3/b^2)^{-2} = a^{-6}/b^{-4} = b^4/a^6$.

35. A If distance = rate $\times$ time, and both rate and time are quadrupled, then distance is increased 16-fold.

36. B $1/x + 1/y - 1/2 = 1/4 + 8 - 3/8 = 7\tfrac{7}{8}$.

37. A If David (D) = (5/4) Mark (M) = 2 Susan (S), then S = (5/8)M = 110 lb.

38. E Set the equation so that \$180 = x + (5/4)x, so \$180 = (9/4)x and x = \$80.

39. A A line perpendicular to another line will have a slope that when multiplied by the other slope will equal −1. The perpendicular line to the line with slope = 3 and will be −1/3. With this new line, consider x = 3 and adjust for y so that the line will pass through 3, −1. In this case, when x = 3, y = −1, so no change in the equation is needed.

40. E Convert all fractions to the lowest common denominator, and −21/24 + 4/24 + −18/24 = −35/24 = $-1^{11}/_{24}$.

Standard Score to Raw Score Conversion Chart

Standard Score	QRT	RCT	Biology	General Chemistry	Organic Chemistry	SNS (Total Science)	PAT
30	40	50	–	–	30	100	90
29	39	–	40	–	–	99	89
28	–	49	–	30	29	98	88
27	–	–	–	–	–	97	–
26	38	48	39	–	–	96	87
25	37	47	–	29	28	95	85–86
24	36	–	38	–	–	94	84
23	35	46	–	28	27	92–93	81–83
22	33–34	43–45	37	–	–	89–91	78–80
21	31–32	40–42	35–36	27	26	86–88	74–77
20	29–30	37–39	34	26	25	81–85	70–73
19	27–28	34–36	32–33	24–25	23–24	76–80	68–69
18	24–26	31–33	30–31	22–23	21–22	70–75	59–64
17	22–23	26–30	27–29	20–21	19–20	63–69	52–58
16	19–21	24–25	24–26	18–19	17–18	56–62	46–51
15	16–18	20–23	21–23	16–17	15–16	48–55	39–45
14	14–15	18–19	18–20	13–15	13–14	41–47	32–38
13	11–13	16–17	15–17	11–12	11–12	33–40	26–31
12	9–10	13–15	12–14	9–10	8–10	27–32	21–25
11	7–8	10–12	10–11	7–8	7	21–26	17–20
10	6	9	8–9	6	5–6	17–20	13–16
9	5	7–8	6–7	4–5	4	13–16	10–12
8	4	–	5	3	3	10–12	7–9
7	3	6	4	–	–	7–9	6
6	2	4–5	3	2	2	5–6	4–5
5	–	–	2	–	–	4	3
4	–	3	–	1	1	3	2
3	1	2	1	–	–	2	–
2	–	–	–	–	–	–	–
1	0	1	0	0	0	0–1	0–1

Answer Sheet 1
MODEL EXAMINATION B

Survey of the Natural Sciences

1 Ⓐ Ⓑ Ⓒ Ⓓ Ⓔ	26 Ⓐ Ⓑ Ⓒ Ⓓ Ⓔ	51 Ⓐ Ⓑ Ⓒ Ⓓ Ⓔ	76 Ⓐ Ⓑ Ⓒ Ⓓ Ⓔ
2 Ⓐ Ⓑ Ⓒ Ⓓ Ⓔ	27 Ⓐ Ⓑ Ⓒ Ⓓ Ⓔ	52 Ⓐ Ⓑ Ⓒ Ⓓ Ⓔ	77 Ⓐ Ⓑ Ⓒ Ⓓ Ⓔ
3 Ⓐ Ⓑ Ⓒ Ⓓ Ⓔ	28 Ⓐ Ⓑ Ⓒ Ⓓ Ⓔ	53 Ⓐ Ⓑ Ⓒ Ⓓ Ⓔ	78 Ⓐ Ⓑ Ⓒ Ⓓ Ⓔ
4 Ⓐ Ⓑ Ⓒ Ⓓ Ⓔ	29 Ⓐ Ⓑ Ⓒ Ⓓ Ⓔ	54 Ⓐ Ⓑ Ⓒ Ⓓ Ⓔ	79 Ⓐ Ⓑ Ⓒ Ⓓ Ⓔ
5 Ⓐ Ⓑ Ⓒ Ⓓ Ⓔ	30 Ⓐ Ⓑ Ⓒ Ⓓ Ⓔ	55 Ⓐ Ⓑ Ⓒ Ⓓ Ⓔ	80 Ⓐ Ⓑ Ⓒ Ⓓ Ⓔ
6 Ⓐ Ⓑ Ⓒ Ⓓ Ⓔ	31 Ⓐ Ⓑ Ⓒ Ⓓ Ⓔ	56 Ⓐ Ⓑ Ⓒ Ⓓ Ⓔ	81 Ⓐ Ⓑ Ⓒ Ⓓ Ⓔ
7 Ⓐ Ⓑ Ⓒ Ⓓ Ⓔ	32 Ⓐ Ⓑ Ⓒ Ⓓ Ⓔ	57 Ⓐ Ⓑ Ⓒ Ⓓ Ⓔ	82 Ⓐ Ⓑ Ⓒ Ⓓ Ⓔ
8 Ⓐ Ⓑ Ⓒ Ⓓ Ⓔ	33 Ⓐ Ⓑ Ⓒ Ⓓ Ⓔ	58 Ⓐ Ⓑ Ⓒ Ⓓ Ⓔ	83 Ⓐ Ⓑ Ⓒ Ⓓ Ⓔ
9 Ⓐ Ⓑ Ⓒ Ⓓ Ⓔ	34 Ⓐ Ⓑ Ⓒ Ⓓ Ⓔ	59 Ⓐ Ⓑ Ⓒ Ⓓ Ⓔ	84 Ⓐ Ⓑ Ⓒ Ⓓ Ⓔ
10 Ⓐ Ⓑ Ⓒ Ⓓ Ⓔ	35 Ⓐ Ⓑ Ⓒ Ⓓ Ⓔ	60 Ⓐ Ⓑ Ⓒ Ⓓ Ⓔ	85 Ⓐ Ⓑ Ⓒ Ⓓ Ⓔ
11 Ⓐ Ⓑ Ⓒ Ⓓ Ⓔ	36 Ⓐ Ⓑ Ⓒ Ⓓ Ⓔ	61 Ⓐ Ⓑ Ⓒ Ⓓ Ⓔ	86 Ⓐ Ⓑ Ⓒ Ⓓ Ⓔ
12 Ⓐ Ⓑ Ⓒ Ⓓ Ⓔ	37 Ⓐ Ⓑ Ⓒ Ⓓ Ⓔ	62 Ⓐ Ⓑ Ⓒ Ⓓ Ⓔ	87 Ⓐ Ⓑ Ⓒ Ⓓ Ⓔ
13 Ⓐ Ⓑ Ⓒ Ⓓ Ⓔ	38 Ⓐ Ⓑ Ⓒ Ⓓ Ⓔ	63 Ⓐ Ⓑ Ⓒ Ⓓ Ⓔ	88 Ⓐ Ⓑ Ⓒ Ⓓ Ⓔ
14 Ⓐ Ⓑ Ⓒ Ⓓ Ⓔ	39 Ⓐ Ⓑ Ⓒ Ⓓ Ⓔ	64 Ⓐ Ⓑ Ⓒ Ⓓ Ⓔ	89 Ⓐ Ⓑ Ⓒ Ⓓ Ⓔ
15 Ⓐ Ⓑ Ⓒ Ⓓ Ⓔ	40 Ⓐ Ⓑ Ⓒ Ⓓ Ⓔ	65 Ⓐ Ⓑ Ⓒ Ⓓ Ⓔ	90 Ⓐ Ⓑ Ⓒ Ⓓ Ⓔ
16 Ⓐ Ⓑ Ⓒ Ⓓ Ⓔ	41 Ⓐ Ⓑ Ⓒ Ⓓ Ⓔ	66 Ⓐ Ⓑ Ⓒ Ⓓ Ⓔ	91 Ⓐ Ⓑ Ⓒ Ⓓ Ⓔ
17 Ⓐ Ⓑ Ⓒ Ⓓ Ⓔ	42 Ⓐ Ⓑ Ⓒ Ⓓ Ⓔ	67 Ⓐ Ⓑ Ⓒ Ⓓ Ⓔ	92 Ⓐ Ⓑ Ⓒ Ⓓ Ⓔ
18 Ⓐ Ⓑ Ⓒ Ⓓ Ⓔ	43 Ⓐ Ⓑ Ⓒ Ⓓ Ⓔ	68 Ⓐ Ⓑ Ⓒ Ⓓ Ⓔ	93 Ⓐ Ⓑ Ⓒ Ⓓ Ⓔ
19 Ⓐ Ⓑ Ⓒ Ⓓ Ⓔ	44 Ⓐ Ⓑ Ⓒ Ⓓ Ⓔ	69 Ⓐ Ⓑ Ⓒ Ⓓ Ⓔ	94 Ⓐ Ⓑ Ⓒ Ⓓ Ⓔ
20 Ⓐ Ⓑ Ⓒ Ⓓ Ⓔ	45 Ⓐ Ⓑ Ⓒ Ⓓ Ⓔ	70 Ⓐ Ⓑ Ⓒ Ⓓ Ⓔ	95 Ⓐ Ⓑ Ⓒ Ⓓ Ⓔ
21 Ⓐ Ⓑ Ⓒ Ⓓ Ⓔ	46 Ⓐ Ⓑ Ⓒ Ⓓ Ⓔ	71 Ⓐ Ⓑ Ⓒ Ⓓ Ⓔ	96 Ⓐ Ⓑ Ⓒ Ⓓ Ⓔ
22 Ⓐ Ⓑ Ⓒ Ⓓ Ⓔ	47 Ⓐ Ⓑ Ⓒ Ⓓ Ⓔ	72 Ⓐ Ⓑ Ⓒ Ⓓ Ⓔ	97 Ⓐ Ⓑ Ⓒ Ⓓ Ⓔ
23 Ⓐ Ⓑ Ⓒ Ⓓ Ⓔ	48 Ⓐ Ⓑ Ⓒ Ⓓ Ⓔ	73 Ⓐ Ⓑ Ⓒ Ⓓ Ⓔ	98 Ⓐ Ⓑ Ⓒ Ⓓ Ⓔ
24 Ⓐ Ⓑ Ⓒ Ⓓ Ⓔ	49 Ⓐ Ⓑ Ⓒ Ⓓ Ⓔ	74 Ⓐ Ⓑ Ⓒ Ⓓ Ⓔ	99 Ⓐ Ⓑ Ⓒ Ⓓ Ⓔ
25 Ⓐ Ⓑ Ⓒ Ⓓ Ⓔ	50 Ⓐ Ⓑ Ⓒ Ⓓ Ⓔ	75 Ⓐ Ⓑ Ⓒ Ⓓ Ⓔ	100 Ⓐ Ⓑ Ⓒ Ⓓ Ⓔ

Answer Sheet

Perceptual Ability Test

1 Ⓐ Ⓑ Ⓒ Ⓓ Ⓔ　　24 Ⓐ Ⓑ Ⓒ Ⓓ Ⓔ　　47 Ⓐ Ⓑ Ⓒ Ⓓ Ⓔ　　70 Ⓐ Ⓑ Ⓒ Ⓓ Ⓔ
2 Ⓐ Ⓑ Ⓒ Ⓓ Ⓔ　　25 Ⓐ Ⓑ Ⓒ Ⓓ Ⓔ　　48 Ⓐ Ⓑ Ⓒ Ⓓ Ⓔ　　71 Ⓐ Ⓑ Ⓒ Ⓓ Ⓔ
3 Ⓐ Ⓑ Ⓒ Ⓓ Ⓔ　　26 Ⓐ Ⓑ Ⓒ Ⓓ Ⓔ　　49 Ⓐ Ⓑ Ⓒ Ⓓ Ⓔ　　72 Ⓐ Ⓑ Ⓒ Ⓓ Ⓔ
4 Ⓐ Ⓑ Ⓒ Ⓓ Ⓔ　　27 Ⓐ Ⓑ Ⓒ Ⓓ Ⓔ　　50 Ⓐ Ⓑ Ⓒ Ⓓ Ⓔ　　73 Ⓐ Ⓑ Ⓒ Ⓓ Ⓔ
5 Ⓐ Ⓑ Ⓒ Ⓓ Ⓔ　　28 Ⓐ Ⓑ Ⓒ Ⓓ Ⓔ　　51 Ⓐ Ⓑ Ⓒ Ⓓ Ⓔ　　74 Ⓐ Ⓑ Ⓒ Ⓓ Ⓔ
6 Ⓐ Ⓑ Ⓒ Ⓓ Ⓔ　　29 Ⓐ Ⓑ Ⓒ Ⓓ Ⓔ　　52 Ⓐ Ⓑ Ⓒ Ⓓ Ⓔ　　75 Ⓐ Ⓑ Ⓒ Ⓓ Ⓔ
7 Ⓐ Ⓑ Ⓒ Ⓓ Ⓔ　　30 Ⓐ Ⓑ Ⓒ Ⓓ Ⓔ　　53 Ⓐ Ⓑ Ⓒ Ⓓ Ⓔ　　76 Ⓐ Ⓑ Ⓒ Ⓓ Ⓔ
8 Ⓐ Ⓑ Ⓒ Ⓓ Ⓔ　　31 Ⓐ Ⓑ Ⓒ Ⓓ Ⓔ　　54 Ⓐ Ⓑ Ⓒ Ⓓ Ⓔ　　77 Ⓐ Ⓑ Ⓒ Ⓓ Ⓔ
9 Ⓐ Ⓑ Ⓒ Ⓓ Ⓔ　　32 Ⓐ Ⓑ Ⓒ Ⓓ Ⓔ　　55 Ⓐ Ⓑ Ⓒ Ⓓ Ⓔ　　78 Ⓐ Ⓑ Ⓒ Ⓓ Ⓔ
10 Ⓐ Ⓑ Ⓒ Ⓓ Ⓔ　　33 Ⓐ Ⓑ Ⓒ Ⓓ Ⓔ　　56 Ⓐ Ⓑ Ⓒ Ⓓ Ⓔ　　79 Ⓐ Ⓑ Ⓒ Ⓓ Ⓔ
11 Ⓐ Ⓑ Ⓒ Ⓓ Ⓔ　　34 Ⓐ Ⓑ Ⓒ Ⓓ Ⓔ　　57 Ⓐ Ⓑ Ⓒ Ⓓ Ⓔ　　80 Ⓐ Ⓑ Ⓒ Ⓓ Ⓔ
12 Ⓐ Ⓑ Ⓒ Ⓓ Ⓔ　　35 Ⓐ Ⓑ Ⓒ Ⓓ Ⓔ　　58 Ⓐ Ⓑ Ⓒ Ⓓ Ⓔ　　81 Ⓐ Ⓑ Ⓒ Ⓓ Ⓔ
13 Ⓐ Ⓑ Ⓒ Ⓓ Ⓔ　　36 Ⓐ Ⓑ Ⓒ Ⓓ Ⓔ　　59 Ⓐ Ⓑ Ⓒ Ⓓ Ⓔ　　82 Ⓐ Ⓑ Ⓒ Ⓓ Ⓔ
14 Ⓐ Ⓑ Ⓒ Ⓓ Ⓔ　　37 Ⓐ Ⓑ Ⓒ Ⓓ Ⓔ　　60 Ⓐ Ⓑ Ⓒ Ⓓ Ⓔ　　83 Ⓐ Ⓑ Ⓒ Ⓓ Ⓔ
15 Ⓐ Ⓑ Ⓒ Ⓓ Ⓔ　　38 Ⓐ Ⓑ Ⓒ Ⓓ Ⓔ　　61 Ⓐ Ⓑ Ⓒ Ⓓ Ⓔ　　84 Ⓐ Ⓑ Ⓒ Ⓓ Ⓔ
16 Ⓐ Ⓑ Ⓒ Ⓓ Ⓔ　　39 Ⓐ Ⓑ Ⓒ Ⓓ Ⓔ　　62 Ⓐ Ⓑ Ⓒ Ⓓ Ⓔ　　85 Ⓐ Ⓑ Ⓒ Ⓓ Ⓔ
17 Ⓐ Ⓑ Ⓒ Ⓓ Ⓔ　　40 Ⓐ Ⓑ Ⓒ Ⓓ Ⓔ　　63 Ⓐ Ⓑ Ⓒ Ⓓ Ⓔ　　86 Ⓐ Ⓑ Ⓒ Ⓓ Ⓔ
18 Ⓐ Ⓑ Ⓒ Ⓓ Ⓔ　　41 Ⓐ Ⓑ Ⓒ Ⓓ Ⓔ　　64 Ⓐ Ⓑ Ⓒ Ⓓ Ⓔ　　87 Ⓐ Ⓑ Ⓒ Ⓓ Ⓔ
19 Ⓐ Ⓑ Ⓒ Ⓓ Ⓔ　　42 Ⓐ Ⓑ Ⓒ Ⓓ Ⓔ　　65 Ⓐ Ⓑ Ⓒ Ⓓ Ⓔ　　88 Ⓐ Ⓑ Ⓒ Ⓓ Ⓔ
20 Ⓐ Ⓑ Ⓒ Ⓓ Ⓔ　　43 Ⓐ Ⓑ Ⓒ Ⓓ Ⓔ　　66 Ⓐ Ⓑ Ⓒ Ⓓ Ⓔ　　89 Ⓐ Ⓑ Ⓒ Ⓓ Ⓔ
21 Ⓐ Ⓑ Ⓒ Ⓓ Ⓔ　　44 Ⓐ Ⓑ Ⓒ Ⓓ Ⓔ　　67 Ⓐ Ⓑ Ⓒ Ⓓ Ⓔ　　90 Ⓐ Ⓑ Ⓒ Ⓓ Ⓔ
22 Ⓐ Ⓑ Ⓒ Ⓓ Ⓔ　　45 Ⓐ Ⓑ Ⓒ Ⓓ Ⓔ　　68 Ⓐ Ⓑ Ⓒ Ⓓ Ⓔ
23 Ⓐ Ⓑ Ⓒ Ⓓ Ⓔ　　46 Ⓐ Ⓑ Ⓒ Ⓓ Ⓔ　　69 Ⓐ Ⓑ Ⓒ Ⓓ Ⓔ

Answer Sheet 2

MODEL EXAMINATION B

Reading Comprehension Test

1 Ⓐ Ⓑ Ⓒ Ⓓ Ⓔ   14 Ⓐ Ⓑ Ⓒ Ⓓ Ⓔ   27 Ⓐ Ⓑ Ⓒ Ⓓ Ⓔ   40 Ⓐ Ⓑ Ⓒ Ⓓ Ⓔ
2 Ⓐ Ⓑ Ⓒ Ⓓ Ⓔ   15 Ⓐ Ⓑ Ⓒ Ⓓ Ⓔ   28 Ⓐ Ⓑ Ⓒ Ⓓ Ⓔ   41 Ⓐ Ⓑ Ⓒ Ⓓ Ⓔ
3 Ⓐ Ⓑ Ⓒ Ⓓ Ⓔ   16 Ⓐ Ⓑ Ⓒ Ⓓ Ⓔ   29 Ⓐ Ⓑ Ⓒ Ⓓ Ⓔ   42 Ⓐ Ⓑ Ⓒ Ⓓ Ⓔ
4 Ⓐ Ⓑ Ⓒ Ⓓ Ⓔ   17 Ⓐ Ⓑ Ⓒ Ⓓ Ⓔ   30 Ⓐ Ⓑ Ⓒ Ⓓ Ⓔ   43 Ⓐ Ⓑ Ⓒ Ⓓ Ⓔ
5 Ⓐ Ⓑ Ⓒ Ⓓ Ⓔ   18 Ⓐ Ⓑ Ⓒ Ⓓ Ⓔ   31 Ⓐ Ⓑ Ⓒ Ⓓ Ⓔ   44 Ⓐ Ⓑ Ⓒ Ⓓ Ⓔ
6 Ⓐ Ⓑ Ⓒ Ⓓ Ⓔ   19 Ⓐ Ⓑ Ⓒ Ⓓ Ⓔ   32 Ⓐ Ⓑ Ⓒ Ⓓ Ⓔ   45 Ⓐ Ⓑ Ⓒ Ⓓ Ⓔ
7 Ⓐ Ⓑ Ⓒ Ⓓ Ⓔ   20 Ⓐ Ⓑ Ⓒ Ⓓ Ⓔ   33 Ⓐ Ⓑ Ⓒ Ⓓ Ⓔ   46 Ⓐ Ⓑ Ⓒ Ⓓ Ⓔ
8 Ⓐ Ⓑ Ⓒ Ⓓ Ⓔ   21 Ⓐ Ⓑ Ⓒ Ⓓ Ⓔ   34 Ⓐ Ⓑ Ⓒ Ⓓ Ⓔ   47 Ⓐ Ⓑ Ⓒ Ⓓ Ⓔ
9 Ⓐ Ⓑ Ⓒ Ⓓ Ⓔ   22 Ⓐ Ⓑ Ⓒ Ⓓ Ⓔ   35 Ⓐ Ⓑ Ⓒ Ⓓ Ⓔ   48 Ⓐ Ⓑ Ⓒ Ⓓ Ⓔ
10 Ⓐ Ⓑ Ⓒ Ⓓ Ⓔ   23 Ⓐ Ⓑ Ⓒ Ⓓ Ⓔ   36 Ⓐ Ⓑ Ⓒ Ⓓ Ⓔ   49 Ⓐ Ⓑ Ⓒ Ⓓ Ⓔ
11 Ⓐ Ⓑ Ⓒ Ⓓ Ⓔ   24 Ⓐ Ⓑ Ⓒ Ⓓ Ⓔ   37 Ⓐ Ⓑ Ⓒ Ⓓ Ⓔ   50 Ⓐ Ⓑ Ⓒ Ⓓ Ⓔ
12 Ⓐ Ⓑ Ⓒ Ⓓ Ⓔ   25 Ⓐ Ⓑ Ⓒ Ⓓ Ⓔ   38 Ⓐ Ⓑ Ⓒ Ⓓ Ⓔ
13 Ⓐ Ⓑ Ⓒ Ⓓ Ⓔ   26 Ⓐ Ⓑ Ⓒ Ⓓ Ⓔ   39 Ⓐ Ⓑ Ⓒ Ⓓ Ⓔ

Quantitative Reasoning Test

1 Ⓐ Ⓑ Ⓒ Ⓓ Ⓔ   11 Ⓐ Ⓑ Ⓒ Ⓓ Ⓔ   21 Ⓐ Ⓑ Ⓒ Ⓓ Ⓔ   31 Ⓐ Ⓑ Ⓒ Ⓓ Ⓔ
2 Ⓐ Ⓑ Ⓒ Ⓓ Ⓔ   12 Ⓐ Ⓑ Ⓒ Ⓓ Ⓔ   22 Ⓐ Ⓑ Ⓒ Ⓓ Ⓔ   32 Ⓐ Ⓑ Ⓒ Ⓓ Ⓔ
3 Ⓐ Ⓑ Ⓒ Ⓓ Ⓔ   13 Ⓐ Ⓑ Ⓒ Ⓓ Ⓔ   23 Ⓐ Ⓑ Ⓒ Ⓓ Ⓔ   33 Ⓐ Ⓑ Ⓒ Ⓓ Ⓔ
4 Ⓐ Ⓑ Ⓒ Ⓓ Ⓔ   14 Ⓐ Ⓑ Ⓒ Ⓓ Ⓔ   24 Ⓐ Ⓑ Ⓒ Ⓓ Ⓔ   34 Ⓐ Ⓑ Ⓒ Ⓓ Ⓕ
5 Ⓐ Ⓑ Ⓒ Ⓓ Ⓔ   15 Ⓐ Ⓑ Ⓒ Ⓓ Ⓔ   25 Ⓐ Ⓑ Ⓒ Ⓓ Ⓔ   35 Ⓐ Ⓑ Ⓒ Ⓓ Ⓔ
6 Ⓐ Ⓑ Ⓒ Ⓓ Ⓔ   16 Ⓐ Ⓑ Ⓒ Ⓓ Ⓔ   26 Ⓐ Ⓑ Ⓒ Ⓓ Ⓔ   36 Ⓑ Ⓑ Ⓒ Ⓓ Ⓔ
7 Ⓐ Ⓑ Ⓒ Ⓓ Ⓔ   17 Ⓐ Ⓑ Ⓒ Ⓓ Ⓔ   27 Ⓐ Ⓑ Ⓒ Ⓓ Ⓔ   37 Ⓐ Ⓑ Ⓒ Ⓓ Ⓔ
8 Ⓐ Ⓑ Ⓒ Ⓓ Ⓔ   18 Ⓐ Ⓑ Ⓒ Ⓓ Ⓔ   28 Ⓐ Ⓑ Ⓒ Ⓓ Ⓔ   38 Ⓐ Ⓑ Ⓒ Ⓓ Ⓔ
9 Ⓐ Ⓑ Ⓒ Ⓓ Ⓔ   19 Ⓐ Ⓑ Ⓒ Ⓓ Ⓔ   29 Ⓐ Ⓑ Ⓒ Ⓓ Ⓔ   39 Ⓐ Ⓑ Ⓒ Ⓓ Ⓔ
10 Ⓐ Ⓑ Ⓒ Ⓓ Ⓔ   20 Ⓐ Ⓑ Ⓒ Ⓓ Ⓔ   30 Ⓐ Ⓑ Ⓒ Ⓓ Ⓔ   40 Ⓐ Ⓑ Ⓒ Ⓓ Ⓔ

Model Examination B

 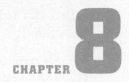

SURVEY OF THE NATURAL SCIENCES   TIME LIMIT: 90 MINUTES

The following items are questions or incomplete statements. Read each item carefully, then choose the best answer.

1. If 120 amino acids form a protein, the gene for that protein contains _____ nucleotides.

    A. 60
    B. 40
    C. 240
    D. 360
    E. 120

2. In the process of respiration, oxygen

    A. combines with carbon to form CO2
    B. produces energy in the form of ATP as it passes through the respiratory chain
    C. acts as the final electron acceptor
    D. is a cofactor for glycolytic enzymes
    E. bonds to lactic acid to form pyruvic acid

3. Mitosis and meiosis share several characteristics. Which of the following processes occurs in mitosis but does NOT occur in meiosis?

    A. Genetically identical daughter cells are produced.
    B. Spindle fibers form.
    C. Centromeres divide.
    D. Sex chromosomes segregate.
    E. Homologous pairs come together to form tetrads.

4. Organisms that obtain energy from light are

    A. heterotrophic
    B. lytic
    C. hydrophilic
    D. heliotrophic
    E. autotrophic

5. In association with reproductive organs, the follicle

    A. secretes androgen to the testes
    B. is a sac that protects and nourishes the egg
    C. fuses to the yolk sac to form the umbilical cord
    D. later becomes the digestive tract
    E. has the same function as the zygote

6. The process of fermentation

    A. converts ethanol into fructose
    B. yields glucose as an end product
    C. occurs only if oxygen is present
    D. takes place in the endoplasmic reticulum
    E. is less efficient than aerobic respiration in producing energy

7. Which of the following organelles is absent from fungi?

   A. Secretory vesicles
   B. Mitochondria
   C. Chloroplasts
   D. Golgi bodies
   E. Ribosomes

8. The liver has several functions. One of those functions is to

   A. convert ammonia into urea
   B. remove salts from filtrates
   C. return filtered blood to the circulatory system
   D. secrete antidiuretic hormone
   E. return sugars and amino acids to the blood

9. In the testes, the _____ respond to the leutinizing hormone by producing steroids.

   A. Gametes
   B. Germ cells
   C. Interstitial cells
   D. Tubules
   E. Endometrial cells

10. Which of the following terms best describes a bacteriophage?

    A. Prokaryote
    B. Virus
    C. Organelle
    D. Bacterium
    E. Eukaryote

11. In the absence of oxygen, aerobic organisms obtain their energy from

    A. oxidative phosphorylation
    B. the Krebs cycle
    C. glycolysis
    D. respiration
    E. photosynthesis

12. Eukaryotic cell membranes

    A. invaginate to form cristae, on which are arranged the electron transport systems
    B. are single layers of molecules approximately 75 angstroms in thickness
    C. are composed exclusively of phospholipids
    D. form rigid layers that prevent the cell from expanding
    E. are selectively permeable

13. Research into a new drug reveals that one of its side effects is to destroy the ectodermal germ layer of developing embryos. If this drug were administered to a pregnant woman, which of the following would be absent in the fetus?

    A. Spinal cord
    B. Femur
    C. Stomach
    D. Heart
    E. Iliac vein

14. _____ synthesizes complementary nucleic acid strands in a process called transcription.

    A. DNA polymerase
    B. DNA ligase
    C. RNA polymerase
    D. Helicase
    E. Toposiomerase

15. _____ phosphorylation occurs in glycolysis, while _____ phosphorylation occurs in the electron transport chain.

    A. Oxidative, substrate-level
    B. Oxidative, photo
    C. Photo, substrate-level
    D. Substrate-level, photo
    E. Substrate-level, oxidative

16. Crossing over occurs in which of the following phases of meiosis:

    I. Prophase I
    II. Metaphase I
    III. Prophase II

    A. I
    B. II
    C. III
    D. I and II
    E. I and III

17. Which of the following organelles is enclosed by a single membrane?

    A. Peroxisome
    B. Secretory vesicle
    C. Nucleus
    D. Centriole
    E. Chloroplast

18. Disulfide bridges that help hold the three-dimensional shape of a protein are part of its

    A. primary structure
    B. secondary structure
    C. tertiary structure
    D. quaternary structure
    E. overall structure

19. A population of rabbits is in Hardy-Weinberg equilibrium, with 9 percent of the population homozygous recessive for the albino trait. The percent of the population that is heterozygous for the albino trait is

    A. 3
    B. 42
    C. 18
    D. 27
    E. 36

20. Corals are in the same phylum as

    A. sponges
    B. giant squid
    C. starfish
    D. jellyfish
    E. tapeworms

21. Darwin's theory of natural selection states that evolution "selects" for traits that

    A. increase an organism's ability to survive in an environment
    B. decrease the number of deleterious genes
    C. increase the number of viable offspring for an individual
    D. result in longer life spans
    E. lead to improved social behavior

22. The term *saltatory conduction* describes

    A. the process by which neurotransmitters are inhibited in a chemical synapse
    B. the transmission of impulses between the dendrites of a gap junction
    C. changes in the sodium concentrations of the axon
    D. the processing of information by a nerve cell
    E. the propagation of an impulse along an insulated axon

23. Albinism is inherited as an autosomal recessive trait. If a man and a woman are both heterozygous for albinism, what is the probability that their child will also be heterozygous for this trait?

    A. 0
    B. .25
    C. .5
    D. .75
    E. 1

24. During the process of neurulation,

    A. the ectoderm begins to develop into the notochord
    B. the endoderm begins to develop into the notochord
    C. the mesoderm begins to develop into the notochord
    D. the neural tube opens and begins to develop into the spinal column
    E. the third and fourth cleavages take place

25. Within a eukaryotic cell, the site for chemical modification of proteins is the

    A. secretory vesicles
    B. Golgi apparatus
    C. mitochondria
    D. ribosomes
    E. nucleolus

26. Cholesterol is an example of

    A. a steroid
    B. a carbohydrate
    C. a polysaccharide
    D. an amino acid
    E. a protein

27. The following statements describe different aspects of a cell's cytoskeleton. Which statement is FALSE?

    A. The cytoskeleton is associated with three different classes of filaments.
    B. Cilia and flagella terminate in structures known as basal bodies.
    C. Intermediate filaments are about 10 nm in diameter.
    D. Microtubules are composed of two types of lipids.
    E. One function of the cytoskeleton is to maintain the shape of the cell.

28. Which of the following does (do) NOT belong to the peripheral nervous system?

    A. Afferent neurons
    B. Efferent neurons
    C. Optic nerve
    D. Spinal cord
    E. Olfactory bulbs

29. During a menstrual cycle, hormone levels vary according to a programmed sequence. Which of the following describes the correct sequence of events?

    A. Increase in FSH, decrease in LH, increase in estrogen
    B. Increase in estrogen, increase in FSH, decrease in progesterone
    C. Decrease in LH, increase in FSH, increase in progesterone
    D. Increase in FSH, increase in estrogen, decrease in progesterone
    E. Increase in estrogen, increase in FSH, increase in progesterone

30. If an individual is heterozygous for five independently assorting genes, how many genetically different gametes can he produce?

    A. 5
    B. 10
    C. 50
    D. 5^2
    E. 2^5

31. Measles, herpes, and smallpox are caused by the activity of viruses. Yet the debate continues as to whether viruses are even alive. Which statement best supports the argument that viruses are NOT alive?

    A. Viruses are not eukaryotic cells.
    B. Viruses are primitive and extremely small.
    C. Viruses need other cells in order to reproduce.
    D. Viruses are parasitic.
    E. Viruses can lie dormant for long periods of time.

32. Sucrose is a

    A. subunit of starch
    B. subunit of cellulose
    C. trisaccaharide of fructose, galactose, and glucose
    D. disaccharide of glucose and fructose
    E. sugar produced in glycolysis

33. Muscle contractions are triggered by

   A. calcium
   B. phosphorus
   C. sodium
   D. potassium
   E. myofibrils

34. Which of the following is NOT consistent with a humoral immune response?

   A. B-cell production of antibodies
   B. T-cell destruction of foreign cells
   C. Decrease in B-cell production after infection is controlled
   D. Storage of memory cells in the spleen
   E. Removed by phagocytic cells of complexes of antigen

35. Which of the following glands has both an endocrine and an exocrine function?

   A. Adrenal
   B. Pancreas
   C. Pituitary
   D. Pineal
   E. Thyroid

36. In which of the following phyla are only bilaterally symmetrical animals found?

   A. Chordata
   B. Echinodermata
   C. Mollusca
   D. Ctenophora
   E. Platyhelminthes

37. In an experiment to better understand bird speciation, a researcher placed a mesh fence in the middle of a large bird cage. The fence prevented birds on one side from mating with birds on the other side. This experiment simulates

   A. parapatric speciation
   B. genetic drift
   C. sympatric speciation
   D. allopatric speciation
   E. Hardy-Weinburg equilibrium

38. On a remote island, a new spider species is discovered. The spider strongly resembles a well-known poisonous species, but is harmless. The spider is an example of

   A. mutualism
   B. parasitism
   C. Batesian mimicry
   D. Mullerian mimicry
   E. intraspecific competition

39. If a segment of a DNA base sequence is CAT, what is the complementary portion of mRNA?

   A. CAT
   B. TAC
   C. ATC
   D. GTU
   E. GUA

40. Which of the following characteristics does NOT describe an *r*-selected species?

   A. Occurs more often in stable environments
   B. Has a high birth rate
   C. Has a short life span
   D. Tends to stay below carrying capacity
   E. Maximizes population growth

41. In which of the following compounds is the oxidation number of sulfur equal to +2?

   A. H_2S
   B. S_8
   C. SCl_2
   D. Na_2SO_3
   E. SO_4^{2-}

42. Which of the following molecular species is trigonal pyramidal?

   A. SO_2
   B. BF_3
   C. CH_4
   D. NH_3
   E. HCO_3

43. In the reaction below, which compound is acting like a conjugate acid?

    $$H_2C_2O_4(aq) + H_2O(l) \leftrightarrow HC_2O_4^-(aq) + H_3O^+(aq)$$

    A. $H_2C_2O_4$
    B. H_2O
    C. $HC_2O_4^-$
    D. H_3O^+
    E. None of the above

44. The numbers of protons and neutrons, respectively, in $_8^{17}O^{2-}$ are

    A. 8 and 10
    B. 9 and 8
    C. 8 and 9
    D. 17 and 8
    E. 8 and 17

45. In which of the following species does phosphorus exhibit its highest oxidation number?

    A. P_2O_5
    B. PH_3
    C. H_3PO_3
    D. P_4
    E. PCL_3

46. In the nuclear reaction below, what is X?

    $$X + proton \rightarrow {}^{22}Mg + neutron$$

    A. ^{21}Ne
    B. ^{23}Mg
    C. ^{21}Mg
    D. ^{22}Na
    E. ^{23}Na

47. Precipitation of a solution will occur when

    A. ion product $> K_{sp}$
    B. ion product $= K_{sp}$
    C. ion product $< K_{sp}$
    D. ion product will always cause precipitation.
    E. ion product will never cause precipitation.

48. If ΔG has a negative value, the reaction

    A. is at equilibrium
    B. is nonspontaneous, but its reverse reaction is spontaneous
    C. is spontaneous and forward
    D. is exothermic
    E. is endothermic

49. Which of the following types of bonds is characterized by being brittle, a poor conductor of electricity, and held together by electrostatic forces?

    A. Metallic
    B. Ionic
    C. Covalent
    D. Molecular
    E. Hydrogen

50. The point of a phase diagram at which the gas and liquid states are indistinguishable is known as the

    A. critical point
    B. triple point
    C. equivalence point
    D. titration point
    E. point of neutrality

51. In an experiment 25 g of HCl (g) is dissolved in water to make 100 mL of an acidic solution. Assuming that the acid completely ionized, what is the pH of the solution?

    A. $-\log[25/(0.1 \times 2)]$
    B. $-\log[25 \times 0.1/36]$
    C. $-\log[25/(0.1 \times 36)]$
    D. $-\log[36/(0.1 \times 25)]$
    E. $-\log[0.1/25]$

52. If a balloon is filled with gas until the pressure equals 43 atmospheres at 200 K, what temperature will have to be reached for the balloon pressure to reach 55 atmospheres?

    A. 256 K
    B. 1,200 K
    C. 131 K
    D. 2,500 K
    E. 1,813 K

53. In which two compounds does sulfur have the same oxidation state?

    A. SO_4 and Na_2SO_4
    B. SO_2 and Na_2SO_4
    C. SO_3 and H_2SO_4
    D. SO_2 and SO_3
    E. SO_4 and H_2S_2

54. What is the percent by mass of bromine in BrO_4^-?

    A. 39.5
    B. 24.8
    C. 49.3
    D. 55.5
    E. 16.3

55. What mass of styrene (molar mass = 104.1) will contain 4.5×10^{20} molecules of styrene?

    A. 0.00778 g
    B. 7.78×10^{-4} g
    C. 7.78×10^3 g
    D. 7.78×10^{-2} g
    E. 7.78×10^4 g

56. As carbon dioxide undergoes sublimation, which physical transformation occurs?

    A. Gas to solid
    B. Solid to gas
    C. Solid to liquid
    D. Solid to liquid to gas
    E. Gas to liquid

57. Which of the following compounds consistently have the highest melting points?

    A. Dipoles
    B. Alkanes
    C. Molecular crystals
    D. Salts
    E. Metals

58. Which of the following is NOT a correct chemical formula?

    A. $SrBr_2$
    B. CaO_2
    C. Mg_3N_2
    D. Na_2S
    E. AlI_3

59. When ammonium oxalate, $(NH_4)_2C_2O_4$, is dissolved in water, the ions formed are

    A. $2N^{3-}(aq) + 8H^+(aq) + 2C^{4+}(aq) + 4O^{2-}(aq)$
    B. $(NH_4)^{2+}(aq) + C_2O_4^{2-}(aq)$
    C. $2NH_4^+(aq) + C_2O_4^{2-}(aq)$
    D. $NH_4^{2+}(aq) + C_2O_4^{2-}(aq)$
    E. $2NH_4^+(aq) + 2CO_2^-(aq)$

60. A solution of KNO_3 is known to have a 0.564 molar concentration. To calculate the concentration of this solution in terms of molarity, which of the following must be specified?

    A. The density of the solution
    B. The volume of the solution
    C. The temperature of the solution
    D. The solubility product of KNO_3
    E. The K_a of nitric acid

61. A 10.0-g sample of ethane, C_2H_6, is burned in an enclosed vessel with 40.0 grams of oxygen. Which of the following best describes the mixture when the reaction is complete?

    A. The mass of the system is 50.0 g.
    B. The limiting reactant is C_2H_6.
    C. The theoretical yield of CO_2 is 29.33 g.
    D. 2.67 g of oxygen is left over.
    E. All of the above statements are correct.

62. Which of the following sets of quantum numbers is IMPOSSIBLE?

A. 4, 3, 1, +1/2
B. 3, 2, −2, −1/2
C. 5, 0, 0, −1/2
D. 2, 2, −1, +1/2
E. 3, 2, 0, +1/2

63. A compound consisting of carbon, hydrogen, and oxygen is known by quantitative analysis to have 38.71 % carbon and 9.68 % hydrogen. What is the empirical formula of this compound?

A. CHO
B. CH_2O
C. CH_3O
D. $C_2H_6O_2$
E. CH_3

64. A substance that acts as both a Brönsted acid and a Brönsted base in an aqueous solution is

A. $HClO$
B. H_2SO_4
C. PO_4^{3-}
D. HSO_3^-
E. ClO_4^-

65. The percent composition, by weight, of nitrogen in the compound $(NH_4)_2Cr_2O_7$ is

A. $\left[\dfrac{14}{[14 + 4(1) + 2(52) + 7(16)]} \right] \times 100$

B. $\left[\dfrac{(2)14}{[2(14) + 8(1) + 2(52) + 7(16)]} \right] \times 100$

C. $\left[\dfrac{14}{(14 + 1 + 52 + 16)} \right] \times 100$

D. $\left[\dfrac{(2)14}{[2(14) + 4(1) + 2(52) + 7(16)]} \right] \times 100$

E. $\left[\dfrac{(2)14}{[8(1) + 2(52) + 7(16)]} \right] \times 100$

66. Which reaction has the most positive value of ΔS?

A. $2NO_2\ (g) \rightarrow N_2O_4\ (l)$
B. $2NO_2\ (g) \rightarrow N_2O_4\ (g)$
C. $N_2O_4\ (l) \rightarrow 2NO_2\ (g)$
D. $N_2O_4\ (g) \rightarrow 2NO_2\ (g)$
E. $N_2O_4\ (l) \rightarrow 2NO_2\ (l)$

67. Which is the correct set of coefficients to balance the equation for the oxidation of ammonia?

$$NH_3 + O_2 \rightarrow NO + H_2O$$

A. 2, 3, 2, 3
B. 3, 2, 3, 2
C. 4, 5, 4, 6
D. 2, 2, 2, 3
E. 4, 6, 4, 6

68. A liter of solution contains 0.00001 mole of HCl. What is the pH of this solution?

A. 1.0
B. 4.0
C. −4.0
D. −5.0
E. 5.0

69. Which trend in the halogen family occurs with increasing atomic number?

A. Decreasing ionic radius
B. Increasing first ionization potential
C. Decreasing electronegativity
D. Decreasing covalent radius
E. Decreasing melting points

70. How many liters of 5.0 molar ethyl alcohol (C_2H_5OH) can be prepared by dissolving 460 g of ethyl alcohol in water? (Molecular weight of ethyl alcohol = 46)

A. 1.0
B. 1.5
C. 2.0
D. 2.5
E. 5.0

71. In a double-bonded carbon atom

    A. hybridization between one *s* orbital and one *p* orbital occurs

    B. hybridization between one *s* orbital and two *p* orbitals occurs

    C. hybridization between one *s* orbital and three *p* orbitals occurs

    D. hybridization between two *s* orbitals and two *p* orbitals occurs

    E. no hybridization occurs

72. Given the structures of D-mannose and D-galactose below, what is the most specific relationship between the two molecules?

CHO   CHO
HO — H   H — H
HO — H   HO — H
H — OH   HO — H
H — OH   H — OH
CH_2OH CH_2OH

    D-mannose   D-galactose

    A. Structural isomers

    B. Conformers

    C. Epimers

    D. Enantiomers

    E. Diastereomers

73. What is the correct assignment of bond angles in the structure below?

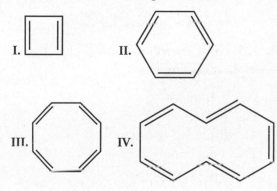

    A. $a = 90°, b = 90°$

    B. $a = 180°, b = 109.5°$

    C. $a = 120°, b = 120°$

    D. $a = 180°, b = 120°$

    E. $a = 180°, b = 180°$

74. The most acidic hydrogen in the following compound is

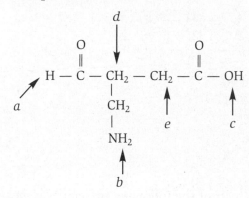

    A. *a*

    B. *b*

    C. *c*

    D. *d*

    E. *e*

75. Which of the following is aromatic?

    A. II only

    B. II, III, and IV only

    C. I, II, and IV only

    D. II and IV only

    E. All of the above

76. How many chiral centers are present in isoleucine below?

$$H_3C - CH - CH_2CH_3$$
$$H_2N - CH - COOH$$

A. 0
B. 1
C. 2
D. 3
E. 4

77. Which of the following molecules is most likely to be formed in abundance by a free-radical bromination reaction?

A. CH_3Br
B. $BrC(CH_3)_3$
C. $CH_3-CHBr-CH_2$
D. $CH_3-(CH_2)_8-CH_2Br$
E. None of these substances can be created by this reaction.

78. Which of the following will have the highest boiling point?

A. 1-butanol
B. pentane
C. 3-methyl-1-butanol
D. 1-pentanol
E. 2-methyl-propane

79. How many peaks does CH_4 have in its ^1H NMR spectrum?

A. 1
B. 4
C. 12
D. 16
E. The number of peaks depends on the phase of methane in the sample.

80. In the reaction

$$C_2H_5OH + CH_3O^- \rightleftharpoons C_2H_5O^- + CH_3OH$$

the Brönsted-Lowry bases are

A. C_2H_5OH and CH_3O^-
B. $C_2H_5O^-$ and CH_3OH
C. C_2H_5OH and CH_3OH
D. $C_2H_5O^-$ and CH_3O^-
E. None of the above

81. Which reaction below is a possible initiation step in the free-radical chlorination of $CH_3CH_2CH_2CH_3$ by Cl_2?

A. $Cl\bullet + CH_3CH_2CH_2CH_3 \rightarrow$ $HCl + CH_3CH_2CH\bullet CH_3$
B. $Cl_2 \rightarrow 2Cl\bullet$
C. $Cl\bullet + CH_3CH_2CH_2CH_2\bullet \rightarrow$ $CH_3CH_2CH_2CH_2Cl$
D. $Cl\bullet + CH_3CH_2CH_2CH_3 \rightarrow$ $CH_3CH_2CH_2CH_2\bullet + HCl$
E. $Cl_2 + CH_3CH_2CH\bullet CH_3 \rightarrow$ $CH_3CH_2CHClCH_3 + Cl\bullet$

82. Which of the following alkyl halides would you expect to be most reactive by an S_N2 mechanism?

A.
$$CH_3$$
$$CH_3 - C - CH_2 - Br$$
$$CH_3$$

B. $CH_3 - CH - CH_2 - CH_3$
$$Br$$

C. $CH_3 - CH_2 - CH_2 - CH_2 - Br$

D.
$$CH_3$$
$$CH_3 - C - Br$$
$$CH_3$$

E. $CH_3 - CH - CH - CH_3$
$$CH_3 \quad I$$

83. Which of the following compounds has the highest boiling point?

A. CH_3CH_3

B.

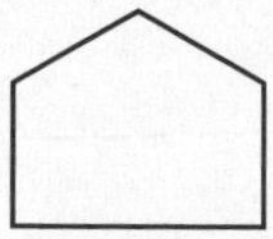

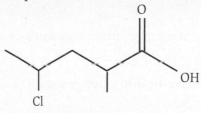

C. $CH_3CH_2CH_2CH_3$
D. $CH_3CH_2CH(CH_3)CH_3$
E. $CH_3CH_2CH_2CH_2CH_3$

84. Which of the following molecules is the LEAST soluble in water?

A. $CH_3 — CH_2 — CH_2 — \overset{\overset{O}{\|}}{C} — H$

B. $CH_3 — CH_2 — CH_2 — CH_2 — NH_2$

C. $CH_3 — CH_2 — O — CH_2 — CH_3$

D. $CH_3 — \overset{\overset{O}{\|}}{C} — CH_3$

E. $CH_3 — CH_2 — CH_2 — CH_3$

85. What is the principal product of the following reaction?

$$CH_3 — CH = CH_2 + HCl \longrightarrow ?$$

A. $CH_3 — \underset{\underset{Cl}{|}}{CH} — \underset{\underset{H}{|}}{CH_2}$

B. $CH_3 — \underset{\underset{H}{|}}{CH} — \underset{\underset{Cl}{|}}{CH_2}$

C. $CH_3 — CH = C\overset{H}{\underset{Cl}{\diagdown}}$

D. $CH_3 — C\,(Cl) = CH_2$

E. $CH_2 = Br = CH_2$

86. Which mechanism is used in the degradation of 2-pentanol to form 1-pentene and 2-pentene?

A. $S_N 1$
B. $S_N 2$
C. E1
D. E2
E. Oxidation

87. Which of the following carbocations is (are) the most stable?

A. R_2HC^+
B. R_3C^+
C. H_3C^+
D. RH_2C^+
E. B and C are equally stable

88. A Grignard reagent (RMgX) functions in a Grignard reaction as a

A. weak nucleophile.
B. strong nucleophile.
C. weak electrophile.
D. strong electrophile.
E. weak nucleophile or a weak electrophile.

89. What is the IUPAC name of the following compound?

A. 4-chloro-2-methylpentanoic acid
B. 5-chlorohexanoic acid
C. 2-chloro-4-methylpentanoic acid
D. 4-chloro-2-methyl-1-carbonyl-1-pentanol
E. None of the above

90. Which of the following alkyl halides is most likely to have formed by an S_N1 mechanism?

   A. 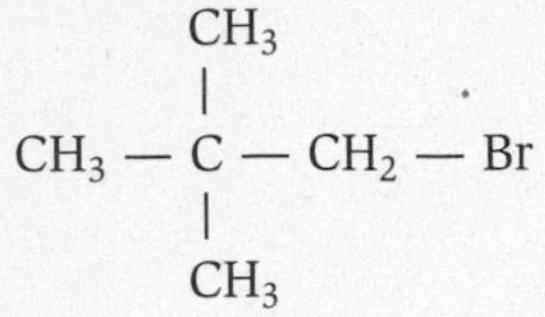
$$CH_3 - \underset{\underset{CH_3}{|}}{\overset{\overset{CH_3}{|}}{C}} - CH_2 - Br$$

   B. 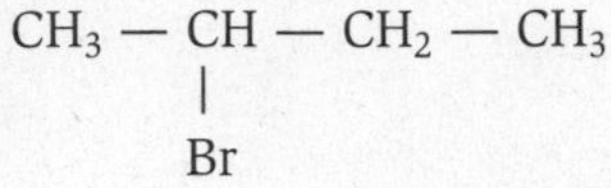
$$CH_3 - \underset{\underset{Br}{|}}{CH} - CH_2 - CH_3$$

   C. $CH_3 - CH_2 - CH_2 - CH_2 - Br$

   D. 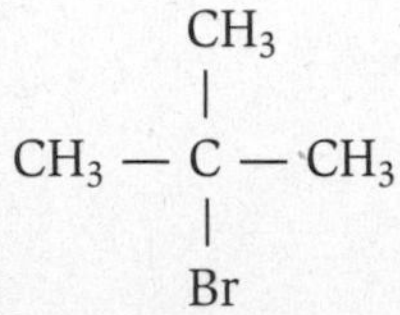
$$CH_3 - \underset{\underset{Br}{|}}{\overset{\overset{CH_3}{|}}{C}} - CH_3$$

   E. 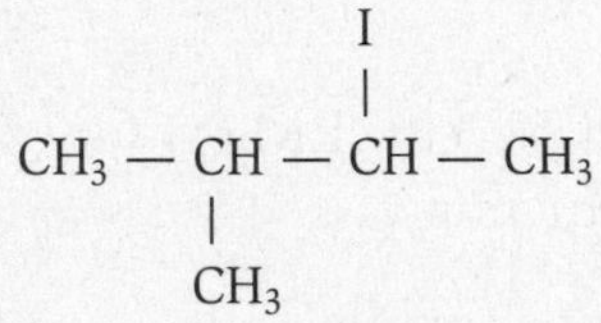
$$CH_3 - CH - \underset{\underset{CH_3}{|}}{\overset{\overset{I}{|}}{CH}} - CH_3$$

91. Which of the following compounds would be the best solvent for an S_N2 reaction?

   A. H_20
   B. CH_3CH_2OH
   C. CH_3SOCH_3
   D. $CH_3CH_2CH_2CH_2CH_3$
   E. NH_3

92. S_N1 reactions show first-order kinetics because

   A. the rate-limiting step is the first step in the reaction
   B. the rate-limiting step involves only one molecule
   C. there is only one rate-limiting step
   D. the reaction involves just one molecule
   E. none of the above

93. The product of a Diels-Alder reaction is a(n)

   A. carboxylic acid
   B. alcohol
   C. aldehyde
   D. ketone
   E. cyclical compound

94. Which of the following represents the product obtained in the reaction below?

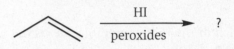

   A.

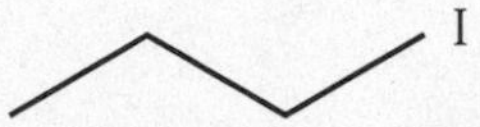

   B.

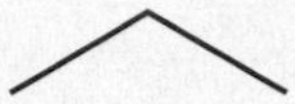

   C.

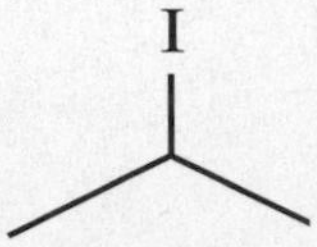

   D.

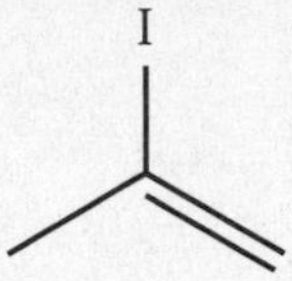

   E. None of the above

95. The products of the following reaction:

$$CH_3-CH_2-C^-\equiv C-\underset{\underset{CH_3}{|}}{\overset{\overset{CH_3}{|}}{CH}} \xrightarrow[\text{2) H}^+]{\text{1) } \Delta,\text{ KMnO}_4,\text{ OH}^-} ?$$

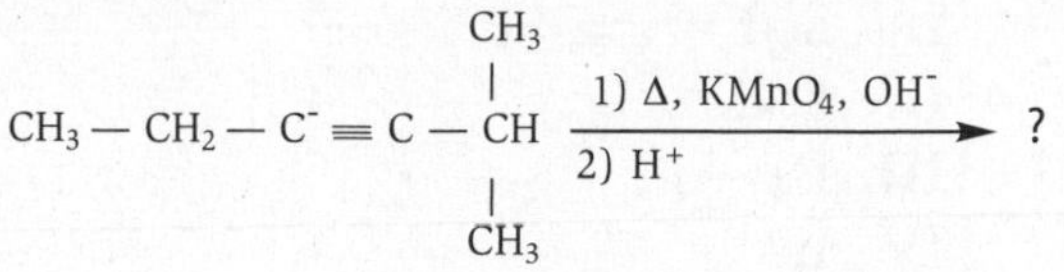

are

A.

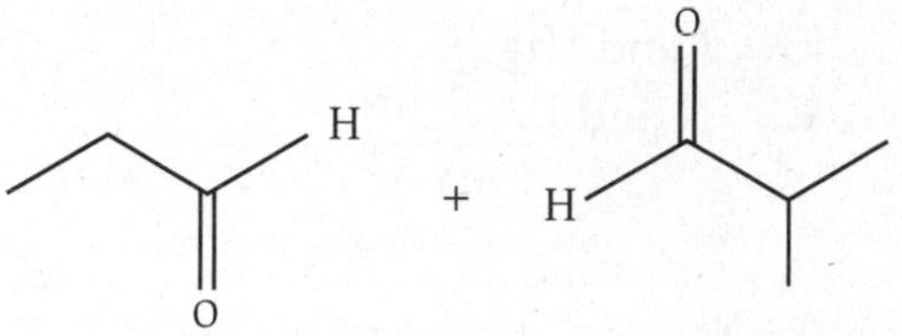

B.

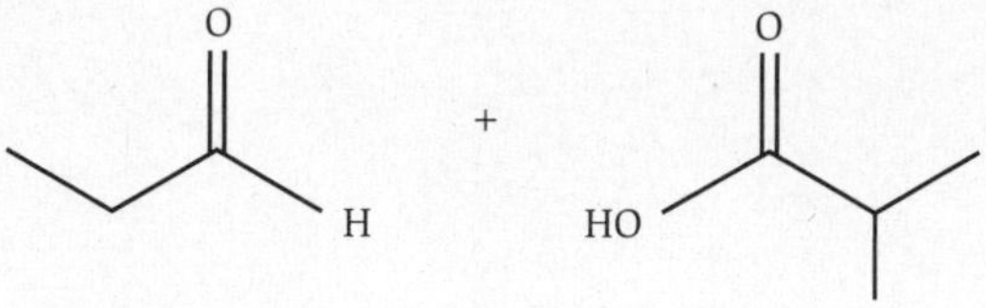

C.

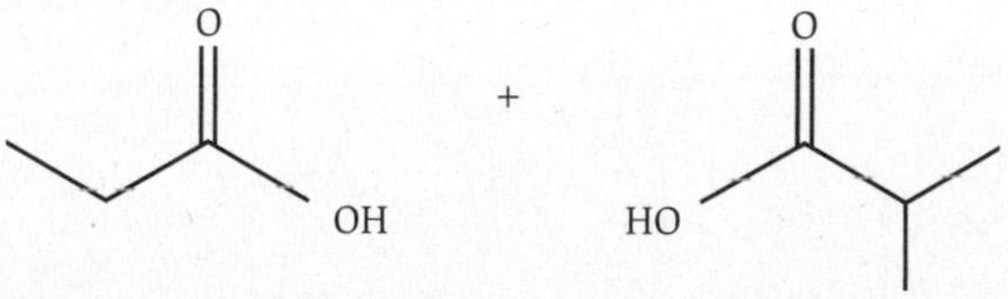

D.

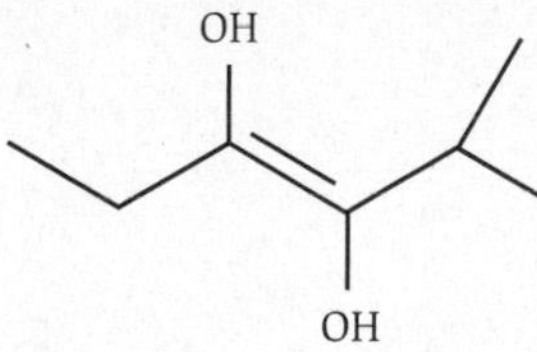

E. none of the above

96. The products of the following reaction:

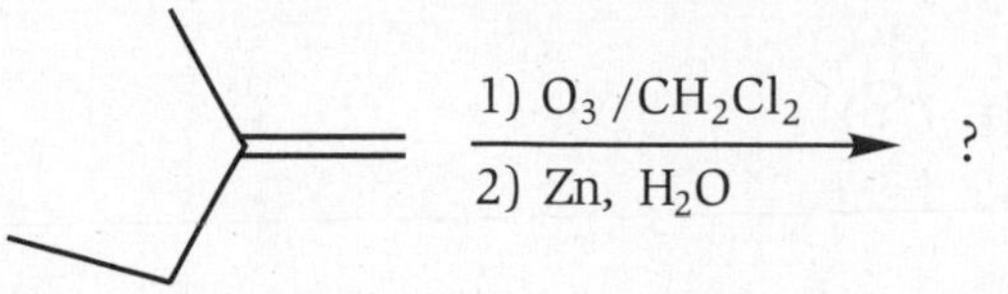

$\xrightarrow[\text{2) Zn, H}_2\text{O}]{\text{1) O}_3\text{ /CH}_2\text{Cl}_2} ?$

are

A.

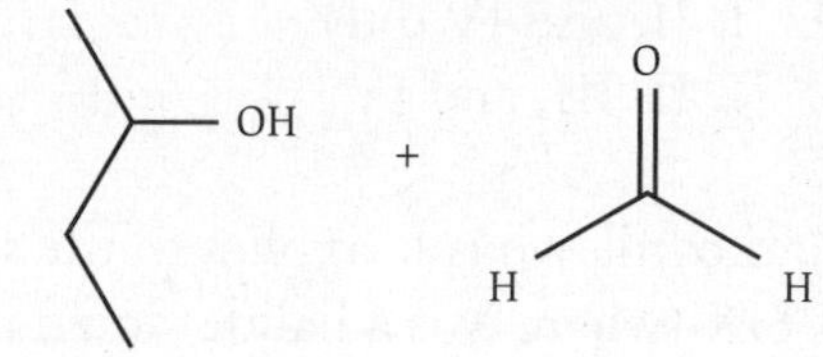

B.

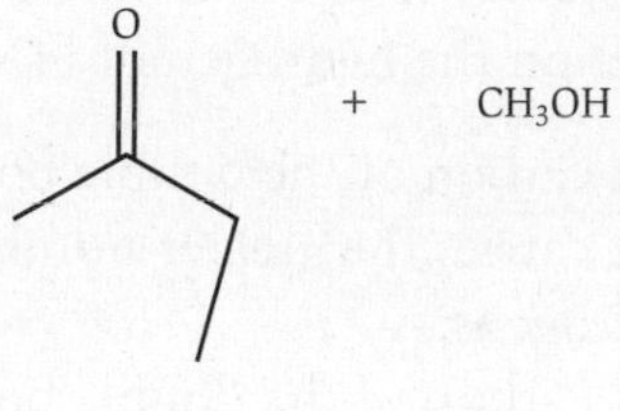

+ CH_3OH

C.

+ CO_2

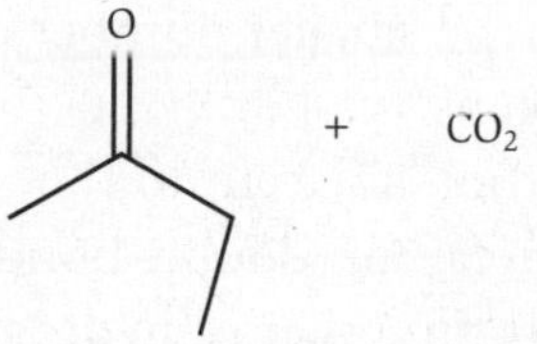

D.

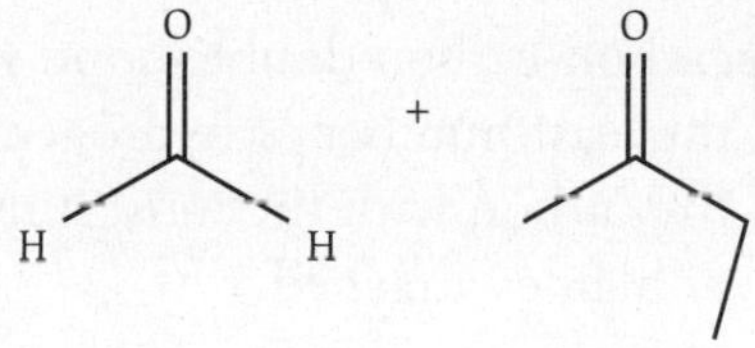

E. A and C

97. A Wittig reaction will produce an

A. alkane
B. alkene
C. alkyne
D. aldehyde
E. alcohol

98. Complete combustion of C_3H_8 will yield

I. CO_2
II. H_2O
III. CO
IV. heat

A. I only
B. I and II only
C. I, II, and III only
D. I, II, and IV only
E. I, II, III, and IV

99. Markovnikov's rule applies to the addition of HX (where X is a halide) to an unsymmetrical carbon-carbon double bond. In this addition the hydrogen of HX goes to

A. that carbon of the double bond that carries the greater number of hydrogens.
B. that carbon of the double bond that carries the smaller number of hydrogens.
C. the carbon adjacent to the carbon-carbon double bond with the most number of hydrogens.
D. the carbon adjacent to the carbon-carbon double bond with the least number of hydrogens.
E. the carbon with the most number of halides attached.

100. Which of the following reactions is(are) two step, unimolecular, and first-order?

I. S_N1
II. S_N2
III. E1
IV. E2

A. I only
B. II only
C. III only
D. I and III
E. II and IV

PERCEPTUAL ABILITY TEST   TIME LIMIT: 60 MINUTES

Part 1: Aperture Passing

For questions 1 through 15:

This section of the exam consists of 15 items similar to the example below. In each item, a three-dimensional object is shown on the left, followed by outlines of five apertures to its right.

The task is the same for each item. Conceptualize how the three-dimensional object looks from each possible side (in addition to the side shown). Then, pick the outline in which the three-dimensional object could pass if the proper side were inserted. Choose the letter corresponding to the correct aperture.

Here are rules for Part 1, the aperture section:

1. The irregular solid three-dimensional object on the left can be rotated in any direction prior to passing through the aperture.
2. The object may not be twisted or rotated in any way once it has started to be passed through the aperture. The correct answer is the exact representation of the external outline of the object viewed from the appropriate side.
3. The objects and the outlines are drawn to the same scale.
4. There are no irregularities in hidden portions of the objects. If the figure has symmetric indentations, it is assumed that the hidden portion is symmetric with the portion shown.
5. There is only one correct answer.

EXAMPLE

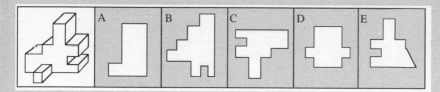

The correct answer is C.

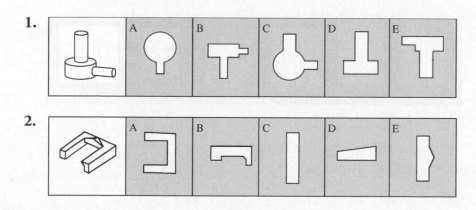

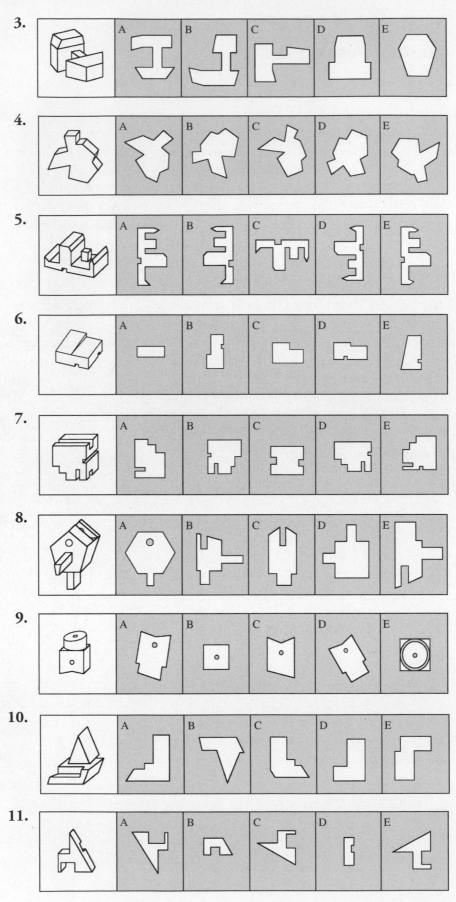

12.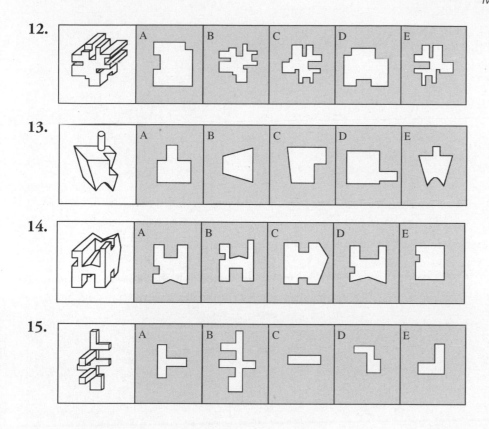

13.

14.

15.

Part 2: Orthographic Projections

For questions 16 through 30:

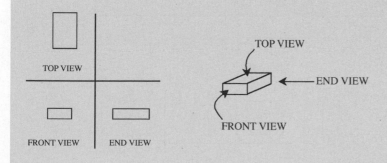

The pictures that follow are representations of solid objects from three different views: top, front, and end views. The pictures are views drawn without perspective: the surface viewed is along parallel lines of vision. The projection that is labeled TOP VIEW is shown looking DOWN on its top surface and is pictured in the upper-left corner. The projection labeled FRONT VIEW is shown looking at the object from the FRONT and is pictured in the lower-left corner. The projection labeled END VIEW is shown looking at the object from the END (or side) and is pictured in the lower-right corner. These three views are always in their respective corners and labeled accordingly.

TOP VIEW

FRONT VIEW   END VIEW

TOP VIEW

END VIEW

FRONT VIEW

If there were a hole in the figure, it would be represented like this:

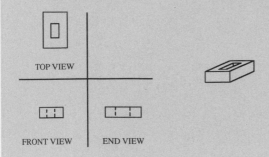

DOTTED lines indicate lines that exist but cannot be seen in the perspective shown.

In the following problems, TWO of the previous three views discussed will be shown with four alternatives to the right. Choose the correct letter that represents the correct view that completes the set.

EXAMPLE

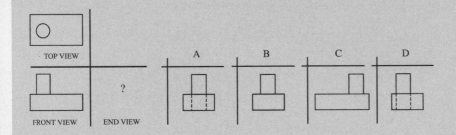

The FRONT VIEW shows that there is a smaller block on top of a larger block and there is no hole. The TOP VIEW shows that the top block is round and is centered on a rectangular block. From this information gathered in the two views given, the correct answer must be B.

In the following problems, one of the three views will be omitted; it is not always the END VIEW as shown in the example.

16. Choose the correct TOP VIEW.

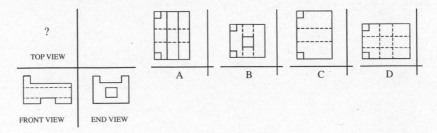

17. Choose the correct END VIEW.

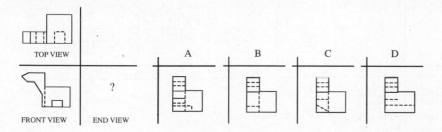

18. Choose the correct FRONT VIEW.

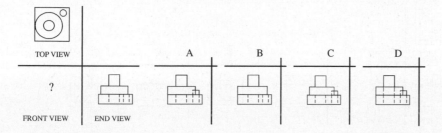

19. Choose the correct FRONT VIEW.

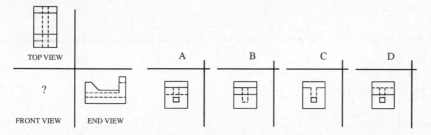

20. Choose the correct END VIEW.

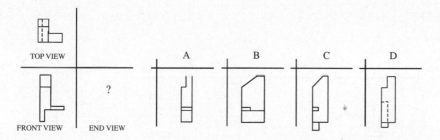

21. Choose the correct TOP VIEW.

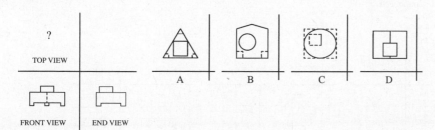

22. Choose the correct TOP VIEW.

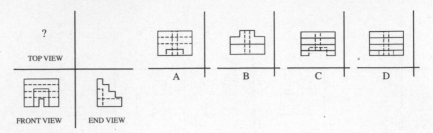

23. Choose the correct END VIEW.

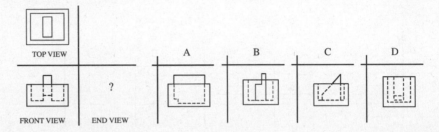

24. Choose the correct TOP VIEW.

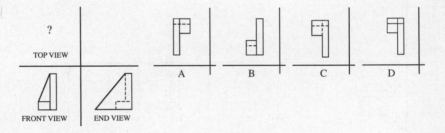

25. Choose the correct FRONT VIEW.

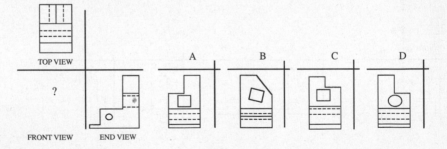

26. Choose the correct END VIEW.

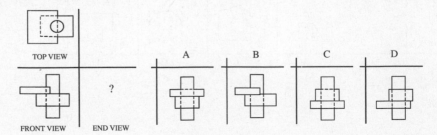

27. Choose the correct TOP VIEW.

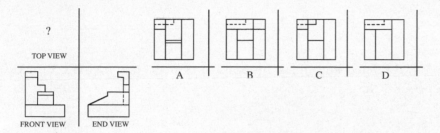

28. Choose the correct FRONT VIEW.

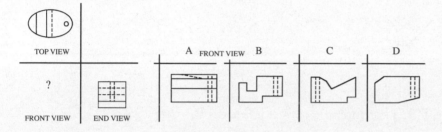

29. Choose the correct TOP VIEW.

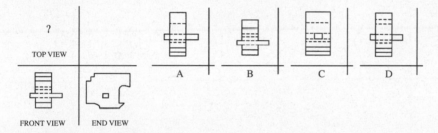

30. Choose the correct FRONT VIEW.

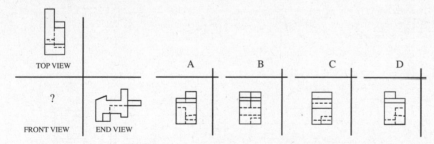

Part 3: Angle Discrimination

For questions 31 through 45:

Examine the INTERNAL ANGLES and rank them in terms of degrees from SMALL to LARGE. Select the alternative that represents the correct ranking.

EXAMPLE

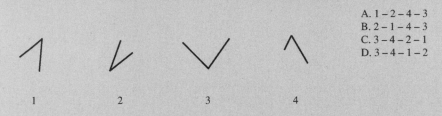

A. 1 – 2 – 4 – 3
B. 2 – 1 – 4 – 3
C. 3 – 4 – 2 – 1
D. 3 – 4 – 1 – 2

The correct ranking is 2–1–4–3. Therefore, the correct answer is B.

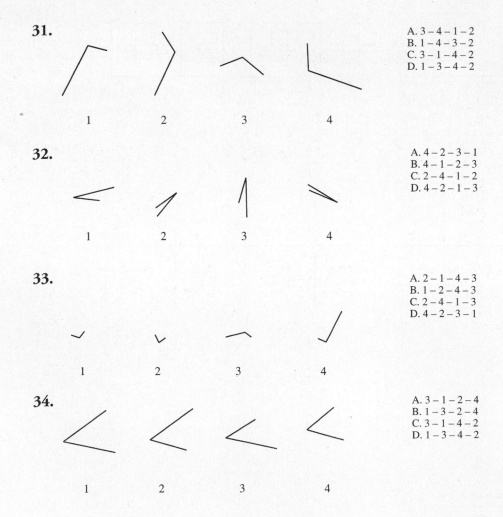

31.

A. 3 – 4 – 1 – 2
B. 1 – 4 – 3 – 2
C. 3 – 1 – 4 – 2
D. 1 – 3 – 4 – 2

32.

A. 4 – 2 – 3 – 1
B. 4 – 1 – 2 – 3
C. 2 – 4 – 1 – 2
D. 4 – 2 – 1 – 3

33.

A. 2 – 1 – 4 – 3
B. 1 – 2 – 4 – 3
C. 2 – 4 – 1 – 3
D. 4 – 2 – 3 – 1

34.

A. 3 – 1 – 2 – 4
B. 1 – 3 – 2 – 4
C. 3 – 1 – 4 – 2
D. 1 – 3 – 4 – 2

35.

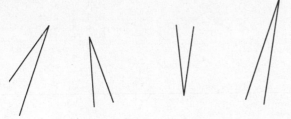

1   2   3   4

A. 3 – 2 – 1 – 4
B. 3 – 1 – 2 – 4
C. 2 – 4 – 1 – 3
D. 4 – 3 – 2 – 1

36.

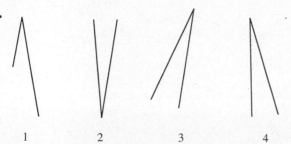

1   2   3   4

A. 2 – 4 – 3 – 1
B. 2 – 4 – 1 – 3
C. 4 – 2 – 3 – 1
D. 4 – 3 – 2 – 1

37.

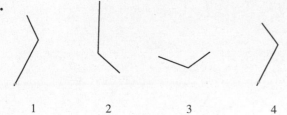

1   2   3   4

A. 4 – 3 – 1 – 2
B. 3 – 1 – 4 – 2
C. 3 – 4 – 2 – 1
D. 4 – 2 – 3 – 1

38.

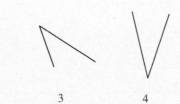

1   2   3   4

A. 4 – 3 – 2 – 1
B. 2 – 4 – 3 – 1
C. 2 – 4 – 1 – 3
D. 4 – 2 – 3 – 1

39.

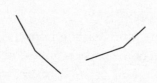

1   2   3   4

A. 1 – 3 – 2 – 4
B. 1 – 4 – 3 – 2
C. 4 – 1 – 2 – 3
D. 1 – 4 – 2 – 3

40.

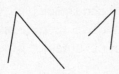

1   2   3   4

A. 3 – 2 – 1 – 4
B. 2 – 3 – 1 – 4
C. 2 – 3 – 4 – 1
D. 3 – 2 – 4 – 1

41.

1   2   3   4

A. 1 – 2 – 4 – 3
B. 4 – 1 – 3 – 2
C. 1 – 4 – 3 – 2
D. 4 – 1 – 2 – 3

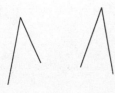
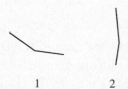

Model Examination B

42.

A. 4 – 1 – 3 – 2
B. 4 – 1 – 2 – 3
C. 1 – 4 – 3 – 2
D. 4 – 3 – 2 – 1

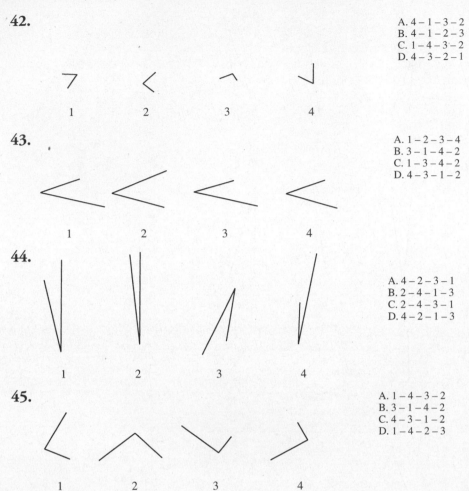

43.

A. 1 – 2 – 3 – 4
B. 3 – 1 – 4 – 2
C. 1 – 3 – 4 – 2
D. 4 – 3 – 1 – 2

44.

A. 4 – 2 – 3 – 1
B. 2 – 4 – 1 – 3
C. 2 – 4 – 3 – 1
D. 4 – 2 – 1 – 3

45.

A. 1 – 4 – 3 – 2
B. 3 – 1 – 4 – 2
C. 4 – 3 – 1 – 2
D. 1 – 4 – 2 – 3

Part 4: Paper Folding

For questions 46 through 60:

A flat, square piece of paper is folded one or more times starting from the left, proceeding stepwise to the illustrations to the right. The original position of the paper is represented by broken lines. The solid line indicates edges of the folded paper. The piece of paper is never twisted or turned and always remains within the outline of the original square. There may be ONE FOLD, TWO FOLDS, or THREE FOLDS in each item. After the last fold, a hole is punched in the paper. Your task is to unfold the paper in your mind and determine the placement of the holes on the original flat, square piece of paper. There is only one correct pattern of hole punches for each item. The black circles indicate hole punches. Choose the pattern that indicates the correct pattern of hole punches in the unfolded paper.

PRACTICE ILLUSTRATIONS

Figure 1   Figure 2   Figure 3   Figure 4

Model Examination B

In this example Figure 1 shows the original flat, square piece of paper. Figure 2 shows the first fold. Figure 3 shows the location of the hole punch in the folded paper. The black circles in Figure 4 show the pattern of the hole punches on the unfolded paper. The answer has two holes since the paper was two layers thick in the position where the hole was punched.

EXAMPLE

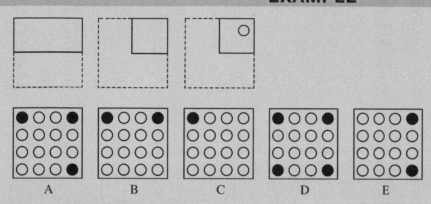

The correct answer is D. The paper was four thicknesses and therefore has four hole punches. The punch was made in the corner, so the four hole punches in the four corners are shown in black in the correct pattern.

46.

47.

48.

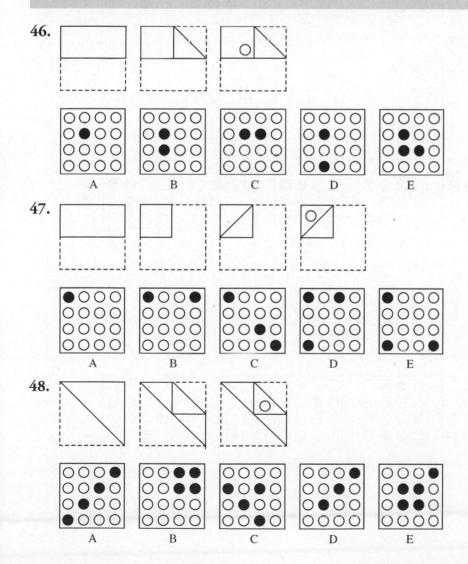

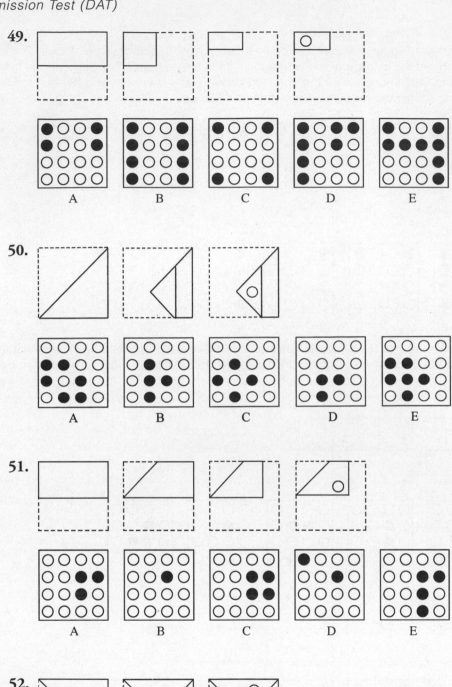

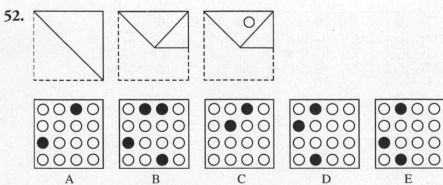

53.

54.

55.

56.

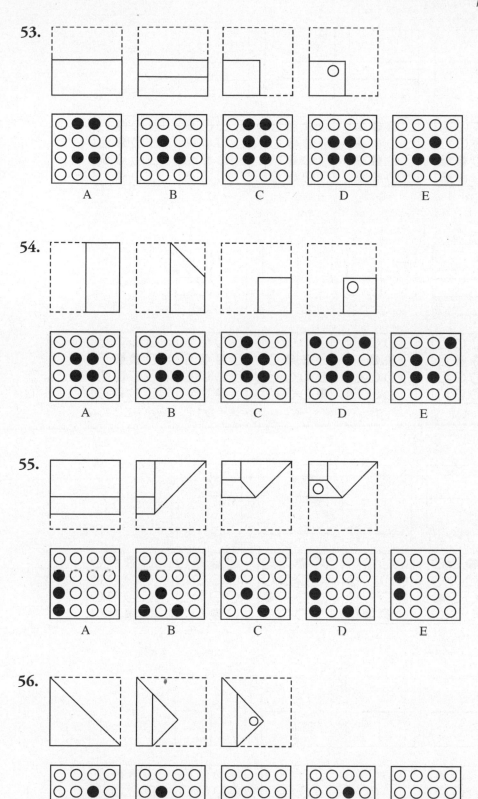

Model Examination B

57.

58.

59.

60.

Part 5: Cubes

For questions 61 through 75:

Each of the figures in this section is representative of cubes of the same size that have been cemented together. After the the cubes were cemented, the group of cubes were painted on each of the exposed sides WITH EXCEPTION TO THE BOTTOM SIDE ON WHICH THE FIGURE IS RESTING. Some illustrations contain hidden cubes. The only hidden cubes are cubes that are necessary to support other cubes.

In each item you are to determine how many cubes have

- ONE side painted,
- TWO sides painted,
- THREE sides painted,
- FOUR sides painted, or
- FIVE sides painted.

There are no problems that will ask for the number of cubes that have none (zero) of their sides painted.

EXAMPLE

In Figure A, how many cubes have two of their sides painted?

A. 1 cube
B. 2 cubes
C. 3 cubes
D. 4 cubes
E. 5 cubes

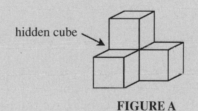

hidden cube

FIGURE A

There are four cubes in Figure A (one is hidden supporting the top cube). The top cube has five sides painted. The hidden cube supporting it has two sides painted. The cubes in the foreground and to the left each have four sides painted. Therefore, there is only one cube that has just two sides painted and the correct answer is A.

Choose the letter that corresponds to the correct number of cubes with the given number of sides painted. Remember that THE BOTTOM OF THE CUBE IS NOT PAINTED.

61. In Figure A, how many cubes have one of their exposed sides painted?
 A. 1 cube
 B. 2 cubes
 C. 3 cubes
 D. 4 cubes
 E. 5 cubes

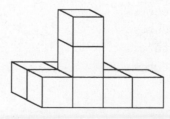

FIGURE A

62. In Figure A, how many cubes have two of their exposed sides painted?
- **A.** 1 cube
- **B.** 2 cubes
- **C.** 3 cubes
- **D.** 4 cubes
- **E.** 5 cubes

63. In Figure A, how many cubes have three of their exposed sides painted?
- **A.** 1 cube
- **B.** 2 cubes
- **C.** 3 cubes
- **D.** 4 cubes
- **E.** 5 cubes

64. In Figure A, how many cubes have four of their exposed sides painted?
- **A.** 1 cube
- **B.** 2 cubes
- **C.** 3 cubes
- **D.** 4 cubes
- **E.** 5 cubes

65. In Figure B, how many cubes have two of their exposed sides painted?
- **A.** 1 cube
- **B.** 2 cubes
- **C.** 3 cubes
- **D.** 4 cubes
- **E.** 5 cubes

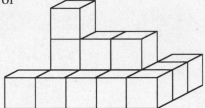

FIGURE B

66. In Figure B, how many cubes have three of their exposed sides painted?
- **A.** 1 cube
- **B.** 2 cubes
- **C.** 3 cubes
- **D.** 4 cubes
- **E.** 5 cubes

67. In Figure C, how many cubes have one of their exposed sides painted?
- **A.** 1 cube
- **B.** 2 cubes
- **C.** 3 cubes
- **D.** 4 cubes
- **E.** 5 cubes

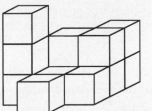

FIGURE C

68. In Figure C, how many cubes have two of their exposed sides painted?
  A. 1 cube
  B. 2 cubes
  C. 3 cubes
  D. 4 cubes
  E. 5 cubes

69. In Figure C, how many cubes have four of their exposed sides painted?
  A. 1 cube
  B. 2 cubes
  C. 3 cubes
  D. 4 cubes
  E. 5 cubes

70. In Figure D, how many cubes have two of their exposed sides painted?
  A. 1 cube
  B. 2 cubes
  C. 3 cubes
  D. 4 cubes
  E. 5 cubes

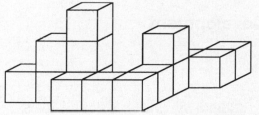

FIGURE D

71. In Figure D, how many cubes have four of their exposed sides painted?
  A. 1 cube
  B. 2 cubes
  C. 3 cubes
  D. 4 cubes
  E. 5 cubes

72. In Figure D, how many cubes have five of their exposed sides painted?
  A. 1 cube
  B. 2 cubes
  C. 3 cubes
  D. 4 cubes
  E. 5 cubes

73. In Figure E, how many cubes have one of their exposed sides painted?
  A. 1 cube
  B. 2 cubes
  C. 3 cubes
  D. 4 cubes
  E. 5 cubes

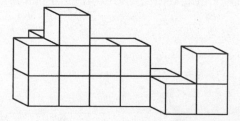

FIGURE E

Model Examination B

74. In Figure E, how many cubes have two of their exposed sides painted?
   A. 1 cube
   B. 2 cubes
   C. 3 cubes
   D. 4 cubes
   E. 5 cubes

75. In Figure E, how many cubes have four of their exposed sides painted?
   A. 1 cube
   B. 2 cubes
   C. 3 cubes
   D. 4 cubes
   E. 5 cubes

Part 6: Form Development

For questions 76 through 90:

A flat pattern will be presented in the box to the left. Your task is to mentally fold this pattern into a three-dimensional figure and choose the correct representation from the choices to the right. There is only one correct choice for each item.

EXAMPLE

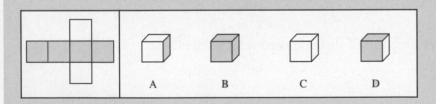

Folding the pattern in the left-most box can form only one of the figures to the right. The only figure that accurately represents the shaded areas once the pattern is folded is D.

Choose the letter that represents the three-dimensional object that correctly represents the folded pattern.

76.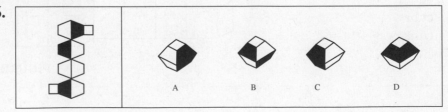

77.

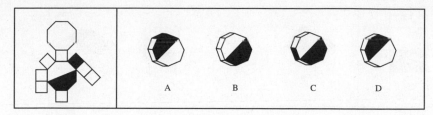

A   B   C   D

78.

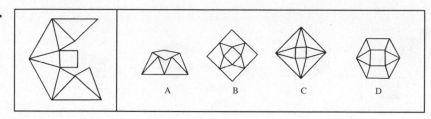

A   B   C   D

79.

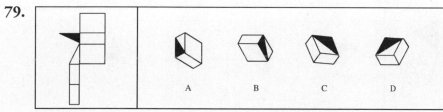

A   B   C   D

80.

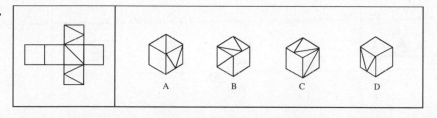

A   B   C   D

81.

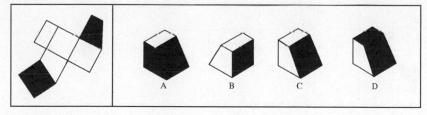

A   B   C   D

82.

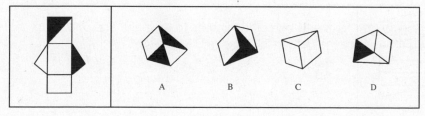

A   B   C   D

83.

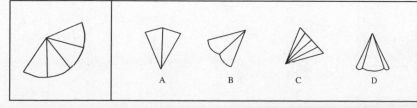

A   B   C   D

84.

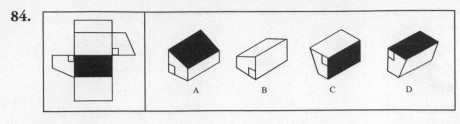

85.

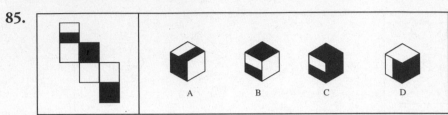

86.

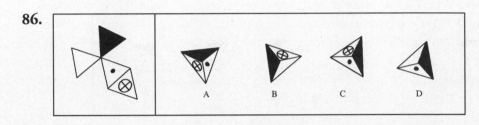

87.

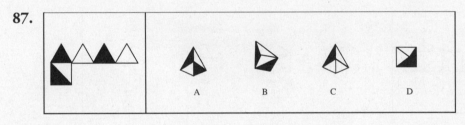

88.

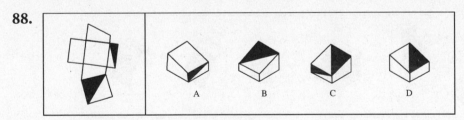

89.

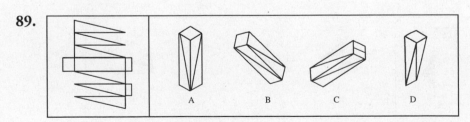

90.

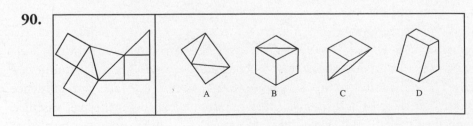

READING COMPREHENSION TEST   TIME LIMIT: 60 MINUTES

This section consists of three passages, with questions and/or incomplete statements following each passage. Read each passage; then read the questions and/or incomplete statements and answer choices carefully. For each question and/or incomplete statement, choose the best answer and blacken the corresponding space on the answer sheet. This section contains 50 items.

Fundamentals of Tooth Movement

Clinical tooth movement requires a periodontal ligament. Forces applied to teeth are mediated through the periodontal ligament and result in remodeling of the periodontal tissues. When an appliance is attached to a tooth and the tooth is moved, the entire surface of the socket is affected. The pressure side of the tooth root compresses the periodontal ligament and alveolar bone, which results in bone resorption. On the opposite surface of the root, the movement stretches the ligament fibers, which causes tension to occur. This situation is, of course, similar in the case of a single or multi-rooted tooth, although it is more complex in the latter.

Sites of Remodeling

On the compression side of the ligament, collagen fiber bundles initially are disorganized and compacted. Vascular flow decreases and cell death may occur. On the tension side of the ligament, the collagen fibers are stretched. The fibroblasts become more spindle-shaped and appear oriented with their long axis in the direction of the fiber bundles. A two-rooted tooth has two or more zones of compression as well as two or more zones of tension. The bifurcation zone has a region of tension toward the left root and a region of compression toward the right root. The apical areas demonstrate transition from tension to compression and are vulnerable locations during tooth movement because too much pressure can cause death of the pulp tissue by interfering with the tooth's vascular supply.

The initial response to physical force is displacement of the tooth; permanent structural changes follow. The histological features accompanying the changes include changes in cell type and number, vascular changes, and changes in the extracellular matrix.

Transduction

The mechanism of transduction—that is, the conversion of physical force into biologic response—is not known, but numerous hypotheses have been introduced. Some of the mechanical and chemical signals proposed as initiators of metabolic changes are altered blood and lymphatic flow; pressure and volume changes within the periodontal space; distortion of matrix molecules, cell membranes, and cell cytoskeleton; stress-generated bioelectric effects from alveolar bone bending; hormonal influences; and inflammatory phenomena and other nervous and immune cellular events. The explanations propose ways for local and systemic factors to influence alveolar bone, periodontal and gingival fiber bundles, cells (mesenchymal, vascular, neural gingival epithelial), and tissue fluids. However, more investigation is needed to elucidate the cascade of changes involved in remodeling of the periodontium during tooth movement.

Force Variables

Time is an important variable in the response of alveolar bone to tooth movement. As might be expected, the histology of the compression and tension zones will change with time. Alveolar bone resorption allows for the gradual movement of the tooth into the space provided and begins on the compression front. On the tension side, bone formation compensates for tooth movement away from the bone under tension. Direct or frontal resorption is a desirable clinical goal because it is not a destructive process.

Osteoclasts appear a few hours after tooth movement begins as they are recruited from monocytes arising from blood vessels. Both osteoclasts and osteoblasts stain with oxidative enzymes. Fibroblasts proliferate, synthesize new matrix in tension sites, and participate in the degradation of necrotic periodontal ligament in areas of compression along with osteoclasts and macrophages.

Histologic Changes

The tissue response to mechanical forces in tooth movement will vary with force magnitude (light, heavy), duration (continuous, intermittent), direction, and point of application. Should the force be too great in magnitude or the movement too rapid, hyalinization of the periodontal ligament may occur. Hyalinization results in the loss of cell activity and vascularity in the pressure zone of the ligament. This zone of the ligament may appear grasslike; hence, the origin of the term. Loss of cells interrupts bone resorption, and tooth movement stops temporarily.

Another feature of hyalinization is its association with undermining resorption. Because resorption cannot occur on the compressed surface of the alveolar bone, osteoclasts are activated in the marrow spaces opposite the compressed alveolar bone surface. When the osteoclasts finish removing the intervening bone, the tooth will move again. As the osteoclasts are destroyed and resorption relieves the compression, new cells from adjacent tissues rebuild the destroyed zone. It is not yet known why compression of the ligament and alveolar bone results in undermining resorption, but lack of blood supply and cell death in the hyalinized zone may contribute. Also, changes in bioelectric potential may signal the onset of resorption.

In addition to delaying orthodontic treatment, undermining resorption of alveolar bone is potentially more damaging to the alveolar process than is direct resorption, as it may result in extensive bone loss and root resorption. What protects the root surface from damage during routine tooth movement is not known. Undermining resorption is not easily controlled, and the extent of damage is unpredictable.

Forces applied to the teeth can also produce distant changes, such as those in periosteum, endosteum, sutures, and possibly even mandibular condyles. A complete explanation of tooth movement must include mechanisms for bone remodeling in alveolar bone marrow spaces, alteration of the gingiva, and transmission of forces to distant sites. Intermittent force and continuous force cause different histological appearances. When the tissues are temporarily relieved of stress, circulation is partially restored, cell activity is restored, and repair takes place. Tooth mobility may be increased, however, which can become a problem.

A lower level of cellularity in the periodontal ligament is found in older individuals and may be related to an initial slower rate of response during tooth movement. Increased age, however, does not reduce the prospect of a successful clinical outcome.

Tipping and Bodily Movement

Tipping of a tooth results in nonuniform alteration of the sockets, whereas bodily movement affects the entire socket in a more constant fashion. When the crown tips to the left, the root apex moves to the right, producing zones of compression and tension on opposite sides of the tooth apex relative to the cervical region. Likewise, both bone resorption and bone deposition occur on the same side of a tooth as it is tipped.

In the case of a short, incompletely developed root, tipping causes resorption at two sites and tension at the opposite two sites. The root apex of a young, completely formed tooth tips in a direction opposite to the crown. In the adult, tipping is complicated by strong apical fibers that resist movement and a narrow ligament space. In this case, tipping causes less movement at the root apex, but causes resorption along most of the length of bone on the compressed side.

A micrograph of the cemental surface reveals the activity of oxidative enzymes during tooth movement in the cementoblasts adjacent to the cementum. Observe the bundles of collagen fibers projecting from the cementum. The stain indicates that the cementocytes, probably newly differentiated, have high functional activity. This is also true for the osteoblasts in the adjacent alveolar bone. New cementum will be deposited, and attachment fiber bundles will be formed in response to the tension.

Both the cementum and the alveolar bone may undergo resorption. If compression is great and occurs over a long period, both opposing surfaces will be affected.

1. If a specimen were stained with oxidative enzymes, what could be seen under a microscope?

    A. Osteoclasts
    B. Osteocytes
    C. Periodontal ligament
    D. Macrophages
    E. Alveolar bone

2. How is tipping different from bodily movement?

    A. Tipping affects the entire socket.
    B. With tipping, resorption and deposition occur on opposite sides of the tooth.
    C. Bodily movement is nonuniform.
    D. Tipping does not involve osteoclasts.
    E. With tipping, resorption and deposition occur on the same side of the tooth.

3. In the bifurcation zone of a multirooted tooth there is a region of compression toward

    A. the crown
    B. the right root
    C. the root apex
    D. the left root
    E. the gingiva

4. Hyalinization may result in

    A. enamel resorption
    B. root formation
    C. excessive tooth movement
    D. extensive bone loss
    E. too much force being placed on the tooth

5. In which of the following does resorption occur?

    A. Cementum
    B. Alveolar bone
    C. Dentin
    D. Periodontal ligament
    E. A and B

6. The visible change due to physical force on the tooth is

    A. tooth displacement
    B. a permanent structural change
    C. bone resorption
    D. pulp death
    E. bone formation

7. If a tooth is moved too quickly what may occur?

    A. Tooth movement may accelerate.
    B. Tooth movement may stop.
    C. Vascularity may increase.
    D. Cell activity may increase.
    E. Resorption may increase.

8. The conversion of a physical force into a biological force is known as

    A. a force variable
    B. a mechanical force
    C. transformation
    D. an intermittent force
    E. transduction

9. The passage suggests that in a child most resorption due to tipping occurs

    A. along the length of the root
    B. near the crown
    C. at the apex
    D. nowhere; no resorption occurs
    E. This information is not given in the passage.

10. What prevent(s) the root surface from being damaged during routine tooth movement?

    A. Osteoclasts
    B. An unknown structure or mechanism
    C. Osteoblasts
    D. Hyalinization
    E. The periodontal ligament

11. What function(s) do fibroblasts serve?

    A. They synthesize bone.
    B. They synthesize matrix.
    C. They aid in periodontal ligament degradation.
    D. They resorb bone.
    E. B and C

12. What may result if too much pressure is placed on a tooth?

    A. Death of enamel
    B. Death of dentin
    C. Death of cementum
    D. Death of pulp
    E. All of the above

13. What may occur if pressure is applied and then temporarily removed from a tooth?

A. Tooth mobility may increase.
B. The tooth will return to its original position.
C. The gingiva will be altered.
D. Bone resorption will continue.
E. Cell death may occur.

14. Metabolic change may be initiated by

A. pressure changes in the periodontal space
B. inflammation
C. altered blood flow
D. altered lymphatic flow
E. all of the above

15. Direct resorption is

A. a destructive process
B. resorption of bone on the tension side
C. not a destructive process
D. not clinically desirable
E. B and C

16. What is required for movement of a tooth to occur?

A. Cementum
B. Dentin
C. Viable pulp
D. Periodontal ligament
E. Bodily movement

Alveolar Process

The alveolar processes are those portions of the maxilla and mandible that support the roots of the teeth. They are composed of the alveolar bone proper and the supporting bone. The alveolar bone proper is the bone that lines the socket. In radiographic terms, it is referred to as the lamina dura. This process is the bony site of attachment of the periodontal ligament fibers. The supporting bone includes the remainder of the alveolar process, specifically the compact cortical plates on the outer surfaces of the alveolar processes and the spongy bone between the cortical plates and the alveolar bone proper.

The alveolar process develops as a result of tooth root elongation and tooth eruption. Alveolar bone matures as the teeth gain functional occlusion; later, if the teeth are lost, the alveolar process disappears. Thus, the teeth are important in the development and maintenance of the alveolar bone. The alveolar bone proper is attached to the supporting cancellous and compact alveolar bone. Bone marrow containing blood vessels, nerves, and adipose tissue fills the space between the cortical plates and the alveolar bone proper. The coronal border of the alveolar process is termed the alveolar crest. It is located about 1 to 1.5 mm below the cemento-enamel junction, and is rounded in the anterior region and nearly flat in the molar area. If the teeth are in buccal or lingual position, the alveolar process will be very thin or partially missing. The area of an apical root penetrating the bone is known as a fenestration, and its occurrence at the coronal root zone is termed dehiscence.

Alveolar Bone Proper

On a histological basis, there are two types of bone: cancellous (spongy) and compact. Alveolar bone proper is a modification of compact bone, as it contains perforating fibers (Sharpey's fibers). These collagen fibers pierce the alveolar bone proper at right angles or obliquely to the surface of the long axis of the tooth. This is the means of attachment for the periodontal ligament to the tooth. The fiber bundles originating from bone are much larger than the fiber bundles inserting in cementum. Perforating fibers occur elsewhere in the skeleton, wherever ligaments and tendons insert. Purely elastic perforating fibers are also found, but not in alveolar bone proper. Because the bone of the alveolar process is regularly penetrated by collagen bundles, it has been appropriately named bundle bone or alveolar bone proper. When this bone is viewed radiographically, it is referred to as the lamina dura. The lamina dura appears more dense than does the adjacent supportive bone, but this radiographic density may be due to the mineral orientation around the fiber bundles and the apparent lack of nutrient canals. Actually, there may be no difference in mineral content between the lamina dura and the supporting bone. The lamina dura is evaluated clinically for periapical or periodontal pathology. Tension created by occlusal forces is believed to be important in the maintenance of this bone. In physiological movement of teeth, this bone is readily resorbed in zones of compression and readily formed in zones of tension. Not all alveolar bone proper appears as bundle bone. At times, there are no apparent perforating fibers in the socketlining bone. Supporting bone constantly undergoes modification in adapting to minor tooth movements, and therefore fibers may be lost or replaced from time to time in some areas of root.

Compact Supporting Bone

The compact or dense bone of the alveolar process is like that found elsewhere in the human body. Compact bone in the alveolar process extends from the alveolar crest labially or bucally to the lower border of the sockets. The cortical bone contains Haversian systems, radiating lamellae with lacunae, and canaliculi. The nutrient canals run in the direction of the long axis of the teeth and anastomose with "perforating canals" (Volkmann's canals) that pierce the bone at right or oblique angles. These canals establish a continuous system that houses the nerves and blood vessels of the bone. A sagittal view of the mandible demonstrates the vascular network in cortical bone. Compact bone comprises the bulk of the interdental alveolar process; cancellous bone is located more apically between the alveolar process proper and the cortical bone. Situated between osteons at the microscopic level are more irregular layers of bone, termed interstitial lamellae. Bone cells (osteocytes) fill the oval lacunae situated in or between the lamellae. Minute canaliculi interconnect with adjacent lacunae; they contain processes of the osteocytes that contact other cells by a system of "gap" junctions.

Cancellous Supporting Bone

The cancellous or spongy bone of the alveolar process is generally composed of heavy trabeculae. The purpose of this supporting bone is to strengthen the alveolar bone proper with struts that pass to the cortical bone. Cancellous bone contains osteocytes in the interior and osteoblasts or osteoclasts on the surface of the trabeculae. Between the bony struts that anastomose between the alveolar bone proper and the cortical bone are medullary cavities containing osteogenic cells, adipose tissue, and mature and immature blood cells. The maxillae are particularly rich in marrow tissue, such as megakaryocytes and immature white and red blood cells.

Physiological Tooth Movement

The eruptive process involves major remodeling of the alveolar processes to compensate for tooth growth and changes in position of the teeth. Repositioning of the teeth involves outward (facial and/or buccal) movement of the teeth as the face enlarges. Root growth results in growth in the height of the alveolar processes, which is compensatory for the increase in the length of the root. Although the two growth processes—tooth eruption and an increase in facial size—have different origins, both relate to positioning of the teeth and to modifications of the fine structures of Haversian and cancellous bone of the alveolar process.

There are several causative factors of alveolar bone changes. First, the increase in the height of the alveolar process associated with root lengthening is "tooth controlled." In the absence of teeth, this change does not occur. Change is especially evident in an older person whose teeth may have been lost, resulting in loss of the bone. Second, facial development involving condylar, maxillary, and mandibular growth also results in movement of the teeth. Because this process is not generated by the tooth, malformations of the face may result in tooth malalignment. Third, there will be further growth of the alveolar process unrelated to tooth eruption. This is part of the facial growth process. The teeth definitely control modifications of the alveolar process because, as a tooth moves, the alveolar bone responds with necessary compensatory changes. In this case, the resorption and deposition of bone around the teeth are a result, not the cause, of tooth movement. Thus, the alveolar process is guided in growth by tooth-related factors and extrinsic growth factors; the effects of these factors are difficult to separate as growth occurs.

Aging of Alveolar Bone

A comparison of young and old alveolar bone reveals a shift with age from alveolar processes with smoothly lined sockets, and active bone formation with numerous viable cells, to alveolar sockets that appear jagged and uneven with fewer cells. The perforating fibers are inserted in an uneven pattern. Marrow appears to have a fatty infiltration, and osteoporosis indicates loss of some bony elements.

Edentulous Jaws

The changes in the jaws resulting from tissue loading, compression, tissue conditioning, and denture retention coupled with the aging processes have not been clearly elucidated. It is apparent, however, that with age the alveolar process in edentulous jaws decreases in size; loss of maxillary bone is accompanied by an increase in the size of the maxillary sinus. The internal trabecular arrangement is more open, indicating bone loss. From a common radiographic viewpoint the locations of various structures such as glands, fatty zones, muscle masses, and blood vessels vary little in the edentulous jaws.

17. How is the periodontal ligament attached to the tooth?

   A. By perforating canals
   B. By lacunae
   C. By canaliculi
   D. By Haversian fibers
   E. By perforating fibers

18. Where is bone marrow located?

   A. In the alveolar bone proper
   B. Between the cortical plates and alveolar bone proper
   C. In the cortical plates
   D. In the coronal border of the alveolar process
   E. In the compact bone

19. As the root of a tooth grows, what happens to the alveolar process?

   A. It decreases in height.
   B. It grows thicker.
   C. It grows thinner.
   D. It grows higher.
   E. It remains unchanged.

20. What is another name for bone cells?

   A. Osteocytes
   B. Osteoblasts
   C. Lacunae
   D. Lamellae
   E. Canaliculi

21. Why is alveolar bone proper considered modified compact bone?

   A. It contains Sharpey's fibers.
   B. It contains Volkmann's canals.
   C. It contains fenestrations.
   D. It contains canaliculi.
   E. It contains lacunae.

22. The alveolar process develops in response to which of the following?

   A. Root elongation
   B. Enamel formation
   C. Tooth eruption
   D. A and B
   E. A and C

23. If all teeth are lost, what, if anything, will happen to the alveolar process?

   A. It will increase in size.
   B. It will increase in density.
   C. It will decrease in density.
   D. It will decrease in size.
   E. It will remain the same.

24. What helps to maintain the lamina dura?

   A. Spongy bone
   B. Tension due to occlusal forces
   C. Compact bone
   D. Nutrient canals
   E. Supporting bone

25. The bone that lines the tooth socket is called

   A. alveolar bone proper
   B. Haversian bone
   C. supporting bone
   D. cancellous bone
   E. Sharpey's bone

26. Where are osteoblasts located?

   A. Inside trabeculae
   B. On the alveolar bone proper
   C. On the surface of the trabeculae
   D. In the lamina dura
   E. In "gap" junctions

27. What is the term for a coronal root penetrating the bone?

   A. Fenestration
   B. Perforating fiber
   C. Volkmann's canal
   D. Lamina dura
   E. Dehiscence

28. The nerves and blood vessels of compact bone are contained in

  A. the lamina dura
  B. cancellous bone
  C. Volkmann's canals
  D. the root
  E. the pulp

29. The growth of the alveolar process is guided by

  A. extrinsic growth factors
  B. tooth-related factors
  C. calcium intake
  D. bone density
  E. A and B

30. Where is the alveolar crest located?

  A. 1–1.5 mm above the cemento-enamel junction
  B. 2–2.5 mm below the cemento-enamel junction
  C. 1–1.5 mm below the cemento-enamel junction
  D. At the cemento-enamel junction
  E. 1–1.5 mm below the dentin-enamel junction

31. Where are immature red blood cells found in abundance?

  A. Bundle bone of maxillae
  B. Cancellous bone of maxillae
  C. Lamina dura of maxillae
  D. Compact bone of maxillae
  E. Cortical plates of maxillae

32. What is the function of spongy bone?

  A. To strengthen the alveolar bone proper
  B. To strengthen the cancellous bone
  C. To provide flexibility to the alveolar bone proper
  D. To carry nutrients to the alveolar bone proper
  E. To strengthen the compact bone

33. What are contained in compact bone?

  A. Lacunae
  B. Lamellae
  C. Haversian systems
  D. Canaliculi
  E. All of the above

Types of Cementum

Cementum is the calcified mesenchymal tissue that forms the outer covering of the anatomic root. There are two main types of root cementum: acellular (primary) and cellular (secondary). Both consist of a calcified interfibrillar matrix and collagen fibrils.

There are two sources of collagen fibers in cementum: Sharpey's (extrinsic) fibers, which are the embedded portion of the principal fibers of the periodontal ligament and are formed by the fibroblasts; and fibers that belong to the cementum matrix per se (intrinsic) and are produced by the cementoblasts. Cementoblasts also form the noncollagenous components of the interfibrillar ground substance, such as proteoglycans, glycoproteins, and phosphoproteins.

Acellular cementum is the first to be formed and covers approximately the cervical third or half of the root; it does not contain cells. This cementum is formed before the tooth reaches the occlusal plane, and its thickness ranges from 30 to

230 µm. Sharpey's fibers make up most of the structure of acellular cementum, which has a principal role in supporting the tooth. Most of the fibers are inserted at approximately right angles into the root surface and penetrate deep into the cementum, but others enter from several different directions. Their size, number, and distribution increase with function. Sharpey's fibers are completely calcified, with the mineral crystals oriented parallel to the fibrils, as they are in dentin and bone, except in a 10- to 50-µm-wide zone near the cementodentinal junction, where they are only partially calcified. The peripheral portions of Sharpey's fibers in actively mineralizing cementum tend to be more calcified than the interior regions, according to evidence obtained by scanning electron microscopy. Acellular cementum also contains other collagen fibrils that are calcified and irregularly arranged or parallel to the surface.

Cellular cementum, formed after the tooth reaches the occlusal plane, is more irregular and contains cells (cementocytes) in individual spaces (lacunae) that communicate with each other through a system of anastomosing canaliculi. Cellular cementum is less calcified than the acellular type. Sharpey's fibers occupy a smaller portion of cellular cementum and are separated by other fibers that are arranged either parallel to the root surface or at random. Sharpey's fibers may be completely calcified or partially calcified or may have a central, uncalcified core surrounded by a calcified border.

Both acellular and cellular cementum are arranged in lamellae separated by incremental lines parallel to the long axis of the root. These lines represent periods in cementum formation and are more mineralized than the adjacent cementum. In addition, loss of the cervical part of the reduced enamel epithelium at the time of tooth eruption may place portions of mature enamel in contact with the connective tissue, which will then deposit over it an acellular afibrillar type of cementum.

Based on these findings, Schroeder has classified cementum as follows: Acellular afibrillar cementum (AAC) contains neither cells nor extrinsic or intrinsic collagen fibers, apart from a mineralized ground substance. It is a product of cementoblasts and in humans is found in coronal cementum.

Acellular extrinsic fiber cementum (AEFC) is composed almost entirely of densely packed bundles of Sharpey's fibers and lacks cells. It is a product of fibroblasts and cementoblasts and in humans is found in the cervical third of roots but may extend further apically.

Cellular mixed stratified cementum (CMSC) is composed of extrinsic (Sharpey's) and intrinsic fibers and contains cells. It is a coproduct of fibroblasts and cementoblasts, and in humans it appears primarily in the apical third of the roots and the apices and in furcation areas.

Cellular intrinsic fiber cementum (CIFC) contains cells but no collagen fibers. It is formed by cementoblasts, and in humans it fills resorption lacunae.

Intermediate cementum is an illdefined zone near the cementodentinal junction of certain teeth that appears to contain cellular remnants of Hertwig's sheath embedded in calcified ground substance.

The inorganic content of cementum (hydroxyapatite) is 45% to 50%, which is less than that of bone (65%), enamel (97%), or dentin (70%). Opinions differ about whether the microhardness increases or decreases with age, and no relationship has been established between aging and the mineral content of cementum.

Permeability of Cementum

In very young animals, both cellular cementum and acellular cementum are very permeable and permit the diffusion of dyes from the pulp and from the external root surface. In cellular cementum, the canaliculi in some areas are contiguous with the dentinal tubuli. With age, the permeability of cementum diminishes.

Cemento-enamel Junction

The cementum at and immediately subjacent to the cemento-enamel junction is of particular clinical importance in root scaling procedures. Three types of relationships involving the cementum may exist at the cemento-enamel junction. In about 60% to 65% of cases cementum overlaps the enamel; in about 30% there is an edge-to-edge butt joint; and in 5% to 10% the cementum and enamel fail to meet. In the last instance, gingival recession may be accompanied by an accentuated sensitivity because the dentin is exposed.

Thickness of Cementum

Cementum deposition is a continuous process that proceeds at varying rates throughout life. Cementum formation is most rapid in the apical regions, where it compensates for tooth eruption, which itself compensates for attrition. The thickness of cementum on the coronal half of the root varies from 16 to 60 μm, or about the thickness of a hair. It attains its greatest thickness (up to 150 to 200 μm) in the apical third and in the bifurcation areas; it is thicker in distal surfaces than in mesial surfaces, probably because of functional stimulation from mesial drift over time. Between the ages of 11 and 70, the average thickness of the cementum increases threefold, with the greatest increase in the apical region. Average thicknesses of 95 μm at age 20 and 215 μm at age 60 have been reported.

The term hypercementosis (cementum hyperplasia) refers to a prominent thickening of the cementum. It may be localized to one tooth or affect the entire dentition. Because of considerable physiologic variation in the thickness of cementum among different teeth in the same person and also among different persons, it is sometimes difficult to distinguish between hypercementosis and physiologic thickening of cementum.

Hypercementosis occurs as a generalized thickening of the cementum, with nodular enlargement of the apical third of the root. It also appears in the form of spikelike excrescences (cemental spikes) created by either the coalescence of cementicles that adhere to the root or the calcification of periodontal fibers at the sites of insertion into the cementum.

The etiology of hypercementosis varies and is not completely understood. The spikelike type of hypercementosis generally results from excessive tension from orthodontic appliances or from occlusal forces. The generalized type occurs in a variety of circumstances. In teeth without antagonists, hypercementosis is interpreted as an effort to keep pace with excessive tooth eruption. In teeth subject to lowgrade periapical irritation arising from pulp disease, it is considered to be compensation for the destroyed fibrous attachment to the tooth. The cementum is deposited adjacent to the inflamed periapical tissue. Hypercementosis of the entire dentition may occur in patients with Paget's disease.

Cementum Resorption and Repair

The cementum of erupted as well as unerupted teeth is subject to resorption. The resorptive changes may be of microscopic proportion or may be sufficiently extensive to present a radiographically detectable alteration in the root contour. Cementum resorption is extremely common. In one microscopic study, it occurred in 236 of 261 teeth (90.5%). The average number of resorption areas per tooth was 3.5. Of the 922 areas of resorption, 708 (76.8%) were located in the apical third of the root, 177 (19.2%) in the middle third, and 37 (4.0%) in the gingival third. Seventy percent of all resorption areas were confined to the cementum without involving the dentin.

Cementum resorption may be due to local or systemic causes or may occur without apparent etiology (i.e., be idiopathic). Among the local conditions in which it occurs are trauma from occlusion; orthodontic movement; pressure from malaligned erupting teeth, cysts, and tumors; teeth without functional antagonists; embedded teeth; replanted and transplanted teeth; periapical disease; and periodontal disease. Among the systemic conditions mentioned as predisposing to or inducing cemental resorption are calcium deficiency, hypothyroidism, hereditary fibrous osteodystrophy, and Paget's disease.

34. Where is intermediate cementum found?

    A. Near the dentino-enamel junction
    B. Near the cemento-enamel junction
    C. Near the cemento-dentinal junction
    D. In Hertwig's sheath
    E. In acellular cementum

35. Most cementum resorption occurs in the

    A. middle third of the root
    B. gingival third of the root
    C. apical third of the crown
    D. middle third of the crown
    E. apical third of the root

36. Where is cementum the thickest?

    A. In the coronal third
    B. Near the dentino-enamel junction
    C. Near the crown
    D. In bifurcation areas
    E. Near the cemento-enamel junction

37. The part of the periodontal ligament that inserts into cementum is called

    A. Sharpey's fibers
    B. cementoblasts
    C. cementoclasts
    D. fibroblasts
    E. the interfibrillar matrix

38. Some canaliculi in cellular cementum are contiguous with

    A. enamel rods
    B. acellular cementum
    C. the pulp
    D. dentinal tubuli
    E. the gingiva

39. Paget's disease may result in _____

    A. cemental spikes
    B. cementum resorption
    C. hypercementosis
    D. osteodystrophy
    E. B and C

40. A prominent thickening of the cementum is called

   A. hypocementosis
   B. acellular afibrillar cementum
   C. hypercementosis
   D. intermediate cementum
   E. interfibrillar ground substance

41. Cellular cementum generally _____ than acellular cementum.

   A. contains fewer cells
   B. is more irregular
   C. contains more Sharpey's fibers
   D. is more regular
   E. is formed earlier

42. Sensitivity may be accentuated because of

   A. failure of cementum and enamel to meet
   B. cementum and enamel forming an edge-to-edge butt joint
   C. cementum overlapping enamel
   D. enamel overlapping cementum
   E. all of the above

43. Idiopathic cementum resorption is due to

   A. systemic causes
   B. local causes
   C. orthodontic treatment
   D. trauma
   E. no apparent reason

44. In the passage hypercementosis and _____ may be used interchangeably.

   A. cementum resorption
   B. cementum hyperplasia
   C. physiologic thickening of cementum
   D. periodontal disease
   E. calcification of cementum

45. The first cementum formed

   A. is cellular
   B. is extrinsic
   C. is acellular
   D. is multinucleated
   E. B and D

46. When does cementum deposition cease?

   A. After eruption is complete
   B. When root formation is complete
   C. When enamel formation is complete
   D. When dentin formation is complete
   E. Cementum deposition does not stop

47. What is the percent of hydroxyapatite in cementum?

   A. 65%
   B. 97%
   C. 70%
   D. 35%
   E. 45%

48. How are cellular and acellular cementum arranged?

   A. In lamellae
   B. In lacunae
   C. In canaliculi
   D. In a random pattern
   E. In rods

49. In which of the following are completely calcified extrinsic fibers found?

   A. Cellular cementum
   B. Lacunae
   C. Acellular cementum
   D. Canaliculi
   E. A and C

50. The calcification of periodontal fibers at the site of insertion into cementum is called

   A. physiologic thickening of cementum
   B. cemental spikes
   C. dentinal spikes
   D. hypocementosis
   E. Sharpey's fibers

Model Examination B

QUANTITATIVE REASONING TEST   TIME LIMIT: 45 MINUTES

The following items are questions or incomplete statements. Read each item carefully, then choose the best answer or completion. Blacken the corresponding space on the answer sheet. This section contains 40 items.

1. If $4^{\frac{x}{3}} = 64$, then $x = $?

    A. -2
    B. 3
    C. 12
    D. 9
    E. 6

2. $\dfrac{\sqrt{15} \times \sqrt{3}}{\sqrt{10}} = $?

    A. $\dfrac{3}{2}$

    B. $\dfrac{3\sqrt{2}}{2}$

    C. $2\sqrt{5}$

    D. $9\sqrt{5}$

    E. $\dfrac{\sqrt{2}}{2}$

3. What is the probability of obtaining heads in each of five tosses of a fair coin?

    A. $\dfrac{3}{5}$

    B. $\dfrac{5}{32}$

    C. $\dfrac{1}{2}$

    D. $\dfrac{5}{8}$

    E. $\dfrac{2}{5}$

4. $-8 - 6\{3+2[5-(3+4)+1]-2\}+7 =$

    A. 0
    B. 2
    C. 4
    D. 5
    E. -4

5. If an ordinary coin is tossed six times, what is the probability of either all heads or all tails?

    A. $\dfrac{1}{4}$

    B. $\dfrac{1}{32}$

    C. $\dfrac{1}{3}$

    D. $\dfrac{1}{8}$

    E. $\dfrac{1}{16}$

6. The value of $\dfrac{5}{6} + \dfrac{2}{3} + \dfrac{1}{4}$ is

    A. $\dfrac{9}{12}$

    B. $1\dfrac{3}{4}$

    C. $2\dfrac{1}{4}$

    D. $\dfrac{3}{4}$

    E. $1\dfrac{2}{5}$

7. The largest of five consecutive even integers is 2 less than twice the smallest. Which of the following is the largest integer?

    A. 16
    B. 18
    C. 12
    D. 20
    E. 10

8. What is the slope of a line containing points $(-3, 6)$ and $(2, 5)$?

   A. 5

   B. $\dfrac{1}{5}$

   C. -5

   D. $-\dfrac{1}{5}$

   E. 1

9. The angles of a triangle are in the ratio 2:3:5. What is the measure of the smallest angle?

   A. $48°$
   B. $36°$
   C. $45°$
   D. $72°$
   E. $60°$

10. If $3x + 2y = 8$ and $x + y = 2$, then $x - y = ?$

   A. 6
   B. 4
   C. 2
   D. -2
   E. 0

11. Which of the following is equal to $(\tan\theta)(\csc\theta)$?

   A. $\cos\theta$
   B. $\cot\theta$
   C. $\sec\theta$
   D. $\sin\theta$
   E. $\csc\theta$

12. What is the equation of the line that contains point $(-3, 1)$ and has a slope of (-2)?

   A. $y = -2x - 3$
   B. $y = 2x + 5$
   C. $y = -2x + 5$
   D. $y = -2x + 1$
   E. $y = -2x - 5$

13. Simplify: $\sqrt{\dfrac{3x^2}{12} + \dfrac{7x^2}{36}}$.

   A. $\dfrac{2}{3}x$

   B. $\dfrac{2x^2}{3}$

   C. $\dfrac{3}{4}x$

   D. $\dfrac{3x^2}{4}$

   E. $4x$

14. The sum of a number x and 6 equals 2 less than the product of 2 and the number. What is the number?

   A. $x = 6$
   B. $x = 8$
   C. $x = 10$
   D. $x = 9$
   E. $x = 5$

15. Julie has $5.50 in nickels and dimes. She has five more nickels than dimes. How many dimes does she have?

   A. 30
   B. 25
   C. 20
   D. 35
   E. 40

16. There are three consecutive even integers such that the third of the three even integers is 10 more than the sum of the first and second. What is the third integer?

   A. -8
   B. -6
   C. -4
   D. -10
   E. -2

17. Which of the following is identically equal to sin 2*A*?

    A. $1 - \cos 2A$
    B. $2 \sin A$
    C. $1 - \cos^2 2A$
    D. $2 \sin A \cos A$
    E. $\dfrac{1}{\sec 2A}$

18. The five tires that came with Steve's new car were rotated frequently so that each tire was used exactly the same amount of time as the others. The tires were replaced when the odometer read 24,000 miles. For how many miles had each been used?

    A. 30,000 miles
    B. 24,000 miles
    C. 18,000 miles
    D. 20,000 miles
    E. 19,200 miles

19. At a convention of dentists, 1,000 dentists are from the west coast. One hundred dentists are women; 60 of the women are not from the west coast. How many male dentists are from the west coast?

    A. 850
    B. 800
    C. 900
    D. 960
    E. 940

20. Brian received a 10% increase in each of the last 2 years. His present salary is $21,780. What was his starting salary?

    A. $19,000
    B. $21,300
    C. $20,000
    D. $18,000
    E. $26,354

21. A florist bought some plants for $150. She sold enough at 75 cents each to meet the cost and had 100 plants left. How many plants were originally purchased by the florist?

    A. 150
    B. 250
    C. 300
    D. 350
    E. 400

22. An automobile travels at an average speed of 45 miles per hour for 1 hour and then at an average speed of 60 miles per hour for the next half hour. What is the average speed for the entire time period?

    A. 47.5 mph
    B. 50 mph
    C. 52.5 mph
    D. 55 mph
    E. 62.5 mph

23. If $\dfrac{1}{2} + \dfrac{4}{2x - 1} = 6$, then $x = ?$

    A. $-\dfrac{1}{2}$
    B. $\dfrac{13}{22}$
    C. $\dfrac{19}{22}$
    D. $-\dfrac{1}{4}$
    E. $-\dfrac{15}{22}$

24. A box has the shape of a rectangular solid, with a base measuring 16 inches by 10 inches and a height of 8 inches. What is the approximate length of the sides of a cubic container having the same volume?

    A. 9.75 in.
    B. 10.85 in.
    C. 10.00 in.
    D. 12.65 in.
    E. 13.15 in.

25. If $\dfrac{1}{5}$ of 27 = 25% of x, then x = ?

A. 5.4

B. $21\dfrac{3}{5}$

C. 1.35

D. 21

E. 21.5

26. An integer from 1 to 9, inclusive, is selected at random. What is the probability that the integer is a multiple of 3?

A. $\dfrac{1}{9}$

B. $\dfrac{2}{9}$

C. $\dfrac{1}{3}$

D. $\dfrac{2}{3}$

E. 1

27. What is the rate of discount on dental equipment listing at $3,050 and selling for $2,745?

A. 0.1%

B. 9.0%

C. 10.0%

D. 10.3%

E. 11.1%

28. If 10 cubic centimeters of 20% acid is mixed with 20 cubic centimeters of 40% acid, the percent of acid in the resulting solution is

A. 50

B. 30

C. 35

D. $33\dfrac{1}{3}$

E. 60

29. If $x = 3 + 5h$ and $y = 3h - 5$, for what value of h will $x = 2y$?

A. 68

B. 34

C. 13

D. –4

E. –11

30. If 85% of $\dfrac{3}{x}$ = 8, then x = ?

A. 2.17

B. 0.375

C. 0.032

D. 0.300

E. 0.319

31. $2\sqrt{20} + \sqrt{45} =$

A. $5\sqrt{7}$

B. $7\sqrt{5}$

C. $15\sqrt{5}$

D. $7\sqrt{10}$

E. $3\sqrt{65}$

32. A river flows at 3 miles per hour. A man can row at 5 miles per hour in still water. If he rows 1 mile upstream and then floats back to the starting place, how many minutes will be required for the roundtrip?

A. 30

B. 42

C. 50

D. 60

E. 65

33. When 1 is added to the numerator of the fraction $\frac{x}{y}$, the fraction equals $\frac{1}{3}$. When 3 is added to the denominator of $\frac{x}{y}$, the fraction equals $\frac{1}{6}$. What is $\frac{x}{y}$?

    A. $\frac{2}{3}$

    B. $\frac{2}{9}$

    C. $\frac{6}{17}$

    D. $\frac{2}{6}$

    E. $\frac{1}{4}$

34. If $(y + 2)x = \frac{1}{4}$, then $y = ?$

    A. $\frac{1}{4} - 2x$

    B. $\frac{x}{4} - 2$

    C. $\frac{1}{4x + 8}$

    D. $\frac{1}{4x} - 2$

    E. $\frac{1 - 8x}{4}$

35. Perform the indicated operations and simplify: $\dfrac{\frac{4}{3} - \frac{2}{5}}{2 + \frac{5}{3}}$

    A. $\frac{14}{55}$

    B. $-\frac{4}{7}$

    C. $-\frac{41}{15}$

    D. $\frac{14}{11}$

    E. $\frac{154}{45}$

36. The value of $\sin\left(\frac{\pi}{3}\right)$ equals the value of

    A. $\sin\left(\frac{2}{3}\right)$

    B. $\sin\left(\frac{\pi}{3}\right)$

    C. $\sin\left(\frac{-5}{6}\right)$

    D. $\sin\left(\frac{5}{6}\right)$

    E. $\sin\left(\frac{-2}{3}\right)$

37. Solve the following equation: $y = \frac{2x + 1}{x - 3}$ for x in terms of y.

    A. $x = -\frac{1}{2}$

    B. $x = -4$

    C. $x = \frac{2y + 1}{y - 3}$

    D. $x = \frac{3y + 1}{y - 2}$

    E. $x = 3y + \frac{2y + 1}{y}$

38. What are two positive numbers whose sum is 6 and whose product is 4?

    A. $2 + \sqrt{5}, 4 - \sqrt{5}$
    B. $3 + \sqrt{5}, 3 - \sqrt{5}$
    C. $3 + \sqrt{20}, 3 - \sqrt{20}$
    D. 6, 0
    E. 2, 4

39. When 2 is added to the numerator of the fraction $\frac{y}{x}$, the fraction equals $\frac{1}{4}$. When 2 is added to the denominator of $\frac{y}{x}$, the fraction equals $\frac{1}{5}$. What is $\frac{y}{x}$?

A. $\frac{10}{40}$

B. $\frac{10}{48}$

C. $\frac{12}{44}$

D. $\frac{1}{3}$

E. $\frac{1}{2}$

40. If snow is falling to the ground at a rate of 1 inch every half hour and is melting at the rate of 0.75 inch every hour, how many inches deep should the snow be after 8 hours of snowfall?

A. 10
B. 22
C. 12
D. 4
E. 2

Answer Key

MODEL EXAMINATION B

Survey of the Natural Sciences

1. D	14. C	27. D	40. A	53. C	65. B	77. B	89. A
2. C	15. E	28. D	41. C	54. D	66. C	78. D	90. D
3. A	16. A	29. E	42. D	55. D	67. C	79. A	91. C
4. E	17. A	30. E	43. D	56. B	68. E	80. D	92. B
5. B	18. C	31. C	44. C	57. D	69. C	81. B	93. E
6. E	19. B	32. D	45. A	58. B	70. C	82. C	94. A
7. C	20. D	33. A	46. D	59. C	71. B	83. B	95. C
8. A	21. C	34. B	47. A	60. A	72. E	84. E	96. A
9. C	22. E	35. B	48. C	61. E	73. D	85. A	97. B
10. B	23. C	36. E	49. B	62. D	74. C	86. C	98. D
11. C	24. C	37. D	50. A	63. C	75. D	87. B	99. A
12. E	25. B	38. C	51. C	64. D	76. C	88. B	100. A
13. A	26. A	39. E	52. A				

Perceptual Ability Test

1. D	13. D	25. D	36. A	47. E	58. C	69. D	80. D
2. E	14. C	26. A	37. A	48. A	59. B	70. C	81. A
3. D	15. A	27. C	38. C	49. B	60. E	71. C	82. A
4. B	16. D	28. B	39. B	50. C	61. A	72. B	83. B
5. A	17. C	29. D	40. D	51. C	62. B	73. B	84. D
6. E	18. B	30. A	41. C	52. A	63. C	74. B	85. A
7. C	19. A	31. B	42. B	53. C	64. B	75. D	86. D
8. E	20. B	32. A	43. B	54. D	65. E	76. B	87. B
9. B	21. A	33. C	44. B	55. A	66. C	77. B	88. C
10. E	22. D	34. A	45. A	56. D	67. B	78. C	89. C
11. C	23. C	35. D	46. B	57. B	68. A	79. B	90. A
12. C	24. D						

Reading Comprehension Test

1. A	8. E	15. C	21. A	27. E	33. E	39. E	45. C
2. E	9. C	16. D	22. E	28. C	34. C	40. C	46. E
3. B	10. B	17. E	23. D	29. E	35. E	41. B	47. E
4. D	11. E	18. B	24. B	30. C	36. D	42. A	48. A
5. E	12. D	19. D	25. A	31. B	37. A	43. E	49. E
6. A	13. A	20. A	26. C	32. A	38. D	44. B	50. B
7. B	14. E						

Quantitative Reasoning Test

1. D	6. B	11. C	16. C	21. C	26. C	31. B	36. A
2. B	7. B	12. E	17. D	22. B	27. C	32. C	37. D
3. C	8. D	13. A	18. E	23. C	28. D	33. B	38. B
4. D	9. B	14. B	19. D	24. B	29. C	34. D	39. B
5. B	10. A	15. D	20. D	25. B	30. E	35. A	40. A

Answer Key

Answers Explained

SURVEY OF THE NATURAL SCIENCES

1. **D** Each amino acid is encoded by three nucleotides, therefore $120 \times 3 = 360$.

2. **C** Molecular oxygen is the final electron acceptor in cellular respiration.

3. **A** Mitosis produces identical daughter cells, while meiosis produces genetically diverse haploid cells. Mitosis and meiosis both involve formation of spindle fibers and division of centromeres. In meiosis, homologous chromosomes form tetrads and sex chromosomes segregate.

4. **E** Autotrophic organisms are "self-feeders" that produce their own food by obtaining energy from chemicals (chemoautotrophs) or sunlight (photoautotrophs).

5. **B** The ovaries contain hundreds of thousands of follicles, each of which contains an ovum that it protects and nourishes. During each menstrual cycle, one follicle releases its ovum.

6. **E** Glycolysis is the first step of cellular respiration and yields 2 ATP. In the absence of oxygen, pyruvate is then fermented into lactic acid or ethanol without producing any additional ATP. In the presence of oxygen, pyruvate continues down the path of aerobic respiration yielding 36 ATP.

7. **C** Chloroplasts are found only in photosynthetic cells such as plant cells.

8. **A** A main function of the liver is to detoxify the body. Ammonia, a toxic substance, is converted to urea in liver cells.

9. **C** Interstitial Leydig cells produce testosterone in response to leutinizing hormone. Sertoli cells of the seminiferous tubules are the site of spermatogenesis.

10. **B** A bacteriophage is a virus that infects a bacteria.

11. **C** See explanation for question 6.

12. **E** Eukaryotic cell membranes are semipermeable, fluid lipid bilayers studded with protein gates and channels. The electron transport chain occurs in the inner mitochondrial membrane in eukaryotic cells; in prokaryotes, an invaginated portion of the cell membrane is the site.

13. **A** The spinal cord is part of the nervous system, which arises from the ectodermal germ layer.

14. **C** Transcription is the process by which a complementary strand of mRNA is made using DNA as the template. RNA polymerase catalyzes the addition of nucleotides to the mRNA.

15. **E** Substrate-level phosphorylation, the direct enzymatic addition of a phosphate group to an ADP molecule forming ATP, occurs in glycolysis. In oxidative phosphorylation of the electron transport chain, energy stored in the mitochondria is used to make ATP.

16. **A** Chiasmata form between homologous chromosomes during prophase I of meiosis, allowing for crossing over and exchange of genetic material.

17. **A** Many organelles, including the nucleus, are enclosed by a bilayer membrane. Ribosomes and centrioles are not enclosed by a membrane. Peroxisomes have only a single-layered membrane.

18. **C** Primary structure is the sequence of amino acids, secondary structure is the result of hydrogen bonds forming an alpha-helix or a beta-sheet, tertiary structure involves many different types of bonds and is responsible for the three-dimensional structure of the protein, and quaternary structure is the overall structure that results from different protein subunits fitting together.

19. **B** The Hardy-Weinberg equation is $p^2 + 2pq + q^2 = 1$, where p = the frequency of the dominant allele and q = the frequency of the recessive allele. The percentage of the population that is homozygous dominant is p^2, the percentage of heterozygotes is $2pq$, and the percentage of recessive homozygotes is q^2. We are told that $q^2 = 0.09$; therefore, $q = 0.3$. We also know that $p + q = 1$, so we solve that $p = 0.7$. Plugging these numbers into the equation, we see that $2pq = 0.42$; therefore, 42% of the population is heterozygous for the albino trait.

20. **D** Cnidarians include corals, sea anemones, and jellyfish. Cnidarians have a tissue level of design (no organs), are radially symmetrical, and are characterized by the presence of nematocysts (stinging cells).

21. **C** Natural selection favors organisms that have high fitness, or the ability to produce viable offspring.

22. **E** Myelinated axons have portions that are insulated by Schwann cells and parts that are not insulated called Nodes of Ranvier. In saltatory conduction, the impulse "jumps" from node to node, propagating a signal much faster than an unmyelinated axon.

23. **C** A simple Punnett square will show that the probability for a homozygous dominant child is 0.25, the probability of a child being a heterozygote is 0.5, and the probability of a child with albinism is 0.25.

24. **C** Gastrulation is the distinction of cell lines into ectoderm, mesoderm, and endoderm. Neurulation involves cells of the mesoderm forming the notochord, which will later go on to form the skeletal spinal column. Remember that the spinal cord and brain are part of the nervous system, formed by the ectoderm.

25. **B** Ribosomes are the site of protein synthesis. Proteins are modified, stored, and shipped to other destinations by the Golgi apparatus.

26. **A** Cholesterol is a steroid. An example of a simple carbohydrate is glucose, a polysaccharide is glycogen, an amino acid is tyrosine, and a protein is albumin.

27. **D** Microtubules are composed of alpha- and beta-tubulin proteins.

Answers Explained

28. D The spinal cord is part of the central nervous system. Afferent, efferent, and cranial nerves such as the optic nerve and olfactory tract are part of the peripheral nervous system.

29. E A slow and stready release of FSH stimulates the follicle to grow and produce estrogen. Estrogen then builds up and, after reaching a threshold, causes a surge in LH and smaller but noticeable increase in FSH. Once the follicle releases its ovum during ovulation, the corps luteum produces estrogen and progesterone.

30. E In independent assortment, the number of possible gametes can be determined by the formula 2^n, where $n =$ haploid number.

31. C Viruses are composed only of genetic information surrounded by a protein coat. They do not have any cytoplasm or cell membrane and rely on a living cell in order to reproduce.

32. D Glucose and fructose are monosaccharides. Sucrose is composed of one glucose and one fructose joined together.

33. A An influx of calcium allows myosin to bind to actin in the process of muscle contraction.

34. B The humoral immune response involves antibody-producing. B-cells with some assistance from helper T-cells. The cell-mediated immune response utilizes cytotoxic T-cells, also with the assistance of helper T-cells.

35. B The endocrine cells of the pancreas secrete insulin directly into the bloodstream. The exocrine cells of the pancreas secrete protein-digesting enzymes and bicarbonate into the duodenum of the small intestine.

36. E Platyhelminthes demonstrate bilateral symmetry. All other phyla include at least some organisms that are radially symmetric.

37. D Allopatric speciation involves species divergence in the presence of a geographical barrier, in this case, the mesh fence.

38. C In Batesian mimicry, a harmless species resembles a dangerous species: in Mullerian mimicry, two dangerous species look alike.

39. E Cytosine pairs with guanine. Adenine pairs with thymine in DNA, but uracil in DNA. T pairs with adenine. Therefore, complementary mRNA of a DNA strand that reads CAT is GUA.

40. A K selected species tend to invest heavy parental care in the few offspring they produce and have a finite amount of resources, limiting the population growth. However, $r =$ selected species are found in less stable environments; they produce a large number of offspring with little or no parental investment. Only a select few offspring will survive to reproduce.

41. C Each Cl has a -1 charge, so the single S has to have a $+2$ charge.

42. D This is a standard question on the DAT identifying NH_3 as trigonal pyramidal.

43. D $H_2C_2O_4$ is the acid, H_2O is the base, $HC_2O_4^-$ is the conjugate base, and H_3O^+ is the conjugate acid.

44. C If the mass is 17 with 8 protons, then there must be 9 neutrons.

45. A In this case, each P has a charge of +5. The P in all other answers have lower oxidation states.

46. D Addition of a proton to Na and release of a neutron will net ^{22}Mg.

47. A When the ion product exceeds K_{sp}, precipitation results.

48. C A negative ΔG means spontaneous conversion of reactants to products.

49. B The characteristics listed in the stem are inherent in ionic solids. Ionic solids by themselves are not good conductors of electricity. However, some ionic solids are good conductors of electricity when dissolved in water.

50. A The critical point is defined as the temperature at which liquid and gas densities are equal and the phase boundaries disappear.

51. C pH is equivalent to $-\log[H^+]$. In this case $[H^+] = 25/(.1 \times 36)$.

52. A The combination of Boyle's law and Charles's law, $P_1V_1/T_1 = P_2V_2/T_2$, can be used to solve this problem. In this case, the volume remains constant, so $T_2 = T_1P_2/P_1 = 256$ K.

53. C S has an oxidation state of +6 for each compound in answer C.

54. D Bromine has a molecular weight of just under 80, and oxygen has a molecular weight of 16. So 80/144 = 55.5%.

55. D Since there are 6.02×10^{23} molecules per mole, then $104.1(4.5 \times 10^{20})/(6.02 \times 10^{23}) = 0.0778$ g.

56. B Sublimation is the transformation of a solid directly to a gas.

57. D Salts have very high melting points because freeing ions requires large amounts of energy.

58. B Calcium does not have an oxidation state of +4.

59. C Two NH_4^+ ions will be released in addition to a single $C_2O_4^{2-}$.

60. A Molality is defined as moles of solute per 1000 grams of solvent. For conversion to molarity, the density will be needed.

61. E Answers A, B, C, and D are all correct statements.

62. D The quantum number l cannot be equal to the principal quantum number n.

63. C Dividing the percentages by formula weights of each of hydrogen, carbon, and oxygen nets a ratio of 3:1:1, respectively. Hence, the empirical formula is CH_3O.

64. D HSO_4^- is the only molecule in the group that can release a proton and also act as a base.

65. B The percent of nitrogen is equivalent to 100 multiplied by the total grams of nitrogen in a mole of the compound divided by total grams of all components.

66. **C** The conversion of a liquid to a gas is accompanied by a large increase in entropy.

67. **C** Balance H first, then N and finally O.

68. **E** pH $= -\log [H^+] = -\log 0.00001 = 5$.

69. **C** One aspect of halogens is that electonegativity decreases with moving down the group.

70. **C** 460 grams of ethanol is equivalent to 10 moles. If a 5 molar solution is needed, then 2 liters can be made.

71. **B** Carbon double bonds are sp^2 hybridized.

72. **E** A structural isomer only has the same molecular formula. A conformer is the same molecule except for rotation around a carbon-carbon single bond. An epimer is a diastereomer that only differs in the spatial arrangement of groups at one chiral carbon. Enantiomers are non-superimposable mirror images of each other. Answer E, diastereomers, are stereoisomers that are not mirror images of each other and differ at more than one chiral carbon.

73. **D** A carbon-carbon triple bond is linear and 180 degrees. A carbon-carbon double bond is planar and 120 degrees.

74. **C** The carboxylic acid has the most acidic hydrogen.

75. **D** Structures II and IV obey Huckel's rule for aromaticity.

76. **C** C-2 and C-3 are both chiral carbons since they each bond to four different groups.

77. **B** The *t*-butyl compound is the most stable radical.

78. **D** Alcohols have higher boiling points than hydrocarbons of the same lengths. *n*-alcohols have higher boiling points than alcohols with the same number of carbons. The longer the length of the alcohol, the higher the boiling point.

79. **A** Only one peak will result since all four hydrogens are identical.

80. **D** Brönsted-Lowry bases accept protons, and in this case CH_3O^- and $C_2H_5O^-$ are the bases.

81. **B** In initiation, Cl_2 must be split into two radicals.

82. **C** The *n*-butyl halide is the most susceptible to backside attack in an S_N2 mechanism.

83. **B** Cycloalkanes have higher boiling points than *n*-alkanes or iso-alkanes with the same number of carbons.

84. **E** A hydrocarbon will usually be less soluble than a compound with a polar atom in its structure.

85. **A** This is an addition reaction that follows Markovnikov's rule.

86. **C** This appears to be an elimination reaction since an alcohol is being converted to an alkene. Since two products are formed it is likely that the intermediate is a carbocation, and so the reaction must be via an $E1$ mechanism.

‌

87. B Tertiary carbocations are always the most stable.

88. B A Grignard reagent is a very powerful nucleophile, having the power of an RCH_2^- as a nucleophile.

89. A Numbering starts at the acid group carbon for this pentanoic acid.

90. D The *t*-butyl carbocation is the most stable cation to undergo a S_N1 mechanism.

91. C A polar yet nonreactive molecule is best for an S_N2 reaction.

92. B The rate-limiting step in an S_N1 reaction is the formation of a carbocation.

93. E A diene attacked by a dienophile results in a cyclical compound.

94. A This is a radical addition reaction that is anti-Markovnikov.

95. C This is a multioxidation reaction, which results in two carboxylic acid products.

96. A Ozonolysis produces carbonyls at both carbons of a carbon-carbon double bond.

97. B Wittig reactions produce alkenes.

98. D Carbon monoxide (CO) is not produced on complete combustion.

99. A Small hydrocarbons have low boiling points.

100. A S_N1 and S_N2.

PERCEPTUAL ABILITY TEST

1. D Entry-3.

2. E Entry-2.

3. D Entry-2.

4. B Entry-2, after 90 degree rotation counterclockwise.

5. A Entry-2, after 90 degree, counterclockwise, 180 degree rotation. Note small notch.

6. E Entry-3, after 90 degree clockwise and 180 degree rotation.

7. C Entry-3, rotated 90 degrees clockwise, 90 degree rotation. Note notches.

8. E Entry-2, note number of sides and position of side extrusions.

9. B Entry-1, note positions of angular surfaces.

10. E Entry-2, after 90 degree rotation clockwise.

11. C Entry-2, note thickness beneath notch.

12. C Entry-2, note relative positions of notches.

13. D Entry-3, note position of extension.

14. C Entry-2, note positions and sizes of notches.

‌Answers Explained

15. **A** Entry-1, note relative sizes and positions (planes) of notches.

16. **D** Note front and end views show hidden lines.

17. **C** Note front view shows 6 lines (3 hidden), and partial enclosure.

18. **B** Note positions of circles relative to object sides and each other.

19. **A** Note end view shows 6 lines, 3 hidden above full-length enclosure.

20. **B** Note front view shows 5 solid lines, note size of lower extension.

21. **A** Side shows extension toward front and 1 hidden line. Note hidden mid-line.

22. **D** End view shows 5 lines. Note the position of hidden lines.

23. **C** Front view shows 5 lines, 2 hidden.

24. **D** Front view shows 3 lines, all solid.

25. **D** End view shows 9 lines. Note positions of bottom lines, solid, and enclosure.

26. **A** Top view shows 6 lines, 2 hidden. Note relative positions.

27. **C** Front view shows 5 solid lines.

28. **B** Note omissions.

29. **D** Front and end view show 3 lines at top.

30. **A** End view shows 7 lines. Note position of hidden lines.

31. **B** 1 appears smallest (omit A, C), 4 appears smaller than 3 (omit D).

32. **A** 4 appears smallest (omit C), 1 appears largest (omit B, D).

33. **C** 2 appears smallest (omit B, D), 3 appears largest (omit A).

34. **A** 3 appears smallest (omit B, D), 2 appears smaller than 4 (omit C).

35. **D** 4 appears largest and 1 appears smallest (omit A, B, C).

36. **A** 2 appears smallest (omit D, C), 3 appears smaller than 1 (omit B).

37. **A** 4 appears smallest (omit B, C), 2 appears largest (omit D).

38. **C** 2 appears smallest (omit A, D), 3 appears largest (omit B).

39. **B** 1 appears smallest (omit C), 2 appears largest (omit A, D).

40. **D** 3 appears smallest (omit B, C), 1 appears largest (omit A).

41. **C** 1 appears smallest (omit B, D), 2 appears largest (omit A).

42. **B** 3 appears largest (omit A, C, D).

43. **B** 3 appears smallest (omit A, C, D).

44. **B** 3 appears largest (omit A, C), 4 appears smaller than 1 (omit D).

45. **A** 1 appears smallest (omit B, C), 3 smaller than 2 (omit D).

46. **B** 2 folds at final position (omit A, E), 1 unfold identifies B.

47. **E** 3 folds at final position (omit A, B), 2 unfolds identifies E.

48. **A** 4 folds at final position (omit D, E), 2 unfolds identifies A.

49. **B** 8 folds at final position (omit A, C, D), 2 unfolds identifies B.

50. **C** 4 folds at final position (omit A, D, E), 2 unfolds identifies C.

51. **C** 4 folds at final position (omit A, B, D), 2 unfolds identifies C.

52. **A** 2 folds at final position (omit B, D, E), 2 unfolds identifies A.

53. **C** 6 folds at final position (omit A, B, D, E).

54. **D** 6 folds at final position (omit A, B, C, E).

55. **A** 3 folds at final position (omit B, D, E), 1 unfold identifies A.

56. **D** 4 folds at final position (omit A, C, E), 1 unfold identifies D.

57. **B** 8 folds at final position (omit D, E), 2 unfolds identifies B.

58. **C** 4 folds at final position (omit A, B, D, E).

59. **B** 2 folds at final position (omit A, D, E), 1 unfold identifies B.

60. **E** 6 folds at final position (omit A, B, C, D).

61. **A** Notice 2 partially hidden cubes (2, 3 painted surfaces).

62. **B** Notice 2 partially hidden cubes (2, 3 painted surfaces).

63. **C** Notice 2 partially hidden cubes (2, 3 painted surfaces).

64. **B** Notice 2 partially hidden cubes (2, 3 painted surfaces).

65. **E** Notice 3 fully hidden cubes (1, 1, 2 painted surfaces).

66. **C** Notice 3 fully hidden cubes (1, 1, 2 painted surfaces).

67. **B** Notice 1 fully hidden cube (2 painted surfaces).

68. **A** Notice 1 fully hidden cube (2 painted surfaces).

69. **D** Notice 1 fully hidden cube (2 painted surfaces).

70. **C** Notice 2 partially hidden cubes (3, 2 painted surfaces).

71. **C** Notice 2 partially hidden cubes (3, 2 painted surfaces).

72. **B** Notice 2 partially hidden cubes (3, 2 painted surfaces).

73. **B** Notice 2 partially hidden cubes, 1 full hidden cube (4, 4, 3 painted surfaces).

74. **B** Notice 2 partially hidden cubes, 1 full hidden cube (4, 4, 3 painted surfaces).

75. **D** Notice 2 partially hidden cubes, 1 full hidden cube (4, 4, 3 painted surfaces).

76. **B** Focus on adjoining sides.

77. **B** Focus on adjoining sides of eight-sided figure.

78. **C** Focus on all object shapes and proportions.

79. **B** Notice relative positions of shaded and nonshaded three-sided figures.

80. **D** Focus on relative positions of halved square.

81. **A** Focus on relative positions of shaded side (nonsquare).

82. **A** Focus on larger clear three-sided figure.

83. **B** Note number of sides and shape of shorter lines of three-sided figures.

84. **D** Focus on small squares relative to shaded four-sided figure.

85. **A** Focus on relative positions of shaded half-square and shaded square.

86. **D** Focus on positions of sides and joining point.

87. **B** Focus on split square and adjoining shadowed three-sided figure.

88. **C** Focus on split square, adjoining four-sided figure, and split small rectangle.

89. **C** Focus on long rectangle, smaller "end-caps," and positions of "points."

90. **A** Notice the available shapes and number of these shapes.

READING COMPREHENSION TEST

1. **A** Paragraph 6, sentence 2.

2. **E** Paragraph 12.

3. **B** Paragraph 2, sentence 6.

4. **D** Paragraph 9, sentence 1.

5. **E** Last paragraph.

6. **A** Paragraph 3, sentence 1.

7. **B** Paragraph 7, last sentence.

8. **E** Paragraph 4, sentence 1.

9. **C** Paragraph 13. You must take information provided in the first two sentences and deduce that resorption take places "in a direction opposite to the crown," which is the apex.

10. **B** Paragraph 9, sentence 2.

11. **E** Paragraph 6, sentence 3.

12. **D** Paragraph 2, last sentence.

13. **A** Paragraph 10, last two sentences.

14. **E** Paragraph 4, sentence 2.

15. **C** Paragraph 5, last sentence.

16. **D** Paragraph 1, sentence 1.

17. **E** Paragraph 3, sentences 2–4.

18. **B** Paragraph 2, sentences 4–5.

19. **D** Paragraph 6, sentence 3.

20. **A** Paragraph 4, sentence 9.

21. **A** Paragraph 3, sentence 2.

22. **E** Paragraph 2, sentence 1.

23. **D** Last paragraph, sentence 2.

24. **B** Paragraph 3, sentence 13.

25. **A** Paragraph 3, sentence 8.

26. **C** Paragraph 5, sentence 3.

27. **E** Paragraph 2, last sentence.

28. **C** Paragraph 4, sentences 4–5.

29. **E** Paragraph 7, last sentence.

30. **C** Paragraph 2, sentence 7.

31. **B** Paragraph 5, sentence 4.

32. **A** Paragraph 5, sentence 1.

33. **E** Paragraph 4, sentence 3.

34. **C** Paragraph 10.

35. **E** Paragraph 18, sentence 6.

36. **D** Paragraph 14, sentence 4.

37. **A** Paragraph 2, sentence 1.

38. **D** Paragraph 12, sentence 2.

39. **E** Paragraph 17, sentence 6; paragraph 19, last sentence.

40. **C** Paragraph 15, sentence 1.

41. **B** Paragraph 4, sentence 1.

42. **A** Paragraph 13, last two sentences.

43. **E** Paragraph 19, sentence 1.

44. **B** Paragraph 15, sentence 1

45. **C** Paragraph 3, sentence 1.

46. **E** Paragraph 14, sentence 1.

47. **E** Paragraph 11, sentence 1.

48. **A** Paragraph 5, sentence 1.

49. **E** Paragraph 3, sentence 6; paragraph 4, sentence 3.

50. **B** Paragraph 16, sentence 2.

Answers Explained

QUANTITATIVE REASONING TEST

1. **D** If $4^3 = 64$, then $x/3$ must equal 3, and $x = 9$.

2. **B** Multiply the numerator to get $\sqrt{45}/\sqrt{15} = 3\sqrt{5}/5/\sqrt{2}\sqrt{5}) = 3/\sqrt{2} = (3\sqrt{2})/2$.

3. **C** There is a 50% or 1/2 probability of obtaining heads on each toss of a coin.

4. **D** To solve this problem, work from the inside and progress out.

5. **B** The probability of tossing heads six consecutive times is $(1/2)^6 = 1/64$. The probability of tossing tails six consecutive times is the same as heads. The probability of either is the sum of the two probabilities so $1/64 + 1/64 = 1/32$.

6. **B** Find the lowest common denominator, convert each fraction, and then sum. $10/12 + 8/12 + 3/12 = 21/12 = 1\ (3/4)$.

7. **B** The equation to be solved is $2n - 2 = n + 8$, where n is the smallest even integer. Thus, $n = 10$, and the largest integer is $n + 8 = 18$.

8. **D** Slope is y/x, and in this case $y/x = (5 - 6)/(2 - (-3)) = -1/5$.

9. **B** In this case, the sum of ratios $= 10$. Since there are $180°$ in a triangle, each angle of the triangle is equivalent to the ratio of the angle multiplied by $18°$ ($180°/10$). Hence, the smallest angle is $2 \times 18° = 36°$.

10. **A** Multiply the whole equation ($x + y = 2$) by 2 and subtract from $3x + 2y = 8$. From this, $x = 4$. Substitute for x in either equation to get $y = -2$, and $x - y = 6$.

11. **C** If $\tan\theta = y/x$, where y is the side opposite θ, and x is the side adjacent to θ, and $\csc\theta = h/y$, where h is the hypotenuse, then $\tan\theta\ \csc\theta = y/x$ multiplied by $h/y = h/x = \sec\theta$.

12. **E** The equation must be $y = -2x + c$ to have a -2 slope. Substitute -3 for x; and $y = 1$.

13. **A** Convert $3x^2/12$ to $9x^2/36$; then add the latter to $7x^2/36$ to get $\sqrt{16x^2}/36 = 2x/3$.

14. **B** The equation to solve is $x + 6 = 2x - 2$. In this case, $x = 8$.

15. **D** For $N = $ nickels and $D = $ dimes, the two equations from the problem are: $0.05\ N + 0.1D = 5.50$ and $N - 5 = D$. Substitute $D + 5$ for N in the first equation, and $D = 35$.

16. **C** The equation from the problem is $n + n + 2 = (n + 4) - 10$. So $n = -8$ and the third integer is -4.

17. **D** If $\sin(A + B) = \sin A \cos B + \sin B \cos A$, then $\sin(2A) = 2\sin A \cos A$

18. **E** If the tires have all traveled the same amount, then each tire has traveled $4/5$ of 24,000 miles $= 19,200$ miles.

19. D If 60 women dentists are not from the west coast, then 40 are from the west coast. Hence, 960 men dentists are from the west coast.

20. D A 10% increase for two consecutive years is a 21% increase overall. Divide $21,780 by 1.21, and the starting salary is $18,000.

21. C If x plants were sold at 75 cents each to meet the cost of $150, then $x = 200$, and so 300 plants were purchased.

22. B Determine the total miles driven for the time driven, then calculate miles per hour. The automobile traveled 45 miles in the first hour and then 30 miles in the next 30 minutes. This is 75 miles in 90 minutes, and translates to 50 mph.

23. C Multiply both sides of the equation by $2(2x - 1)$ to get $2x - 1 + 8 = 24x - 12$. In this case, $x = 19/22$.

24. B The volume of the box is $16 \times 10 \times 8 = 1280$ cubic inches. For a cube to have a volume of 1280 cubic inches, a side must be a little larger than 10.85 inches.

25. B $(27)/5 = x/4$ so $x = (108)/5 = 21\ 3/5$.

26. C Since 3, 6, and 9 are multiples of 3, there are 3 multiples in 9 numbers. So the probability is $3/9 = 1/3$.

27. C The discount is $3050 - $2745 = 305. The rate of discount is $305/$3050 = 10\%$.

28. D The total solution has $(0.2 \times 10\ \text{cc} + 0.4 \times 20\ \text{cc})/30\ \text{cc} = 1/3 = 33\ 1/3\%$.

29. C Substitute $2y$ for x in the first equation. Multiply the second equation by 2 and subtract from the first equation. In this case, y is eliminated, and h is the only variable remaining.

30. E 85% multiplied by $3/x = 8$, so $x = 2.55/8 = 0.319$.

31. B Convert $2\sqrt{20}$ to $4\sqrt{5}$. Convert $\sqrt{45}$ to $3\sqrt{5}$. The sum is $7\sqrt{5}$.

32. C At a net of 2 miles per hour, it will take 30 minutes to go one mile upstream. It will take 20 minutes to drift the mile downstream, so the total time is 50 minutes.

33. B The two equations from the problem are $(x + 1)/y = 1/3$ and $x/(y + 3) = 1/6$. Cross-multiply and subtract one equation from the other to eliminate y, and then solve for x. Substitute for x in either equation to determine y. Finally, determine x/y.

34. D Rearrange the equation first to $xy + 2x = 1/4$, then to $xy = 1/4 - 2x$, followed by $y = (1/4 - 2x)/x$, and finally $y = 1/4x - 2$.

35. A Calculate the numerator and denominator separately. The numerator is 14/15. The denominator is 11/3. Invert the denominator and multiply the numerator to get 11/55.

36. A At one peak of the oscillating sin curve, sin pi/2 = 1, and sin pi/3 and sin 2pi/3 are equal distances away on either side of the peak and are of equal value.

37. D Rearrange the original equation to $y(x - 3) = 2x + 1$, then $xy - 3y = 2x + 1$, then $xy - 2x = 3y + 1$, then $x(y - 2) = 3y + 1$, and finally $x = (3y + 1)/(y - 2)$.

38. B The two equations from the problem are $x + y = 6$ and $xy = 4$. Substitute for either x or y in the second equation, and use the quadratic equation: $(-b \pm \sqrt{b^2 - 4ac})/2a$.

39. B The two equations are $(2 + y)/x = 1/4$ and $y/(x + 2) = 1/5$. Manipulate the equations so that either x or y can be eliminated by subtraction of one equation from the other, then solve for the other variable. Once a variable has been determined, find the value of the other variable by substitution of the known variable into either original equation.

40. A After every hour, 1.25 in. of snow will accumulate. After 8 hours, 10 in. of snow will accumulate.

Answers Explained

Standard Score to Raw Score Conversion Chart

Standard Score	QRT	RCT	Biology	General Chemistry	Organic Chemistry	SNS (Total Science)	PAT
30	40	50	–	–	30	100	90
29	39	–	40	–	–	99	89
28	–	49	–	30	29	98	88
27	–	–	–	–	–	97	–
26	38	48	39	–	–	96	87
25	37	47	–	29	28	95	85–86
24	36	–	38	–	–	94	84
23	35	46	–	28	27	92–93	81–83
22	33–34	43–45	37	–	–	89–91	78–80
21	31–32	40–42	35–36	27	26	86–88	74–77
20	29–30	37–39	34	26	25	81–85	70–73
19	27–28	34–36	32–33	24–25	23–24	76–80	68–69
18	24–26	31–33	30–31	22–23	21–22	70–75	59–64
17	22–23	26–30	27–29	20–21	19–20	63–69	52–58
16	19–21	24–25	24–26	18–19	17–18	56–62	46–51
15	16–18	20–23	21–23	16–17	15–16	48 55	39–45
14	14–15	18–19	18–20	13–15	13–14	41–47	32–38
13	11–13	16–17	15–17	11–12	11–12	33–40	26–31
12	9–10	13–15	12–14	9–10	8–10	27–32	21–25
11	7–8	10–12	10–11	7–8	7	21–26	17–20
10	6	9	8–9	6	5–6	17–20	13–16
9	5	7–8	6–7	4–5	4	13–16	10–12
8	4	–	5	3	3	10–12	7 9
7	3	6	4	–	–	7–9	6
6	2	4–5	3	2	2	5–6	4–5
5	–	–	2	–	–	4	3
4	–	3	–	1	1	3	2
3	1	2	1	–	–	2	–
2	–	–	–	–	–	–	–
1	0	1	0	0	0	0–1	0–1

Appendix

ACRONYMS

You will come across more acronyms in the application process than you can possibly imagine. Some of the most frequently used acronyms are included here.

AADR	American Association for Dental Research
AADS	American Association of Dental Schools
AADSAS	American Association of Dental Schools Application Service
ADA	American Dental Association
AEGD	Advanced Education in General Dentistry
ASDA	American Student Dental Association
B.A.	Bachelor of Arts
BCP	Biology, Chemistry, Physics (AADSAS application)
B.S.	Bachelor of Science
CDA	Canadian Dental Association
DAT	Dental Admission Test (U.S.), Dental Aptitude Test (Canada)
D.D.S.	Doctor of Dental Surgery (equivalent to D.M.D.)
D.M.D.	Doctor of Dental Medicine (equivalent to D.D.S.)
DMO	Dental Maintenance Organization
EFC	Expected Family Contribution
EFN	Exceptional Financial Need Scholarship
FAF	Financial Aid Form
FAFSA	Free Application for Federal Student Aid
GPA	Grade Point Average
GPR	General Practice Residency
HEAL	Health Education Assistance Loan
HMO	Health Maintenance Organization
HPSL	Health Professions Student Loan
HPTQ	High Probability Test Question
LDS	Loans for Disadvantaged Students
M.A.	Master of Arts
M.D.	Doctor of Medicine
M.S.	Master of Science
NDA	National Dental Association

NIDCR	National Institute of Dental and Craniofacial Research (a division of NIH)
NIH	National Institutes of Health
PASS	Postdoctoral Application Support Service
PAT	Perceptual Ability Test
Ph.D.	Doctor of Philosophy
QRT	Quantitative Reasoning Test
RCT	Reading Comprehension Test
SDS	Scholarships for Disadvantaged Students
SNDA	Student National Dental Association
SNS	Survey of the Natural Sciences
TOEFL	Test of English as a Foreign Language
WHO	World Health Organization

FREQUENTLY ASKED QUESTIONS

The following list includes some of the most frequently asked questions that applicants have. The answers should clear up some of the confusion that you may feel about the exam, the application process, dental school, and the dental profession. The questions are presented in four sections:

- Questions Regarding the DAT

- Questions Regarding the Application Process

- Questions Regarding Dental School

- Questions Regarding the Profession of Dentistry

Questions Regarding the DAT

How Do I Familiarize Myself with the Test Format?

Visit the ADA website (*www.ada.org*), which contains test information as well as sample test questions that you can download.

What Is the Scoring of the DAT?

The highest score is 30, with 18–19 being competitive for admittance. Refer to the *Scoring* section on page 2.

What Is an Average Score?

About 17. This is not very competitive for admission.

What Is the Difference Between a Raw Score and a Standard Score? Do Both Get Sent to the Dental Schools that I Checked on my DAT Application?

A raw score is the number of correctly marked answers on a section. That number is converted to a scaled score called the standard score. The score you and the dental schools will receive is the standard score.

Is the DAT an Aptitude Test or an Achievement Test?

Webster's New World Dictionary defines an aptitude test as a test for determining the probability of a person's success in some activity for which he or she is not yet trained. The Canadian Dental Association considers its DAT to be an aptitude test. The SNS, however, is clearly an achievement test as it tests specific knowledge in the discipline of the natural sciences.

When Should I Begin Studying for the DAT?

Three months is adequate preparation time for most test takers. Schedule your DAT accordingly.

Can I Retake the DAT?

You can take the DAT as many times as you wish. The last four attempts will be reported to dental schools. You must wait at least 90 days between examinations.

How Are the Testing Centers Set Up?

You will take the exam on a personal computer similar to one you may have at home or one that you will find in a computer lab at your undergraduate institution. All computers have high resolution monitors. You will be given erasable boards and markers to work out problems and to use for the reading comprehension test. Although the center should be quiet, you will be provided with ear plugs to prevent any distraction from another examinee's typing or mouse clicking.

Can I Leave the Testing Center During the Test Battery?

You will be allowed a 15-minute break approximately halfway through the examination battery (after both the SNS and the PAT have been completed). During this break you may use the restroom, eat a snack, or leave the building. Make sure, however, that you are ready to resume the exam 15 minutes later. This break is optional.

When Will I Receive my Scores?

When you have finished the test, your score will be printed out at the center. A report will be sent electronically to the ADA Department of Testing Services that day, and dental schools will receive your scores within 3 weeks of your test date.

What Should I Take to the Exam?

Two forms of ID (driver's license, state ID, passport, employee ID card) are required. Both must have your signature, and one must have a current photo. Be sure to arrive 30 minutes before the examination time.

Can I Reschedule my Exam?

Yes. However, you must call by noon two days before your test date.

I Have Taken the MCAT. How Is the DAT Different from the MCAT? How Should I Prepare for the DAT?

Many students taking the DAT either have already taken the MCAT or are preparing for both exams simultaneously. Here are four differences between the two exams:

1. There is no physics section on the DAT.

2. The MCAT does not have an analogous PAT section.

3. No writing sample is required on the DAT.

4. The *formats* of the questions differ.

Here are the four sections on the exam:

- *Medical College Admission Test (MCAT)*
  Verbal Reasoning: humanities-based readings
  Physical Sciences: physics, general chemistry
  Biological Sciences: biology, organic chemistry
  Writing Sample

- *Dental Admission Test (DAT)*
  Natural Sciences: biology, organic chemistry, general chemistry
  Perceptual Ability Test
  Reading Comprehension Test: science-based readings
  Quantitative Reasoning Test

The subjects common to both exams are reading analysis, general chemistry, biology, and organic chemistry. The format of the questions is quite different on the two exams. Also, many students who have taken both examinations consider the MCAT sections on biology, organic chemistry, and general chemistry to be significantly more difficult than their DAT counterparts. Therefore, in preparing for the DAT, you should briefly review the science sections and concentrate on practice for the Perceptual Ability Test, Reading Comprehension Test, and Quantitative Reasoning Test.

Questions Regarding the Application Process

What Is AADSAS?

This acronym stands for American Association of Dental Schools Application Service. AADSAS is a centralized application clearinghouse; its purpose is to simplify the application process by providing one standardized application. All but a few dental schools require that you use AADSAS to initiate the application process. The packet of application materials comes with an instruction booklet that is quite thorough and detailed in regard to filling out the application.

How Can I Check the Status of my AADSAS Application?

Contact the organization.

What Can I Do to Maximize my Chances for Admission?

Send in your completed AADSAS application as soon as possible. AADSAS packets are available during June and July prior to the year of matriculation. As a wise applicant, you will have written your Personal Statement before receiving the AADSAS application. By preparing the Personal Statement in advance, you can minimize the turn-around time as this is the most time-consuming section of the application. As soon as the application is completed and double-checked for accuracy, return the packet to AADSAS, making sure all parts of the application are included.

Many schools have a rolling admissions policy; therefore, the applications received first are given the greatest consideration. When a dental school has received deposits for most of the first year seats in the spring of the year of matriculation, competition for the last few seats becomes exponentially greater. Even though AADSAS and dental schools give dates by which applications must be received for consideration, you can be sure that by March or April about 90% of the first-year class has already been chosen.

Should I Send my DAT Scores to AADSAS?

No. The official report will be sent from the ADA to the dental schools you indicated.

What Percent of Applicants Actually Are Admitted to at Least One Dental School?

Approximately 53% .

How Many Schools Should I Apply to?

More than 12 schools may be excessive and fewer than 5 may not be enough. If you have above-average scores on the DAT and an above-average GPA, however, the lower number may be sufficient if you know where you want to go to school.

Does it Matter What my Undergraduate Degree Was in?

Provided that you have taken the prerequisites for dental school admission, your undergraduate major does not matter at all. Your life will be easier though, once you are in dental school, if you have had some biochemistry, physiology, anatomy, micro-biology, or other advanced biology courses. Approximately 55 % of enrolled dental students have majored in the biological sciences: 15% in chemistry/physical sciences; 13% in pre-health science; 4% in language/arts/architecture; 4% in business; and 3% in engineering.

The DAT reported score is a measure of how you performed in comparison to everyone else who took the exam. Having a background in science limited to the minimum prerequisites may put you at a disadvantage in relation to someone who has taken 60–90 credits in biology and chemistry. It is not unreasonable, however, to think that you can perform above average on the DAT with sufficient preparation. The BCP (Biology, Chemistry, Physics) GPA reported on AADSAS is representative of fewer classes; therefore, excellent grades are needed in these prerequisite courses.

Should I Take Classes Now that I Will Have to Take in Dental School?

Doing so is not mandatory, but it will make your life a lot easier once you start your dental studies. It will be to your advantage to be familiar with the course work prior to your exposure to it in dental school. At that point, you will be expected to make clinical correlations to the basic sciences, a task that will be easier if you start with some foundation. It should be noted, however, that although a strong performance in college in advanced-level sciences will strengthen your application, it does absolutely *no* good to take these courses as an undergraduate but not perform well.

Is it Advantageous to Go Through the Pre-Health Professions Office to Obtain Letters of Recommendation?

Yes. See the section *Letters of Recommendation* (pages 12–14) for more information.

What Is an Average GPA?

Your GPA will actually be reported through AADSAS as four different numbers: the overall GPA, the science GPA, the nonscience GPA, and the BCP GPA. Because of the difficulty of most science classes, the science GPA and BCP GPA figures are typically lower than the overall GPA and nonscience GPA figures.

In general, the following GPA figures can be used to assess your competitiveness as an applicant:

3.0–3.2 → Below average
3.2–3.5 → Average
3.5–4.0 → Above average

If your science GPA or BCP GPA is below 3, you may want to consider taking additional biology and/or chemistry courses to boost this number before applying to dental schools.

My GPA is Average. What Can I Do to Make Myself Stand Out from Other Applicants?

Stellar performance on the DAT. This number can be changed, whereas your GPA is pretty much set in stone. Remember: the two most important components of your application are your GPA and your DAT score. These are the numbers for which you will be screened in the first round of admissions. At this point, your future will hinge on a GPA and a DAT score. That's the reality of the process!

I Am Sure I Want to Go into Orthodontics. Should I Express any Desire to Become an Orthodontist to the Admissions Committee?

You will learn that half of the entering class wants to go into orthodotics. The funny thing is that there are only a few spots for this specialty, and all but a few applicants will have to reevaluate their original plans. Take one step at a time. First, work on admittance to a predoctoral dental program, then concern yourself with choosing a postdoctoral specialty. Although you may have had a memorable experience with your own orthodontist, it is wise to wait until you have bent some wires in an "ortho" class to decide that orthodontics is your destined career.

I Have Been Involved in Many Extracurricular Activities While in College. How Will this Aspect of my Life Play into the Admissions Process?

Besides indicating your involvement on the AADSAS form, you will be able to include your many extracurricular activities and accomplishments in your Personal Statement, the interview, and any supplemental application requested.

I Have Been out of School for a Few Years. How Will this Factor into my Application?

Many schools look favorably on the returning student. Returning to school after being successful in the workforce indicates two important qualities: maturity and motivation.

What Should I Do if I Am Placed on a Waiting List at the School that I Want to Attend?

Be persistent! Let the admissions office know that this school is your first choice. Also, if you know some influential people, this would be a suitable time to get in touch with them. Waiting lists are rarely as structured as schools want you to believe.

What Should I Do if I Am Not Accepted to a Dental School this Year?

Call the director of admissions at the schools to which you applied and ask exactly what aspect of your application causes them to reject you. Often they will be frank and tell you outright why you were not granted admission. Take that information at face value, and do the best you can to fix obvious problems. Remember: persistence shows motivation *and* dedication.

Questions Regarding Dental School

Where Do I Go to Find Out About Scholarships?

When you secure a seat by remitting a deposit to a dental school, the next thing you must consider is how you are going to pay for the next 4 years of your life. Securing scholarship money takes resourcefulness and some persistence. There is a tremendous amount of money available; however, you must take the initiative to get your portion of the funds. Grants are monetary disbursements that need not be repaid, whereas loans must be repaid. About 88% of financial aid to dental students is in the form of loans, and 12% comes from scholarships or grants.

The first step is to call the financial aid office at your dental school. Perhaps a brief meeting to obtain information would be helpful as well. Then contact local and state dental societies. One way successful dentists give back to the community is through financial aid to dental students. With the tremendous cost of dental school, it is also worthwhile trying to locate private foundations that offer loans at very low interest rates (1%–5%).

Go to the library and/or a local bookstore and locate published information regarding established foundations and charitable organizations.

The qualification for private grant money can be quite specific and may even appear ridiculous. To actually receive money for these sources, you will need to be persistent. Know what makes you different from the next dental student and then use these differences to your advantage.

If I Choose to Specialize, Will it Matter what Dental School I Went to when I Apply for Postdoctoral Programs?

Superior performance in comparison to your peers when in dental school is much more important than the school itself. Specialty programs place heaviest emphasis on class rank, GPA, and National Board scores.

How Are Dental Schools Ranked?

There are no official rankings for dental schools; there are simply too many factors that enter into the quality of a dental education. The quality of the education offered at a dental school should be evident in the knowledge and skills of its student body. Therefore, a good measure of a dental school education is the annual scores from the first part of the National Boards. These confidential reports from the ADA are given to the deans of the dental schools. It is made very clear that the intent of the board exams is not to rank schools; the boards are administered for the purpose of licensure. The scores from the boards, however, are the only method of ranking that is worth any consideration. *Proprietary rankings should be totally ignored as their evaluation criteria do not measure the education offered.*

The results on Part I of the boards will give you some idea of the didactic preparation that a school offers in the basic sciences. The ranking on Part II will give you an idea of the clinical education offered by a school. You should also realize that a school's rank on either or both parts can change from year to year. Boards are mentioned as a way to evaluate schools simply because you *will* hear admissions officers refer to their school's rankings on the board exams. The best way to obtain actual ranking information is to directly ask the dean what the school's ranks were for the past 3 or so years.

In selecting the schools to which you apply, figure out what criteria are most important to you. Then rank these schools on these bases as you obtain relevant information.

What Should I Look for When I Tour a Dental School?

If you are invited for an interview, prepare a list of questions that you want answered. The interview is a time for you to get to know that school as well as a time for the school to get to know you. Here are some observations you may want to make and questions you may want to ask:

- Are the dental students mixed in with the medical students?
- When was the dental school last renovated?
- Are there a sufficient number of preclinic stations?
- How is the clinic set up? Are there individual operators?
- Are the lecture halls and audio/visual equipment adequate?
- Is there an adequate patient pool?
- What percentage of students remediate?
- What percentage graduate on time?
- Are there *buildings* dedicated to dental research, or *floors*?
- What do the students wear? Scrubs? Casual clothes?
- What is the atmosphere like? Are students and faculty friendly?

What Is the Average Age of the First-Year Dental Student?

The average age of first-time enrollees is approximately 24.3 years.

Questions Regarding the Profession of Dentistry

I Was not Granted Admission to a Medical School Last Year, and I'm now Pursuing Dentistry as an Alternative Career Choice. Are These Two Professions Really all that Different?

As professions, medicine and dentistry share much in common, and therefore it is not unusual for students pursuing a career in medicine to switch to dentistry. The admission criteria are often less stringent, and dentistry is a fine alternative for those who originally intended to practice medicine. Both are highly respected members of the health care field. Nevertheless, the premedical students who use dental school as a fallback are often the first to drop out of their dental school classes. Why is this the case?

There are differences between medical school and dental school that need to be realized. In dentistry, the psychomotor skills tested through practical examinations require a high degree of manual dexterity and attention to detail. Only after detailed scrutiny of the profession of dentistry and the curricula of dental schools should a premedical student opt for a career in dentistry. An alternative for many would-be students of an allopathic medical school is osteopathy. The training and career options for the D.O. and the M.D. are becoming increasingly similar. Medical students seeking the D.O. designation undergo a thorough training in the diagnostic and therapeutic techniques of conventional medicine with an emphasis in manipulative techniques.

It is not the intention here to discourage premedical students from switching to dentistry; rather, it is to inform these students of the differences in training and practice between these professions. If you are attempting the DAT after a less than satisfactory performance on the MCAT, you should research the field of dentistry before you commit to pursuing a dental degree. Base your decision on a solid foundation of information gathered from personal observation and discussion with physicians and dentists. The most intelligent decision that you can make for yourself is one that is well thought out, is based on first-hand observation, and is most closely aligned with your interests and abilities.

I Know my Dental Education Will Have to Be Paid for Entirely by Loans. Is it Realistic to Assume that I Will Earn Enough Money to Repay These Loans?

Yes. Be aware, however, that most new dentists who borrowed the maximum allowance struggle to make payments on their educational loans.

Once I'm a Dentist, Will it Really Matter what School I Went to?

Maybe a handful of patients over the course of your career will care to know where you were educated. How you perform in comparison to your peers at the school that you choose is much more important.

What Percentage of Dentists Practice General Dentistry, and what Percentage Specializes?

Approximately 20–30% specialize in one of the ADA-recognized specialties. If you think you may want to specialize, be cautious when asking admissions officers how many students go on to residencies; the number will include students opting for GPR (General Practice Residency) and AEGD (Advanced Education in General Dentistry) programs, which do not offer specialty training.

How Many Recognized Dental Specialties Are There?

See the section *The Profession of Dentistry* (pages 26–30) for an explanation of each of the eight recognized specialties.

What Are the Personal Qualities or Characteristics of an Excellent Dentist?

Here are some qualities that are important:

1. Compassion
2. Academic superiority and intellectual curiosity in regard to the biological sciences
3. A detail-oriented personality
4. Highly proficient manual dexterity skills
5. Ability to manage a business and personnel
6. Effective interpersonal skills

PERIODIC TABLE OF THE ELEMENTS

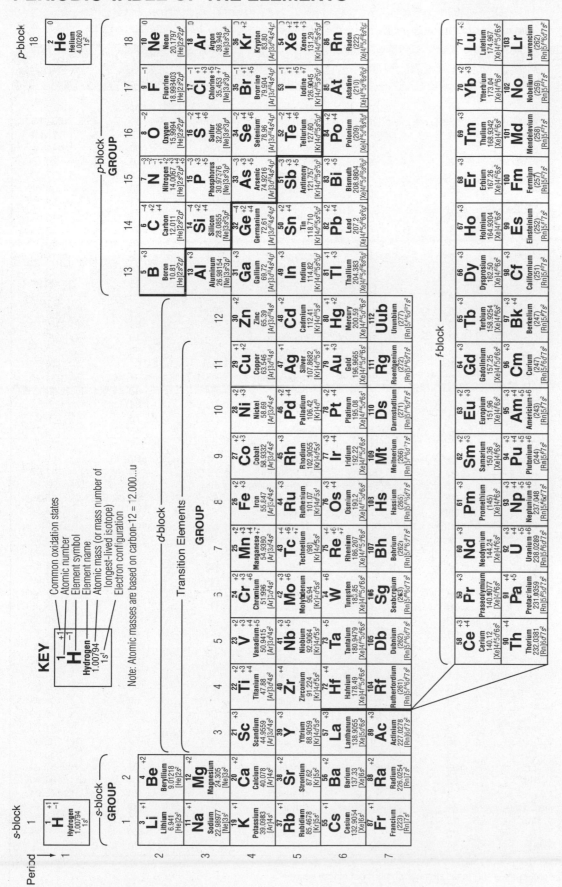

*Due to disputes over the discovery of some of the heavier elements, the International Union for Pure and Applied Chemistry (IUPAC) has devised a systematic naming scheme, based on Greek and Latin roots to temporarily name element 112.

LIST OF ELEMENTS WITH THEIR SYMBOLS

(Atomic masses in this table are based on the atomic mass of carbon-12 being exactly 12.)

Name	Symbol	Atomic Number	Atomic Mass	Name	Symbol	Atomic Number	Atomic Mass
Actinium	Ac	89	(227)	Mendelevium	Md	101	(258)
Aluminum	Al	13	26.98	Mercury	Hg	80	200.59
Americium	Am	95	(243)	Molybdenum	Mo	42	95.94
Antimony	Sb	51	121.75	Neodymium	Nd	60	144.24
Argon	Ar	18	39.95	Neon	Ne	10	20.18
Arsenic	As	33	74.92	Neptunium	Np	93	237.05
Astatine	At	85	(210)	Nickel	Ni	28	58.71
Barium	Ba	56	137.34	Niobium	Nb	41	92.90
Berkelium	Bk	97	(247)	Nitrogen	N	7	14.01
Beryllium	Be	4	9.01	Nobelium	No	102	(259)
Bismuth	Bi	83	208.98	Osmium	Os	76	190.2
Bohrium	Bh	107	(262)	Oxygen	O	8	16.00
Boron	B	5	10.81	Palladium	Pd	46	106.4
Bromine	Br	35	79.90	Phosphorus	P	15	30.97
Cadmium	Cd	48	112.40	Platinum	Pt	78	195.09
Calcium	Ca	20	40.08	Plutonium	Pu	94	(244)
Californium	Cf	98	(251)	Polonium	Po	84	(210)
Carbon	C	6	12.01	Potassium	K	19	39.10
Cerium	Ce	58	140.12	Praseodymium	Pr	59	140.90
Cesium	Cs	55	132.91	Promethium	Pm	61	(145)
Chlorine	Cl	17	35.45	Protactinium	Pa	91	231.04
Chromium	Cr	24	52.00	Radium	Ra	88	(226)
Cobalt	Co	27	58.93	Radon	Rn	86	(222)
Copper	Cu	29	63.55	Rhenium	Re	75	186.2
Curium	Cm	96	(247)	Rhodium	Rh	45	102.91
Darmstadtium	Ds	110	(271)	Roentgenium	Rg	111	(272)
Dubnium	Db	105	(262)	Rubidium	Rb	37	85.47
Dysprosium	Dy	66	162.50	Ruthenium	Ru	44	101.07
Einsteinium	Es	99	(254)	Rutherfordium	Rf	104	(261)
Erbium	Er	68	167.26	Samarium	Sm	62	150.35
Europium	Eu	63	151.96	Scandium	Sc	21	44.95
Fermium	Fm	100	(257)	Seaborgium	Sg	106	(263)
Fluorine	F	9	19.00	Selenium	Se	34	78.96
Francium	Fr	87	(223)	Silicon	Si	14	28.09
Gadolinium	Gd	64	157.25	Silver	Ag	47	107.89
Gallium	Ga	31	69.72	Sodium	Na	11	22.99
Germanium	Ge	32	72.59	Strontium	Sr	38	87.62
Gold	Au	79	196.97	Sulfur	S	16	32.06
Hafnium	Hf	72	178.49	Tantalum	Ta	73	180.95
Hassium	Hs	108	(265)	Technetium	Tc	43	(99)
Helium	He	2	4.00	Tellurium	Te	52	127.60
Holmium	Ho	67	164.93	Terbium	Tb	65	158.92
Hydrogen	H	1	1.008	Thallium	Tl	81	204.37
Indium	In	49	114.82	Thorium	Th	90	232.03
Iodine	I	53	126.90	Thulium	Tm	69	168.93
Iridium	Ir	77	192.2	Tin	Sn	50	118.69
Iron	Fe	26	55.85	Titanium	Ti	22	47.90
Krypton	Kr	36	83.80	Tungsten	W	74	183.85
Lanthanum	La	57	138.91	Uranium	U	92	238.03
Lawrencium	Lr	103	(261)	Vanadium	V	23	50.94
Lead	Pb	82	207.19	Xenon	Xe	54	131.30
Lithium	Li	3	6.94	Ytterbium	Yb	70	173.04
Lutetium	Lu	71	174.97	Yttrium	Y	39	88.91
Magnesium	Mg	12	24.31	Zinc	Zn	30	65.37
Manganese	Mn	25	54.94	Zirconium	Zr	40	91.22
Meitnerium	Mt	109	(266)				

*A number in parentheses is the mass number of the most stable isotope.

REFERENCE TABLES FOR CHEMISTRY

Physical Constants and Conversion Factors

Name	Symbol	Value(s)	Units
Angstrom unit	Å	1×10^{-10} m	meter
Avogadro number	N_A	6.02×10^{23} per mol	
Charge of electron	e	1.60×10^{-19} C	coulomb
electron volt	eV	1.60×10^{-19} J	joule
Speed of light	c	3.00×10^8 m/s	meters/second
Planck's constant	h	6.63×10^{-34} J·s 1.58×10^{-37} kcal·s	joule-second kilocalorie-second
Universal gas constant	R	0.0821 L·atm/mol·K 1.98 cal/mol·K 8.31 J/mol·K	liter-atmosphere/mole-kelvin calories/mole-kelvin joules/mole-kelvin
Atomic mass unit	μ(amu)	1.66×10^{-24} g	gram
Volume standard, liter	L	1×10^3 cm^3 = 1 dm^3	cubic centimeters, cubic decimeter
Standard pressure, atmosphere	atm	101.3 kPa 760 mm Hg 760 torr	kilopascals millimeters of mercury torr
Heat equivalent, kilocalorie	kcal	4.18×10^3 J	joules

Physical Constants for H_2O

Molal freezing point depression .... 1.86°C

Molal boiling point elevation .... 0.52°C

Heat of fusion .... 79.72 cal/g

Heat of vaporization .... 539.4 cal/g

Standard Units

Symbol	Name	Quantity
m	meter	length
kg	kilogram	mass
Pa	pascal	pressure
K	kelvin	thermodynamic temperature
mol	mole	amount of substance
J	joule	energy, work, quantity of heat
s	second	time
C	coulomb	quantity of electricity
V	volt	electric potential, potential difference
L	liter	volume

Selected Prefixes

Factor	Prefix	Symbol
10^6	mega	M
10^3	kilo	k
10^{-1}	deci	d
10^{-2}	centi	c
10^{-3}	milli	m
10^{-6}	micro	μ
10^{-9}	nano	n

Relative Strengths of Acids in Aqueous Solution at 1 ATM and 298 K

Conjugate Pairs Acid	Base	K_a
$HI = H^+ + I^-$		very large
$HBr = H^+ + Br^-$		very large
$HCl = H^+ + Cl^-$		very large
$HNO_3 = H^+ + NO_3^-$		very large
$H_2SO_4 = H^+ + HSO_4^-$		large
$H_2O + SO_2 = H^+ + HSO_3^-$		1.5×10^{-2}
$HSO_4^- = H^+ + SO_4^{2-}$		1.2×10^{-2}
$H_3PO_4 = H^+ + H_2PO_4^-$		7.5×10^{-3}
$Fe(H_2O)_6^{3+} = H^+ + Fe(H_2O)_5(OH)^{2+}$		8.9×10^{-4}
$HNO_2 = H^+ + NO_2^-$		4.6×10^{-4}
$HF = H^+ + F^-$		3.5×10^{-4}
$Cr(H_2O)_6^{3+} = H^+ + Cr(H_2O)_5(OH)^{2+}$		1.0×10^{-4}
$CH_3COOH = H^+ + CH_3COO^-$		1.8×10^{-5}
$Al(H_2O)_6^{3+} = H^+ + Al(H_2O)_5(OH)^{2+}$		1.1×10^{-5}
$H_2O + CO_2 = H^+ + HCO_3^-$		4.3×10^{-7}
$HSO_3^- = H^+ + SO_3^{2-}$		1.1×10^{-7}
$H_2S = H^+ + HS^-$		9.5×10^{-8}
$H_2PO_4^- = H^+ + HPO_4^{2-}$		6.2×10^{-8}
$NH_4^+ = H^+ + NH_3$		5.7×10^{-10}
$HCO_3^- = H^+ + CO_3^{2-}$		5.6×10^{-11}
$HPO_4^{2-} = H^+ + PO_4^{3-}$		2.2×10^{-13}
$HS^- = H^+ + S^{2-}$		1.3×10^{-14}
$H_2O = H^+ + OH^-$		1.0×10^{-14}
$OH^- = H^+ + O^{2-}$		$< 10^{-36}$
$NH_3 = H^+ + NH_2^-$		very small

Note: $H^+(aq) = H_3O^+$

Sample equation: $HI + H_2O = H_3O^+ + I^-$

Constants for Various Equilibria at 1 ATM and 298 K

$H_2O(\ell) = H^+(aq) + OH^-(aq)$	$K_w = 1.0 \times 10^{-14}$
$H_2O(\ell) + H_2O(\ell) = H_3O^+(aq) + OH^-(aq)$	$K_w = 1.0 \times 10^{-14}$
$CH_3COO^-(aq) + H_2O(\ell) = CH_3COOH(aq) + OH^-(aq)$	$K_b = 5.6 \times 10^{-10}$
$Na^+F^-(aq) + H_2O(\ell) = Na^+(OH)^- + HF(aq)$	$K_b = 1.5 \times 10^{-11}$
$NH_3(aq) + H_2O(\ell) = NH_4^+(aq) + OH^-(aq)$	$K_b = 1.8 \times 10^{-5}$
$CO_3^{2+}(aq) + H_2O(\ell) = HCO_3^-(aq) + OH^-(aq)$	$K_b = 1.8 \times 10^{-4}$
$Ag(NH_3)_2^-(aq) = Ag^+(ag) + 2NH_3(aq)$	$K_{eq} = 8.9 \times 10^{-8}$
$N_2(g) + 3H_2(g) = 2NH_3(g)$	$K_{eq} = 6.7 \times 10^5$
$H_2(g) + I_2(g) = 2HI(g)$	$K_{eq} = 3.5 \times 10^{-1}$

Compound	K_{sp}	Compound	K_{sp}
AgBr	5.0×10^{-13}	Li_2CO_3	2.5×10^{-2}
AgCl	1.8×10^{-10}	$PbCl_2$	1.6×10^{-2}
Ag_2CrO_4	1.1×10^{-12}	$PbCO_3$	7.4×10^{-14}
AgI	8.3×10^{-17}	$PbCrO_4$	2.8×10^{-13}
$BaSO_4$	1.1×10^{-10}	PbI_2	7.1×10^{-9}
$CaSO_4$	9.1×10^{-6}	$ZnCO_3$	1.4×10^{-11}

Standard Energies of Formation of Compounds at 1 ATM and 298 K

Compound	Heat (Enthalpy) of Formation* (ΔH_f°)		Free Energy of Formation* (ΔG_f°)	
	kJ/mol	kcal/mol	kJ/mol	kcal/mol
Aluminum oxide Al_2O_3(s)	−1676.5	−400.5	−1583.1	−378.2
Ammonia NH_3(g)	−46.0	−11.0	−16.3	−3.9
Barium sulfate $BaSO_4$(s)	−1473.9	−352.1	−1363.0	−325.6
Calcium hydroxide $Ca(OH)_2$(s)	−986.6	−235.7	−899.2	−214.8
Carbon dioxide CO_2(g)	−393.9	−94.1	−394.7	−94.3
Carbon monoxide CO(g)	−110.5	−26.4	−137.3	−32.8
Copper(II) sulfate $CuSO_4$(s)	−771.9	−184.4	−662.2	−158.2
Ethane C_2H_6(g)	−84.6	−20.2	−33.1	−7.9
Ethene (ethylene) C_2H_4(g)	52.3	12.5	68.2	16.3
Ethyne (acetylene) C_2H_2(g)	226.9	54.2	209.3	50.0
Hydrogen fluoride HF(g)	−271.3	−64.8	−273.3	−65.3
Hydrogen iodide HI(g)	26.4	6.3	1.7	0.4
Iodine chloride ICl(g)	18.0	4.3	−5.4	−1.3
Lead(II) oxide PbO(s)	−215.6	−51.5	−188.4	−45.0
Methane CH_4(g)	−74.9	−17.9	−50.7	−12.1
Magnesium oxide MgO(s)	−601.9	−143.8	−569.7	−136.1
Nitrogen(II) oxide NO(g)	90.4	21.6	86.7	20.7
Nitrogen(IV) oxide NO_2(g)	33.1	7.9	51.5	12.3
Potassium chloride KCl(s)	−437.0	−104.4	−409.4	−97.8
Sodium chloride $NaCl$(s)	−411.5	−98.3	−384.3	−91.8
Sulfur dioxide SO_2(g)	−296.8	−70.9	−300.1	−71.7
Water H_2O(g)	−242.0	−57.8	−228.6	−54.6
Water H_2O(ℓ)	−285.9	−68.3	−237.3	−56.7

*Minus sign indicates an exothermic reaction.
Sample equations:

$2Al(s) + \frac{3}{2}O_2(g) \rightarrow Al_2O_3(s) + 400.5$ kcal

$2Al(s) + \frac{3}{2}O_2(g) \rightarrow Al_2O_3(s) \quad \Delta H = -400.5$ kcal/mol

How to Use the CD-ROM

The software is not installed on your computer; it runs directly from the CD-ROM. Barron's CD-ROM includes an "autorun" feature that automatically launches the application when the CD is inserted into the CD-ROM drive. In the unlikely event that the autorun feature is disabled, follow the manual launching instructions below.

Windows®

Insert the CD-ROM and the program should launch automatically. If the software does not launch automatically, follow the steps below.

1. Click on the Start button and choose "My Computer."
2. Double-click on the CD-ROM drive, which will be named **DAT.**
3. Double-click **DAT.exe** application to launch the program.

Macintosh®

1. Insert the CD-ROM.
2. Double-click the CD-ROM icon.
3. Double-click the **DAT** icon to start the program.

SYSTEM REQUIREMENTS

The program will run on a PC with:
Windows® Intel® Pentium II 450 MHz
or faster, 128MB of RAM
1024 × 768 display resolution
Windows 2000, XP, Vista
CD-ROM Player

The program will run on a Macintosh® with:
PowerPC® G3 500 MHz
or faster, 128MB of RAM
1024 × 768 display resolution
Mac OS × v.10.1 through 10.4
CD-ROM Player